When Illness Goes Public

When Illness Goes Public

Celebrity Patients and How We Look at Medicine

BARRON H. LERNER

The Johns Hopkins University Press
Baltimore

The Johns Hopkins University Press
2715 North Charles Street
Baltimore, Maryland 21218-4363
www.press.jhu.edu

Library of Congress Cataloging-in-Publication Data
Lerner, Barron H.
When illness goes public : celebrity patients and how we look
at medicine / Barron H. Lerner.
p.   cm.
Includes bibliographical references (p.   ) and index.
ISBN 0-8018-8462-4 (hardover : alk. paper)
1. Celebrities—Diseases. 2. Celebrities—Biography.
3. Medicine—Case studies. I. Title.
R703.L47   2006
610.92′2—dc22   2006005258

A catalog record for this book is available from the British Library.

To Ben and Nina

Anything processed by memory is fiction.

—Wright Morris

In order to be a realist you must believe in miracles.

—David Ben-Gurion

Contents

Family members who have endured not only the sickness of a loved one but the graphic exposure of the event naturally build protective walls around these experiences. One aspect of this process is selective recollection. Certain experiences are remembered and even exaggerated; others are forgotten, either consciously or unconsciously. I am thus especially grateful for the courage and generosity of those relatives and friends of my "celebrity patients" who trusted me to revisit events that they probably hoped had receded into the permanent past. I hope I have done justice to the players in these stories, who, thrust into the public spotlight at most inopportune times, almost always rose to the occasion.

Among those people who provided me with either recollections or relevant materials were Lewis Rowland, Donald Mulder, Ray Robinson, Allan Glaser, Richard Stolley, Jeanne Morris, Steven Teitelbaum, James Holland, Janet Cuttner, Elaina Archer, Caren Roberts-Frenzel, Jed Levine, Lonnie Wollin, Jerome Stone, Ronald Fieve, Donald Olsen, Robert Glickman, Bertrand Bell, Antonia New, Cheryl Bulbach, Lucian Leape, Gary Karton, Susie Zeegen, Philip Pizzo, Judge Barrington Parker, Edie Magnus, James Lovette, Patricia Lovette, James Lovette, Jr., Natalie Robins, Jacqueline Kinlow, and Susan Sarandon. Tom Moore's colleagues at Kramer, Dilloff, Livingston and Moore unearthed and then let me study the transcript of the Libby Zion trial. Sarah Redmond, Pete Hanley, and Mary Ann Della-Bianca from ESPN kindly shared transcripts from interviews they had conducted, thereby saving me a lot of legwork. Joy Piccolo O'Connell and

Kristi Piccolo shared difficult memories of Brian Piccolo's arduous death and hooked me up with Joyce Walsh, who runs the Brian Piccolo Cancer Research Fund (www.brianpiccolofund.org). Ruth and Ann Abram provided candid insights into their father's personality. Yasmin Aga Khan chronicled her mother's painful descent into Alzheimer's disease. And Jeanne Moutoussamy-Ashe and Paul Michael Glaser described what it was like to experience the public disclosure of one's most private information. For more information on Alzheimer's and on HIV in children, see www.alz.org and www.pedaids.org.

Special thanks and admiration go to George Pollack, Eleanor Gehrig's former lawyer, whose management of Lou Gehrig's legacy has raised considerable funds to fight ALS (www.columbiaals.org); Una Loy Clark Farrer, the quite remarkable widow of Barney Clark, who eloquently continues to struggle with her memories; Sidney Zion and the late Elsa Zion, who gave me access to very personal materials about the tragic death of their daughter, Libby; Augusto Odone, the proud father of Lorenzo, who devotes his days to understanding why the loss of protective myelin destroys so many young lives (www.myelin.org); Hugo Moser, who endured numerous e-mails from me about how one can tell whether Lorenzo's Oil really works; and Ron and Paula Brazeal, who continue to run the United Leukodystrophy Foundation (www.ulf.org) twenty years after both of their sons died from adrenoleukodystrophy.

Historians cannot function without librarians and archivists, and many helped greatly with this book. They include Robert Clark and his colleagues at the Franklin D. Roosevelt Library; Anne McFarland of the National Baseball Hall of Fame; Sean Noel of the Howard Gotlieb Archival Research Center of Boston University; Carolyn Davis and Nicolette Schneider of the Special Collections Research Center at Syracuse University Library; Jennifer Cole and the staff of the Seeley G. Mudd Library of Princeton University; Kathy Shoemaker of the Robert W. Woodruff Library of Emory University; Walter Jones, Stan Larson, and Roy Webb of the Manuscripts Division of the University of Utah's Merritt Library; Chris McKay of the Schomburg Center for Research in Black Culture of the New York Public Library; Laura Carroll of the American Medical Association Archives; and Kristine Krueger and Janet Lorenz of the Margaret Herrick Library of the Academy of Motion Picture Arts and Sciences. Permission to quote Wright Morris came from Russell & Volkening, Inc.

Closer to home, a large number of colleagues at Columbia University provided advice and assistance with this project. Steven Shea and Rafael Lantigua of the Division of General Medicine gave me leave time to write the book. Bob Goodman, Deborah Klugman, Nell Eisenberg, Nicolette Brown, and Rita Charon helped take care of my patients, who, for some reason, seemed much healthier when I returned. David Rosner, Amy Fairchild, Ron Bayer, Nitanya Nedd, and the other members of the Center for the History and Ethics of Public Health provided crucial feedback on aspects of the book and a comfortable home base from which to work. David Rothman and Tiffany Rounsville from the Center for the Study of Society and Medicine provided early advice and helped me to obtain funding. Others who provided assistance at Columbia include Gerry and Ruth Fischbach, Daniel Wolfe, Jane Booth, and a series of very talented research assistants: Sara Siris, Valeri Kiesig, Joshua Alexander, Rebecca Nardi, Julie Oh, Irina Vodonos, Alison Bateman-House, and Catherine Trimbur.

Outside funding, of course, is what frees an academic to devote a significant amount of time to a project of this magnitude. Grants from the National Library of Medicine and the Greenwall Foundation (www .greenwall.org) provided a jump start for this book, which began life as a history of informed consent. Bill Stubing of Greenwall was especially helpful and flexible as my direction changed. The Investigators in Health Policy program of the Robert Wood Johnson Foundation, ably run by David Mechanic and Lynn Rogut, provided generous funding and great collegiality. I cannot thank the Robert Wood Johnson Foundation enough. It has, to a substantial extent, bankrolled all three of my books. To the degree that I have contributed valuable research in the world of medicine and health care, it could not have happened without RWJ (www .rwjf.org). Finally, I wish to give warm thanks to Angelica Berrie, Arnold Gold, Sandra Gold, Ann Bruder, and the entire staff of the Arnold P. Gold Foundation. I am proud to be the Berrie-Gold Foundation Associate Professor of Medicine and Public Health at Columbia. Many of the people who populate this book embody the worthy goal of the foundation: to restore humanism to medicine. Please see www.humanism-in-medicine .org for more information.

I have received quite wonderful feedback on this project from many scholars. Jonathan Sadowsky and Susan Lederer plowed through the entire manuscript. Keith Wailoo, Tim Westmoreland, and Bonnie Bermas read portions of the book and made important contributions. It was a privilege to participate in Keith's conference on Jesica Santillan, the unfortunate immigrant girl who died after a mismatched organ transplant; the event provided the first public airing of my Libby Zion chapter. Other excellent feedback came from presentations made at the Institute of the History of Medicine at the Johns Hopkins University, at the Indiana University School of Medicine, and at the Chicago Symposium on Medicine, Ethics and Society. Thank you to Randy Packard, Ellen Dwyer, Ann Carmichael, Bill Schneider, and Audiey Kao for the invitations to speak. Others who have provided me with wise counsel include James Tulsky, Joel Howell, Ken Ludmerer, Rosemary Stevens, and David Cantor. Shelley McKellar is among the most generous colleagues I have met. Thanks also go to Laura Chang, Erica Goode, Barbara Strauch, Kate Phillips, and the other staff of the Science Times section of the *New York Times*, who have kindly run my essays, many on "celebrity patients," over the past few years.

This book ended with a different agent and editor than were there at the beginning. Michele Rubin and Peter Ginna helped to shape things during the conceptual phase. My new agent, Robert Shepard, has been unfailingly enthusiastic and professional, though I sometimes wonder if he could have earned more money per hour working at McDonald's. Jacqueline Wehmueller at the Johns Hopkins University Press believed me when I told her that one could write a meaningful and important book comprised of individual stories. I hope I have not misled her and the Press.

One cannot work for five years on a project without the help of friends and family. I cannot thank all of the friends who contributed an encouraging grunt in response to my complaints, but a few should be singled out for their advice and suggestions: Seth Godin, Helene Godin, Lisa Belkin, Bruce Gelb, Susana Morales, Trip Gulick, Jonathan Sackner-Bernstein, Joanne Levine, Doron Scharf, Amelia Peck, and Michael Altshuler. My parents, Phillip and Ronnie Lerner, sister, Dana Lerner, and mother-in-law, Ellen Seibel, are remarkably supportive people, whatever my mood. Our longtime nanny, Margaret Sefa Frempong, takes my side when I squabble with the kids (usually). As always, my loving wife, Cathy Seibel, provided constant support and dutifully read every word of the manuscript. Any errors or misstatements contained within this book are solely her responsibility.

Finally, one cannot tell stories about heroism and courage without thinking of one's children. This book is dedicated to Ben and Nina, who make me proud every day. May you guys triumph over adversity in your lives, too.

When Illness Goes Public

The most famous modern celebrity patient is surely Lance Armstrong. Diagnosed with far-advanced testicular cancer in 1996 and told he would most likely not survive, the 25-year-old Armstrong beat the odds and lived. Then, resuming his bicycling career, he proceeded to win the sport's most demanding and prestigious race: the Tour de France. Indeed, he won it seven times, more than any other cyclist.

Armstrong has written two books about his life, started the Lance Armstrong Foundation, and made countless public appearances to discuss his personal experiences with cancer and how the disease might best be conquered in the future. Armstrong's first book, published in 2000, was entitled *It's Not About the Bike: My Journey Back to Life*. The title and the book made the important point that Armstrong's battle with cancer was much more important and meaningful than what he had accomplished in cycling or elsewhere in his life.[1]

But of course, it *was* all about the bike. Had Lance Armstrong simply been an anonymous survivor of testicular cancer, his recovery would have been compelling to very few people. The fact that Armstrong won the Tour de France, and subsequently became a celebrity, made his story a reference point for millions of people suffering from cancer or other grave diseases. The juxtaposition of the illness and the victories raised a series of questions. What, if anything, did Armstrong's recovery from cancer and his athletic accomplishments have to do with one another? Did Armstrong possess some type of extraordinary qualities that allowed him to beat his cancer? And, finally, what did his story say to other people who had the bad luck to get cancer?

In trying to answer these questions, and to find out why they were being asked, it is crucial to look back historically. Armstrong is only one of many famous patients over the past seventy-five years whose stories have engendered similar questions. This book explores the phenomenon of celebrity illness, why it has become such a preoccupation for the media and the public, and what it tells us about sickness and health, hope and fear, and truth and myth in American society.[2] It pays especially close attention to the "n of 1" phenomenon, in which specific cases—such as that of Armstrong—assume particular importance, even being seen as the definitive examples of given diseases, their prognoses, and how they should be treated.

Sixty years before Armstrong got sick, another American in his twenties fell ill. He was Franklin D. Roosevelt, Jr., 22-year-old son of President and Eleanor Roosevelt. According to the front page of the December 17, 1936, *New York Times*, administration of a new drug, known as Prontylin, had saved the life of the young Roosevelt, a senior at Harvard University, a devoted member of the crew team, and fiancé of Delaware heiress Ethel Du Pont. Roosevelt had been suffering from pharyngitis, a potentially fatal throat infection caused by bacteria known as streptococci.[3]

Perhaps the most obvious question this story raises for a historian is, Was it true? After all, historians are in the business of recounting past events as accurately as possible. But not all historical questions are answerable. I obtained as much information as I could about Roosevelt's illness at the Franklin D. Roosevelt Library. Franklin Jr. initially had a sinus infection, which was then complicated by the pharyngitis, what is now commonly termed "strep throat." Today, pharyngitis is readily treatable. But in the 1930s, before antimicrobials like Prontylin and penicillin, such infections could spread to the blood. This condition, known as septic sore throat, could lead to death.

Did administration of the new drug save Roosevelt's life? It is impossible to know. Perhaps, had I been able to obtain his medical record, I might have a better guess. The answer, at least for now, is "possibly."

This question, however, may be one of the least interesting that might be asked about the episode. Like the other stories in this book, the Roosevelt anecdote raises a series of far more meaningful and provocative historical questions. Why was the story about Franklin Roosevelt, Jr., on the front page of America's most important newspaper? Why did media coverage of "famous patients" such as Roosevelt increase so dramatically during the twentieth century? How have public versions of celebrity illnesses correlated with actual events? And, most important for this book, what impact have such sick celebrities had on Americans struggling to understand and treat their own illnesses?

This book tells the story of thirteen famous patients diagnosed and treated over the past seventy-five years. Some of these people were famous when they became sick. Others became famous because their illnesses or treatments were unique. The cases highlight, among other subjects, doctor-patient confidentiality, death and dying, medical errors, consent for experimental treatment, and the question of who—patients, families, or doctors—should make decisions at the bedside.

The specific cases I cover in the book were not necessarily representative examples of these topics. Nevertheless, these "extraordinary" stories generated intense interest among "ordinary" Americans who had experienced the same illnesses or controversial clinical situations. And because these illness stories were so compelling and powerful, they had another effect. Their apparent lessons came into direct conflict with a parallel historical trend, the growing dependence on so-called evidence-based medicine (EBM) to guide clinical decisions. Who was right, the celebrity patient who had gone public or the statistician with reams of data? And who got to say so?[4]

To some degree, the focus on famous cases cuts against trends in academic historical scholarship. Before the 1970s, most historians—including medical historians—wrote so-called great man history. These works generally stressed seminal historical figures, such as presidents and generals, attempting to demonstrate how such individuals had advanced their particular fields. But with the rise of social history, scholars began to emphasize the stories of ordinary Americans and how, at times, these people had been victimized by social forces, such as racism and sexism.

This book gently rejects this recent trend that discourages the study of famous individuals and seminal events. These public illnesses—featured in newspapers and magazines, in television news programs and documentaries, and in book-length biographies—were compelling and often heartbreaking tales that Americans followed, discussed, and debated. While not rejecting attempts to understand what actually occurred, the book explores the myths and meanings that came to surround these thirteen examples—a more sophisticated way to understand history than simply recounting actual events.[5]

By the early twentieth century, a series of dramatic changes were taking place in medicine. Scientific advances, most notably the germ theory of disease, had greatly expanded the medical profession's knowledge. Improvements in medical education ensured that medical students were exposed to cutting-edge laboratory medicine as well as patients with a variety of diseases. Hospitals, armed with new diagnostic technologies, such as electrocardiogram machines and x-rays, opened private pavilions to attract paying patients seeking the most up-to-date medical care. Finally, doctors could report a series of exciting breakthroughs: the 1910 synthesis of Salvarsan, the first specific treatment for syphilis; the 1922 isolation and use of insulin, a highly effective treatment for diabetes mellitus; and the 1935 emergence of Prontylin and Prontosil, the first sulfonamide antimicrobials.[6]

This was the setting when Franklin Roosevelt, Jr., took sick in November 1936 with a sinus infection, a collection of pus in the maxillary cavity behind his right cheek. He was admitted to Phillips House, the private portion of the Massachusetts General Hospital, an affiliate of the prestigious Harvard Medical School. Roosevelt's physician was George Loring Tobey, Jr., whom *Time* magazine described as a "fashionable and crackerjack ear, nose and throat specialist." The only specific treatment available in the 1930s for a sinus infection was surgical drainage, and this is what Roosevelt's doctors were contemplating when he developed pharyngitis on or about December 10, 1936.[7]

It was this infection, caused by streptococcal bacteria, that led doctors to consider using Prontylin. Roosevelt had a fever and a high white blood cell count, suggesting that, in Eleanor's words, the infection was "getting into his system." At first, Tobey and his colleagues recommended making a more extensive surgical incision into the infected sinus. But they apparently concluded that Roosevelt's worsening condition stemmed not from his infected sinuses but from a concurrent throat infection.

Prontylin, a pill, and Prontosil, an injectable medication, had been synthesized by a German chemist, Gerhard Domagk, in 1935, and then tested around the world. Early results were encouraging, even amazing. Patients receiving the drugs were being cured of formerly untreatable streptococcal infections, including abdominal peritonitis, childbed fever, and erysipelas, a severe skin infection. At a 1936 meeting of the Southern Medical Association, held the month before Roosevelt became ill, Johns Hopkins University physicians Perrin H. Long and Eleanor A. Bliss had reported on nineteen patients who received the drugs. Several "gravely" ill patients had recovered. But the vast majority of patients with streptococcal infections, including pharyngitis, were still receiving more traditional treatments, such as streptococcal antiserum, which was produced from the blood of other patients who had had streptococcal infections.[8]

The decision to try Prontylin (initially in conjunction with Prontosil) in Roosevelt's case was made by Tobey. The Boston physician was aware of the early research studies and had already used the drug with "marked success" in several other patients. From our modern perspective, administering the new wonder drug to the president's son may seem to have been an obvious decision. Why wouldn't a physician do everything to save the life of his patient, especially such a prominent one whom he believed to be gravely ill?[9]

But at the time, the decision could not have been an easy one. While the value and relative safety of the sulfonamides would be well-established by the end of the 1930s, the data as of 1936 were preliminary. Our modern notion that one needs to take antibiotics to cure bacterial infections did not yet exist. If something had gone wrong with this new treatment, Tobey would have been held responsible and even accused of having used his patient as a guinea pig.

Little is known about how the doctors presented their decision to use Prontylin to Franklin Jr. and his mother, who made numerous visits to Boston during her son's several-week hospitalization. It seems likely that the Roosevelts were told both that the infection was possibly fatal and that a new treatment existed that had saved lives. Eleanor Roosevelt almost certainly contacted her relative through marriage, the renowned Yale University neurosurgeon Harvey Cushing, for advice, as she did throughout her son's illness. Cushing evidently did not put up any roadblocks. When the First Lady had previously asked him about the doctors' plan to make a larger incision into the sinus, Cushing had "advised doing as they suggested."[10]

It was relatively rare in the 1930s for patients to question their physicians' judgment. But the Roosevelts' decision to try the new medication also likely bespoke a growing public faith in the medical profession, which was basking in the glow of its recent successes. In 1937, the year after Roosevelt's illness, Congress established the National Cancer Institute as part of the National Institutes of Health. During World War II, the Committee on Medical Research would sponsor research relevant to the military. And after the war, the NIH would undergo dramatic expansion, funding a growing number of basic science and clinical research projects.[11]

Historians later referred to this era as American medicine's "golden age." Physicians and researchers during these decades were routinely analogized to soldiers and explorers, whose "courage to fail" promised cures for diseases, such as cancer and organ failure, the victims of which had previously been doomed. The damned, in other words, could now be saved. "There are no incurable diseases," financier and Franklin Roosevelt friend Bernard Baruch had been told by his physician father, "only diseases for which no cure has yet been found."[12]

Of course, as of the 1930s, there still remained much official and popular skepticism about "curative" medications such as Prontylin. For decades, organized medicine, represented most forcefully by the American Medical Association, had waged war against quacks and other purveyors of worthless, and even dangerous, nostrums. All this new talk of cures, even coming from reputable physicians, generated uneasiness. Still, as the twentieth century progressed, the NIH's budget increased, and new cures, such as penicillin and streptomycin, emerged, medicine's ability to combat old scourges grew, and so did the public's confidence. Hence it is hardly surprising that the *New York Times* chose to feature the young Roosevelt's recovery on its front page.

But it was not only the novel medical treatment that made Roosevelt's illness newsworthy. The basic nature of what journalists covered was undergoing dramatic changes. In the nineteenth century, most newspapers emphasized local news, but publishers gradually began to realize that national and international news could sell more papers. Some publications stressed serious issues, such as politics and tariffs, but others strived for the lurid. Growing media coverage promoted some of the earliest American celebrities, whom the historian Renee Sentilles defines as "distant social figure[s] with whom spectators perceive themselves as sharing a personal relationship."[13]

The press's obsession with the sensational accelerated during the last decades of the nineteenth century. William Randolph Hearst, publisher of the *New York Journal*, brought his own hyperbolic version of the Spanish-American War to American readers, while Joseph Pulitzer's *New York World* sent journalist Nellie Bly around the world. These newspapers unabashedly presented readers with "the startling, the amazing and the stupefying." A large part of the allure of such coverage was its focus on specific individuals, whether heroes or villains. "Names make news," Hearst announced, and then proved.[14]

By the 1920s, the tabloid was born: publications such as the *New York Daily News* and *Daily Mirror* filled their pages with large photographs that did not necessarily have news value. And the people who most commonly appeared in such images were from the worlds of sports and Hollywood.

Benefiting from the end of World War I, a strong economy, and increased leisure time, sports grew tremendously during the 1920s. Athletes such as baseball slugger Babe Ruth, boxer Jack Dempsey, and tennis star Bill Tilden became bona fide heroes. Meanwhile, Hollywood's output of motion pictures skyrocketed. By 1920, the "star system" had been established, in which studios marketed their actors, such as Greta Garbo, Mary Pickford, and Rudolph Valentino, as much as or more than the films in which they appeared. During the Great Depression of the 1930s, Hollywood stars, whether on screen or in real life, served as important symbols of better times. Of course, the most famous American during these years was neither an athlete nor an actor but Charles Lindbergh, the courageous aviator whose son was kidnapped and killed in 1932.[15]

Such attention validated and, in turn, elevated the status of these public figures, who would later be dubbed celebrities. It was this development that led the historian Daniel Boorstin to attack the culture of celebrity in his famous 1962 book *The Image*. He derisively wrote, in an often-quoted line, that "the celebrity is a person who is known for his well-knownness."[16]

These men and women could not have become so famous so quickly without the rise of communication technologies that could broadcast their accomplishments. Beyond newspapers and tabloids, there was radio. In 1922, several million Americans listened to radio broadcasts of the World Series between the New York Yankees and the New York Giants. Soon, other famous people, ranging from President Franklin D. Roosevelt to actors in serials and comedy shows, would enter private homes via radio. With the expanding distribution of newsreel footage to movie theaters

during the interwar years, important information was increasingly disseminated across the country in hours or days, not weeks or months.[17]

What was the allure of the new celebrities featured in print and on radio?
Critic Richard Schickel believes the explanation lies in dual myths: those
of intimacy and autonomy. Celebrities, in their advocacy of a commercial
product, a charitable cause, or—as we shall see—greater knowledge of disease, could be very compelling figures. The impression that celebrities
truly cared created a bond with members of the public, particularly those
feeling vulnerable. Many people, entertainment historian Neal Gabler
writes, "profess feeling closer to, and more passionate about, [celebrities]
than about their own primary relationships." At the same time, due to his
fame and wealth, the celebrity seemed to be his "own boss," the "master
of his own fate." Such a notion, according to historian Leo Braudy, was
particularly potent in democratic America, which was built on the myth of
the frontier and the individualistic credo that "God helps those who help
themselves." Identification with this apparent power was particularly compelling at a time of stress or crisis.[18]

Press coverage of the famous was not a one-way street. In the late nineteenth century, entertainers such as P. T. Barnum and Buffalo Bill Cody
were relentless self-promoters. The 1920s also saw the birth of public relations, as companies and individuals employed agencies to publicize their
achievements and place them in a positive light. Babe Ruth and his Yankee
teammate Lou Gehrig, for example, hired a writer named Christy Walsh
to handle their public appearances and place them in advertisements.[19]

The "father" of public relations was Edward Bernays, who saw himself
as much more than simply a promoter of talent. For Bernays, public relations meant shaping public thought. In one of his most famous advertising
campaigns, Bernays urged Americans to reach for a Lucky Strike cigarette
instead of a sweet, even though he privately believed that cigarettes were
a health hazard. A good public relations man, according to Bernays, got
the public to behave in a certain way that benefited his clients. Like Barnum and Cody, who blurred fiction and fact to provide superior entertainment, Bernays was more than happy to "redefine reality."[20]

One clear victim of these early efforts at "spin" and the need for tabloids
to attract readers was objectivity. This statement does not imply that all
journalism before the 1920s was truthful. But a major shift occurred during and after this decade as more and more "interested parties" began to

shape the content of the news. Journalism scholars have termed this process "framing," in which the media presented news and features using predictable and formulaic patterns that reinforced cultural beliefs. At one extreme of the spectrum were what Boorstin famously called "pseudo-events," occurrences that seemed newsworthy but were staged for the camera. Historians writing about celebrity must thus be aware of a pitfall: they may not be describing who people actually were but rather who they seemed to be.[21]

An early focus of tabloids that gossiped about the lives of celebrities was scandal or bad luck: messy divorces, crime, bankruptcy, and adultery. But despite their seemingly eventful lives, celebrities, just as other Americans, spent most of their time doing ordinary things. Gradually, these seemingly mundane activities came to be seen as having entertainment value. One such activity was getting sick.

At times, illnesses of celebrities were indubitably newsworthy. Two such examples occurred in 1926. In August, screen idol Rudolph Valentino developed a perforated appendix, which led to peritonitis and, within eight days, death. More than a hundred thousand people came to view Valentino's body, and riots broke out among the distraught mourners. This, surely, was a news event. So was the death of famed magician Harry Houdini, also from peritonitis, two months later. Houdini had been punched in the stomach nine days before he died.

But if Americans had the right to know about this type of unexpected calamity, what about more chronic illnesses among the famous? There were certainly examples in which such stories went public, as with Ulysses S. Grant's death from cancer in 1885. But it was Grant's candor that gave the press access in the first place. In most cases, public discussion of health issues remained taboo. After all, confidentiality had been a central tenet of the physician-patient relationship since the era of the famed Greek physician Hippocrates, more than two thousand years earlier. Indeed, this emphasis on confidentiality at times led physicians to hide medical information that Americans were arguably entitled to know about: the serious illnesses of presidents, such as Woodrow Wilson, who was incapacitated for much of his second term of office.[22]

By the 1930s, however, the press, especially gossip columnists like Walter Winchell, had increasingly begun to cover the illnesses of notable people. One such individual was Thomas Edison, who suffered from kidney disease, intestinal disorders, and confusion during 1930 and 1931. Toward the end of Edison's life, the press camped out near his New Jersey home, chronicling his decline in great detail.

It is not surprising, therefore, that the press, then feasting on the story of King Edward VIII's abdication of the British throne, also chose to cover the hospitalization of Franklin Roosevelt, Jr. During the early days of the illness, the Boston newspapers, the *New York Times*, and the wire services wrote small articles describing his sinus infection, the treatment options, and his potential discharge. But attention increased after Tobey, on December 16, 1936, informed the media about Roosevelt's throat infection and his doctors' decision to use Prontylin. Tobey felt compelled to go to the press when inaccurate rumors surfaced that a new medication had been used to cure Roosevelt's *sinus* problem. He justified his use of Prontylin because Roosevelt's throat condition had been "extremely serious" and the patient had "faced death."[23]

Although they asked numerous questions about Prontylin, the members of the press covering the Roosevelt case never questioned the medical details provided by the doctors, a skill that reporters would later cultivate. Once the story became one about the daring rescue of a president's child, it is not surprising that it received page-one coverage across the country. But it is worth remembering that this type of event, which would immediately be covered today on television, cable, radio, and the Internet, was, in 1936, only beginning to become an acceptable news story. This development had everything to do with the social and cultural changes that were occurring at this time: the growing attention to medical science, the tabloid turn in journalism, the rising cult of the celebrity, and chinks in the armor of physician-patient confidentiality.[24]

Media coverage of Roosevelt's illness, in turn, led to a large response from Americans. Throughout this book, the reactions of the public to celebrity illnesses are recounted and analyzed. These accounts best demonstrate how popular understandings of medicine evolved over the years in question.

In Roosevelt's case, thousands of greeting cards arrived for Phillips House's "most-inquired-about patient." Other letters were sent to the White House. Though only a few of these missives survive, they help to demonstrate which aspects of Roosevelt's story most intrigued Americans.[25]

One interested group was individuals who had experienced similar medical problems. Several former victims of streptococcal infections, for example, volunteered to donate blood for the production of streptococcal antiserum. "If he needs any blood to make him better," wrote a generous 10-year-old boy from New York City, "he can have some of mine." Among the saddest letters was one from an Atlanta judge, which recounted the death of his son, a lawyer, from a streptococcal infection. "My loss was too much," he wrote. "Nothing since has seemed worthwhile."[26]

Between the sinus and throat problems, there was a lot of opportunity for unsolicited advice. Among the purported remedies suggested by writers were borax powder, herbal tea, vitamin A, and chiropractic. Other correspondents requested help for themselves or others. A Wisconsin man, concerned about a friend's son with a streptococcal throat infection, wrote to the president requesting the name of Franklin Jr.'s doctor. A Mississippi woman wrote on behalf of her son, who was a "semi-invalid" from sinus problems, wondering whether Prontylin would be of use. "For heaven's sake let me know if your son has found any relief," she entreated.[27]

These letters signaled a new type of dialogue about medicine. Up through the nineteenth century, Americans had learned about diseases and their treatments from their physicians, from family and friends, from public health campaigns publicizing tuberculosis and other diseases, and from advertisements for patent medicines. But famous discoveries—such as Pasteur's rabies vaccine in the 1880s—had begun to make headlines. By the 1930s, moreover, there were journalists who regularly wrote about medicine. And there were identifiable, famous patients suffering from familiar illnesses and gaining access to the best medical care. It is little wonder that the public took notice.[28]

But the Roosevelt episode also demonstrates the often problematic nature of this new avenue for medical information. First, cases like that of Roosevelt were complicated. For example, Prontylin did nothing for sinus infections, but it was hard to convince the public of this fact. Second, what made its way into the newspapers was variable. Reporters gleaned information from a series of sources, which were at times unreliable. Thus, Tobey did not disclose Roosevelt's throat infection and the use of Prontylin until six days after the crisis, only when he felt obliged to dispel inaccurate statements. Third, there was no guarantee that reports about the illnesses of famous individuals, even when they revealed the "truth," would be remembered as such.

A large body of historical literature has recently argued that the way in which events are remembered may be as significant as the actual events themselves. That is, while historical events surely occur, interpretation of such occurrences begins immediately and cannot be separated from the supposed reality. Recollections, the historian Mark Roseman has written, are a collection of facts, memories, and rumors.[29]

Some have thus viewed the writing of history skeptically. History, Napoleon is said to have remarked, is "a fable agreed upon." Or, as journalist Edwin M. Yoder, Jr., has stated, "When the history fails to fit the myths, we bend the history." To use modern jargon, "spin," whether conscious or unconscious, helpful or misleading, begins as soon as someone first tries to recount an event. Many years later, what we are likely remembering is not the event itself but its first telling by a journalist or eyewitness.[30]

This phenomenon becomes clear when we return to the Roosevelt story. "Cheats Death from Throat," read a *Boston American* headline of December 17, 1936. That same day, on page one, the *New York Times* announced: "Young Roosevelt Saved by New Drug." Three days later, *Times* science reporter Waldemar Kaempffert offered his "moral" of the Roosevelt case: "Consult always with a doctor who keeps up with the medical literature."[31]

Yet, the reality was much more complicated. Roosevelt had been administered a new drug that may have saved his life. But there is no way to know whether he actually was dying. And there is a good chance he was not. For one thing, Eleanor Roosevelt's frequent, fairly detailed comments about Franklin Jr.'s illness in her voluminous correspondence and her "My Day" columns conveyed none of the urgency and danger that supposedly existed. Nor did she make any comment whatsoever about Prontylin, something she likely would have done had she truly believed that a wonder drug had saved her son's life. The story that Eleanor chose to tell thus calls Tobey's account somewhat into question. And even if Franklin Jr. had developed septic sore throat, the more serious variety of the condition, he might have lived anyway. Probably one-quarter to one-half of patients with this condition recovered—even without antimicrobials.

But none of these subtleties made their way into subsequent accounts of the illness. Roosevelt's throat infection and the administration of Prontylin became a mandatory anecdote in the triumphant tale of the sulfonamides. "Desperately ill with a 'strep' infection," one history reported, Roosevelt "was given the drug and quickly recovered."[32]

The point here is not that such accounts are inevitably wrong or misleading. Rather, the way we remember seminal historical events—in this case, illnesses among the famous—can only be fully understood by considering who is telling the story, where it is being recounted, and why it is being reported in a certain way. Memory, cultural historian Marita Sturken writes, "indicates collective desires, needs and self-definitions." What we choose to remember and forget, she argues, is not accidental.[33]

This conclusion becomes even more apparent as illness narratives are told and retold in histories of medicine, in biographies and autobiographies, and on television news shows and documentaries. Although all of these media are nonfiction and thus supposedly an authoritative source of the "truth," there are always distorting factors at play. For example, as we shall see in the case of Steve McQueen, acquaintances of sick celebrities may write biographies. But since these people have generally played a role during the illness, they present events through their own prism. In addition, there is the understandable tendency of friends and family to "airbrush" the dead, converting the complex events of illness into tales of heroism. Similarly, news documentaries must be funded, either by entertainment conglomerates or by industry, a process that fosters subtle or overt slanting of the material.[34]

When stories of illness are fictionalized in Hollywood films, such as *Fear Strikes Out* (1957), *Brian's Song* (1971), and *Lorenzo's Oil* (1992), locating reality becomes even more challenging. For one thing, movies tend to simplify complex stories, blurring characters and events to create more coherent or dramatic story lines. And films tend to elevate one or two characters into heroic roles, portraying them as more powerful than they actually were. Historians caution that such "seamless" narratives, often presented as straightforward cautionary tales, should immediately raise skepticism. In his book *Life: The Movie*, Neal Gabler goes further, arguing that Americans may actually find more meaning in the stories of fictional movie characters than in their own lives.[35]

The stories in this book are not meant to provide a comprehensive history of celebrity patients over the past seventy-five years. Rather, I selected a sample of famous cases that provided me with access to new, interesting materials and the possibility of novel historical interpretations. This decision means that some obvious choices, like Betty Ford, Karen Ann Quinlan, Rock Hudson, and Christopher Reeve, are mentioned only in passing. In addition, the majority of the book's subjects are white and male (though several are women), reflecting the fact that such individuals long dominated politics and sports and thus were more likely than other people to become famous patients. Indeed, there is only one member of a minority group, Arthur Ashe, among my main subjects. Further scholarship should explore the growing importance of African Americans, Hispanics, and people from other minority groups who go public with their illnesses.[36]

But my selection of cases should not be viewed as random. The thirteen celebrity patients are grouped into three roughly chronological categories, underscoring how the study of celebrity is historically contingent. As Renee Sentilles writes, celebrities have served as a "social mirror." Examining who the public adored in given eras illuminates the time periods in question. This book thus provides a coherent explanation of how the phenomenon of the celebrity patient has evolved.[37]

The first group, which includes Lou Gehrig, Jimmy Piersall, Margaret Bourke-White, John Foster Dulles, and Brian Piccolo, consists of well-known individuals from the worlds of sports, politics, and the media who grew sick between 1935 and 1970. People became celebrity patients in this era if they were already famous, became ill, and were willing to go public with their stories. The second group consists of Morris Abram, Steve McQueen, and Rita Hayworth, who were sick between 1970 and 1980, a period when activism was emerging in many aspects of American life. These celebrities became famous patients because they (or their family members) challenged aspects of the medical system and "outed" its apparent deficiencies. Those in the third group, including Barney Clark, Libby Zion, Elizabeth Glaser, Arthur Ashe, and Lorenzo Odone, became sick between 1980 and 1995. Because of unusual or uncommon characteristics, their stories attracted enormous attention, even though these individuals were initially either unknown or reluctant to go public. These five patients thus exemplified the democratization of fame that emerged in Hollywood and throughout America during these years. Illness turned out to be a compelling—and potentially beneficial—way to achieve one's fifteen minutes of fame.

The book's first story, told in chapter 1, begins a few years after Franklin

Roosevelt, Jr., received his Prontylin. It might be argued that New York Yankees' first baseman Lou Gehrig was the first "modern patient," whose mysterious illness was chronicled in newspapers across the country. He had played in more than two thousand consecutive baseball games, setting a record for longevity and earning the moniker "The Iron Horse." Thus, when Gehrig took himself out of the lineup on May 3, 1939, the news spread rapidly across the country via radio, newspaper, and newsreel. The media also covered Gehrig's subsequent trip to the Mayo Clinic and his eventual diagnosis with a progressive neurological disorder, amyotrophic lateral sclerosis (ALS). The press also tracked his subsequent treatment and death, although, as we shall see, in complicated ways.

Americans who discovered the Gehrig story in the press, in biographies, or in *Pride of the Yankees*, Hollywood's 1942 paean to the late slugger, could learn a great deal about a series of subjects: neurological illness, experimental treatment, concealment of a fatal prognosis, and early death. They could then bring this knowledge to their own medical encounters or to those of friends and family. While Gehrig's story was surely unique, it was also universal.

So, too, were the stories of three other famous patients from the 1950s explored in chapters 2 through 4: baseball star Jimmy Piersall, whose tremendous mood swings and bizarre behavior on the field were diagnosed as manic-depression; glamorous *Life* magazine photographer Margaret Bourke-White, who underwent experimental brain surgery to try to cure the Parkinson's disease that had stiffened her limbs; and Secretary of State John Foster Dulles, who struggled with colon cancer as he traveled the globe, battling the "cancer of communism." Thanks to these three individuals, a series of formerly hidden subjects, such as experimentation, risk, and curability, became acceptable fare both for existing media outlets and for a new one, television.

Chapter 5 deals with another prominent individual who developed cancer, Chicago Bears' running back Brian Piccolo, whose short life became the focus of a famous television movie, *Brian's Song*. Piccolo was diagnosed with cancer in 1969, more than a decade after Dulles, but he still largely followed doctors' orders. But by the time prominent lawyer Morris Abram and actor Steve McQueen developed cancer in the 1970s, as described in chapters 6 and 7, things had changed. Both men challenged their doctors, crafting their own experimental treatments and then telling the public that they knew better than their doctors. Viewed together, these three cases demonstrate the transition of the doctor-patient relationship from one controlled by paternalistic physicians to one stressing patient-based autonomy. But as the care of cancer patients took on political dimensions, it only became harder to ascertain the efficacy of various treatments, such as McQueen's controversial mixture of vitamins, enzymes, and enemas.

Chapter 8 focuses on the difficulties of diagnosing disease. Rita Hayworth, the beautiful Hollywood actress, probably had Alzheimer's disease for more than a decade before it was correctly diagnosed in the late 1970s. Although more reluctantly than Abram and McQueen, Hayworth's daughter, Yasmin Aga Khan, publicly discussed her discontent with a medical system that had labeled her mother a chronic alcoholic. Over the next decades, Princess Yasmin used her celebrity to become a prominent activist for the Alzheimer's cause, publicizing the disease and raising millions of dollars for research.

Chapters 9 and 10 tell the stories of two ordinary people who became famous patients in the 1980s: Barney Clark and Libby Zion. In 1983, Clark, a Seattle dentist, became the recipient of the first permanent artificial heart. The resultant media circus at the University of Utah, where the procedure was performed, ensured that a series of medical issues—human experimentation, informed consent, and end-of-life treatment—had permanently arrived on the public's radar screen. But the lessons of the Clark case remained complicated, reflecting more about who was telling the story than about what had actually occurred at the bedside.

The 1984 Zion case put the issue of medical error front and center. The mysterious illness and death of Zion, an 18-year-old girl, would probably have gone unnoticed had her father not been Sidney Zion, a powerful New York lawyer and journalist. Zion embarked on a crusade to blame his daughter's death both on her physicians and on the way young doctors were educated. But the medical establishment told the story differently.

It would be impossible to write a book on the growing relationship of medicine, celebrity, and the media without including HIV and AIDS. In no other instance have patient-activists so angrily—and effectively—combated what they saw as ignorance about a disease and publicized the need to fund better research. Two such activists were Elizabeth Glaser, wife of actor Paul Michael Glaser, and the tennis star Arthur Ashe. Both Glaser and Ashe were outed as HIV-positive by an aggressive media, which had increasingly come to see its role as identifying famous patients. Yet, as discussed in chapter 11, both Glaser and Ashe, once forced to go public, did so eloquently. The fact was that a celebrity who was sick with a disease like AIDS or hepatitis C could make people pay attention to issues of stigma, politics, and, in Ashe's case, race.

The book's last celebrity patient is Lorenzo Odone, a young boy who, like Lou Gehrig a half-century earlier, developed a progressive neurological disorder. In Gehrig's case, it was ALS. In Odone's case, it was ALD, adrenoleukodystrophy, which was diagnosed in 1983. In one sense, the story of Lorenzo Odone demonstrates just how much had changed since the 1930s. When told that their son's condition was untreatable, Lorenzo's parents, Augusto and Michaela Odone, embodying the new disease activism, sprang into action. Within four years, having confounded all odds, they had developed an oil-based remedy that they believed prevented the disease and sometimes stemmed its progression. But some ALD families rejected these claims, questioning the Odones' "celebrity" status that seemingly allowed them to supersede the doctors. And some physicians also disagreed, believing that the oil's purported benefits were mostly wishful thinking. Without better data, it was not clear when, if ever, it would be possible to truly evaluate what the Odones had accomplished.

When I began this book on famous patients, I did not expect that it would so strongly emphasize this last issue—how we establish scientific proof in medicine. Yet this is, I believe, the correct focus. Over the past decade, evidence-based medicine has achieved ascendancy. Its advocates, seeking to establish the true effectiveness of medical and public health interventions, have established a hierarchy of statistical methodologies. At the top of the list are randomized controlled trials and their cousins, meta-analyses, which use data collected from multiple such trials. Lacking these types of sophisticated data, EBM experts argue, it is difficult to establish what in medicine does or does not work.[38]

But when specific patients confront medical decisions, and when policy makers discuss issues such as medical error or the allocation of medical technologies, another type of evidence is available: the anecdotal case, or what is known in statistics as an "n of 1." This is exactly the type of case explored in this book. During a personal health crisis, publicist Amy Doner Schachtel states, "Americans listen to celebrities, not the medical expert who is unknown to them." But it is not fame alone that can make a particular case important to a sick person. The past experiences of a relative, a friend, or the patient himself or herself may have a tremendous impact on decision-making.[39]

What should we make of such individual medical stories? EBM experts, not surprisingly, decry their significance, correctly noting that what happens to one sick person with a given disease likely has no medical relevance for a second person with the same condition. In addition, the growing tendency of celebrities to accept reimbursement for their disease advocacy may make their claims particularly suspect.

Relying on such stories, moreover, may be not only bad medicine but bad history. There is a tendency to judge such accounts retrospectively, using the known outcome to evaluate what happened. Thus, because he suffered greatly for 112 days and then died, Barney Clark made the wrong decision in opting for an artificial heart. And because Morris Abram survived his leukemia, he was right to have demanded experimental treatment and that all of his hospital visitors wash their hands. Clark's story thus becomes a cautionary tale of medical technology gone awry, Abram's an inspiring tale of how one patient saved his own life.

But the history of individual persons experiencing illness can also be done well. Such scholarship avoids post hoc conclusions, focusing instead on how people struggled with and then made difficult choices. Herein lies the relevance to modern medicine, in which patients rely on numerous types of information as they try to understand their illnesses and then arrive at the best decisions.

In both fields—history and medicine—individual stories remain as powerful as ever, despite what the experts and scholars say. This book asks why this is so.

Chapter 1

The First Modern Patient

The Public Death of Lou Gehrig

Perhaps the most common question that physicians, baseball fanatics, and historians have asked about Lou Gehrig's ALS is, When did it begin? This is surely an interesting topic. It is said that hitting a baseball is the most difficult act in sports. So for how long did Gehrig actually manage to play in the major leagues with a crippling neurological disease like amyotrophic lateral sclerosis?

But the onset of Gehrig's illness raises other questions as well. What were Gehrig, his wife, and his teammates thinking as he grew clumsier and clumsier in 1938 and 1939? Why did it take so long for Gehrig's illness to be properly diagnosed? What role did the media play in either revealing or concealing his true condition? What types of treatment did Gehrig undergo and what were the goals of this therapy? What did the doctors tell him about his fate? Did he know he was dying? Finally, how did the American public come to understand Gehrig's highly unusual and devastating illness?

Answering these questions is not easy. Although authors have found some relevant historical material, there has been much speculation and deduction. Indeed, the story of Gehrig's ALS has been told and retold so many times that it is difficult to trace what the facts really are and from where they originated. As with other remembered illnesses, it has been easier to try to fit the facts into a recognizable historical narrative than to construct a revised narrative from what has been discovered. In this man-

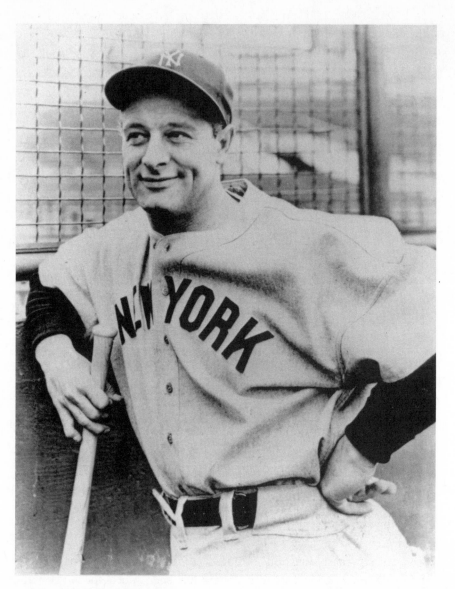

Lou Gehrig as a New York Yankee, in undated photograph from before his illness. TM 2005 Estate of Eleanor Gehrig by CMG Worldwide, www.LouGehrig.com.

ner, Gehrig's illness and death have remained tragic but somehow comfortable in their retelling.

Lou Gehrig was as unlikely a candidate as anyone for a degenerative neurological disease. Gehrig was born in New York City to German immigrant parents on June 19, 1903. The story of Gehrig's childhood and subsequent baseball career is well known. He was shy and unassuming, letting his bat speak for him, first at the New York High School of Commerce and then at Columbia University. After two years in the minor leagues, Gehrig became a Yankee in 1925. On June 1, he pinch hit. When he started at first base the next day, he replaced Everett Scott, who then held the record for the most consecutive games played in the major leagues: 1,307.[1]

Gehrig quickly became a formidable hitter. He was a clumsy fielder at first, but worked hard at mastering his position. Gehrig was also impressive physically, standing six feet, one inch, tall and blessed with a sturdy, muscular build. Over the next dozen years, as part of several championship teams, Gehrig racked up Hall of Fame statistics. In 1934 he won the Triple Crown, leading the American League in home runs, runs batted in, and batting average. Although overshadowed by his talented and flamboyant teammate Babe Ruth, Gehrig was perhaps even more feared by pitchers.

On August 17, 1933, Gehrig broke Scott's endurance record and, on May 31, 1938, he played in his two-thousandth consecutive game. There were a few games in which Gehrig, hurt, had played only a few innings, but he forged ahead despite broken bones, muscle strains, blisters, and chronic back pain. The media dubbed him "The Iron Horse," comparing his strength and reliability to the steam locomotive. Lou Gehrig, wrote biographer Stanley W. Carlson, was the "most durable athlete of all time." In 1938 Gehrig was only 36 years old. There was no telling how many consecutive games he would play.[2]

But Gehrig began the 1938 season in a terrible slump. Despite having a particularly strong August, batting .400 and knocking in 23 runs, he finished with statistics that were far below his usual output: 29 home runs, 114 runs batted in, and a batting average of .295.

In a 1989 article, neurologist Edward J. Kasarskis analyzed Gehrig's 1938 season. Based on statistics, photographs, the 1938 movie *Rawhide*, in which Gehrig had appeared, and a series of interviews with baseball players from the 1930s, Kasarskis concluded that Gehrig's ALS began before the 1938 season. Some of the facts clash with this conclusion, notably

Gehrig's productive August. Still, it seems likely that Gehrig's disease began sometime in 1938, making his subsequent accomplishments at the
plate and in the field even more remarkable than what he had achieved
when healthy.[3]

If Kasarskis is correct, another question emerges. Why didn't anyone in
1938 figure out that Gehrig was seriously ill? One person who is often
quoted as having done so is James Kahn, a reporter for the *New York Sun*,
who supposedly said, "I think there is something wrong with [Gehrig]. I
mean something physically wrong . . . I don't know what it is, but I'm satisfied that it goes far beyond his ball playing." Recent research, however,
has revealed that this statement came from an April 25, 1939, article that
Kahn wrote for the *New York Graphic*. Over time, evidently, the date of the
statement got pushed back to 1938.[4]

Why might this new date have emerged? Once Gehrig's grim fate and
the long period his illness had remained undiagnosed became known, it
was probably natural to try to find some retrospective proof that at least
one person had figured out what was going on. But it made sense that no
one in 1938 would have had an inkling that the powerful Iron Horse was
harboring a degenerative, let alone fatal, illness. Thus, Gehrig passed the
winter of 1938–39 much as he always did, spending time with his wife,
Eleanor, in their Larchmont, New York, home. Gehrig had met Eleanor
Twitchell, the daughter of a wealthy Chicago businessman, in 1929. She
was everything that Gehrig was not: outgoing, cultured, and socially well-
connected. Gehrig preferred watching movies alone, playing bridge, and
going eel fishing. But opposites attracted, and the couple married in 1933.
By all accounts, the marriage was especially close. Gehrig, who unabashedly called Eleanor "the sweetest girl in the world," much preferred to
return to Larchmont after home games than to go out drinking with his
teammates.

Eleanor Gehrig's account of what transpired between the 1938 and 1939
seasons is itself susceptible to false recollection. She discussed her husband's deterioration publicly only after his death, most notably in a 1976
book, *My Luke and I*, written with *New York Times* sportswriter Joseph
Durso. Still, her recollections remained quite consistent over time and may
thus be believable.[5]

During the winter of 1938–39, Eleanor Gehrig reported, her husband
became very clumsy. He stumbled over curbstones and fell while ice-

skating. "And at home," she noted, "he began to drop things, as though he'd lost some of his reflexes."[6]

The Gehrigs consulted several physicians, one of whom was M. W. Norton of New Rochelle, New York. Norton's diagnosis: gallbladder disease. Again, such a conclusion, meaning that Gehrig had stones in his gallbladder that caused pain when he ate, seems perplexing from our current perspective. How could a physician confuse a neurological disease with a gallbladder problem?

Yet the practice of medicine in the late 1930s was quite different from its modern counterpart. Illness, at least chronic illness, was much less of an emergency than it is today. Most physicians were not specialists but general practitioners, who relied largely on a patient's history and physical examination to reach a diagnosis. Today, a patient suspected of having gallbladder disease immediately receives an ultrasound or CAT scan of the abdomen. If no stones are present, the physician likely reconsiders the diagnosis. But in 1939, gallbladder disease was a clinical diagnosis invoked for a wide range of symptoms.[7]

Gehrig was placed on a gallbladder diet, told to avoid fried foods, sweets, and eggs. It made little difference. Eager to get back into shape, Gehrig arrived early at the Yankees' spring training camp in St. Petersburg, Florida.

What transpired during spring training in 1939 made Gehrig's earlier problems seem trivial. Joe DiMaggio, Gehrig's teammate, later wrote: "Poor Lou. He couldn't hit a loud foul. He stood up there once in batting practice and missed nineteen straight swings—all on good fast balls that he ordinarily would have smacked into the next county." Sportswriters covering the Yankees agreed. Rud Rennie of the *New York Herald-Tribune* termed Gehrig "the Yankees' No. 1 problem" and the "crumbling iron man." "He can't hit and he can't move around the bag," noted Joe Williams of the *New York World Telegram*. "All spring," Williams wrote, "the customers have been reading about how bad he looked in the field and at the bat."[8]

What did the sportswriters and, by proxy, the fans think was happening? There were other baseball players who had been stricken with severe medical problems. In 1911, Addie Joss of the Cleveland Indians died from tubercular meningitis, and the St. Louis Browns' first baseman George Sisler missed the 1923 season with sinusitis and blurred vision. But for the most part, the difficulties of baseball players—who were, after all, young and healthy—were characterized in terms of their performance on the diamond. Players having trouble performing, for whatever reason, were said to be in a slump.

From our modern perspective, it may seem incredible that Gehrig's contemporaries did not realize he was severely ill. During one game, Gehrig let two balls go through his legs that, according to one reporter, "your eight-year-old kid would have handled with his eyes closed." At least once, Gehrig apparently fell over in the locker room when attempting to tie his shoes. Yet, as the historian Leo Braudy writes, fate always seems more rigid when we look backward. Since no one knew what tragedy was looming, it made sense that Gehrig was seen not as diseased but as "ball shy."[9]

"Has the time come to turn the Iron Horse out to pasture?" Joe Williams asked. "We don't think so. We think he'll have a couple more good years." Yankees' manager Joe McCarthy agreed, at least on the record. "Gehrig's getting stronger, and he'll be better," he told James Kahn in early April 1939. "I'm not worried about him." "Your correspondent discerns no great cause for alarm," Sid Mercer reassured readers of the *New York Journal American*. "He looked bad last Spring, too."[10]

The slump theory gained credence because there was a logical explanation: Gehrig's streak of consecutive games. He had played fourteen years without missing a day. Surely he was entitled to a slump. "We firmly believe," journalist Vincent X. Flaherty would declare after the first baseman left the lineup in May 1939, that "Gehrig's inexorable zeal to perpetuate his consecutive games streak, which ended at 2,130 games, is the direct cause of his present misfortune."[11]

When James Kahn of the *New York Sun* raised this possibility with Gehrig toward the end of spring training, the first baseman demurred. "And those ten or fifteen games a season I might have missed by not playing every day," he stated, "wouldn't have added an hour to my athletic life." But Gehrig did not deny his decline. Eerily, he remarked that "an athlete's life is a short one."[12]

Despite Gehrig's woeful spring training performance, McCarthy started him at first base when the 1939 season began. Gehrig played the first eight games, getting four hits in twenty-eight at-bats for a poor batting average of .143. As the story goes, near the end of the eighth game, when Gehrig made a routine fielding play, the Yankee pitcher Johnny Murphy complimented him. Now feeling patronized as well as incompetent, Gehrig went to McCarthy and asked to be replaced for the good of the team. McCarthy complied, leading to the stunning announcement before the May 3, 1939, Yankees game that Babe Dahlgren would start at first base against the Detroit Tigers.

It is easy to see why this story has retained such currency, given its emphasis on Gehrig's selflessness. In point of fact, McCarthy had been pondering such a substitution and may have forced Gehrig to make the inevitable decision.[13]

Either way, Gehrig was out of the lineup. The degree to which the Yankees believed (or wanted to believe) that Gehrig was just tired is demonstrated by what happened next: nothing. Gehrig continued to travel with the team, even though he was not playing. He was not sent to other physicians. In early June, Gehrig and the Yankees were again in Detroit, where they watched an exhibition game involving former Tigers, including "Wahoo" Sam Crawford, then 59 years old. After he saw Crawford slam several balls into right field, Gehrig remarked: "It doesn't seem logical to me I should have slipped back so swiftly." Reporter Edward T. Murphy of the *New York Sun* agreed, speculating that Gehrig might be "suffering from some kind of organic trouble."[14]

The Crawford incident, evidently, was enough to convince Gehrig to go for a checkup at the Mayo Clinic, something Yankees' president Edward G. Barrow had begun to urge. The world-renowned facility, located in Rochester, Minnesota, was founded by two brothers, Charles and William Mayo, in 1889. Mayo attracted patients, including celebrities and people with confusing conditions, from around the world. One person especially relieved about the Mayo visit was Eleanor Gehrig, who had grown increasingly worried that her husband's physical ailments were due to a brain tumor.

Only a decade earlier, Gehrig's trip would have occurred secretly, or the media might have willingly concealed it. But by 1939, reflecting the gradually changing press coverage, Gehrig's hospitalization was fair game, reported in newspapers across the country. Over the next week, journalists persistently questioned Mayo Clinic officials about Gehrig's condition. As would be the case with Jimmy Piersall, Margaret Bourke-White, John Foster Dulles, and Brian Piccolo, Gehrig became a famous patient because he was a well-known celebrity who became sick in the public's view. Gehrig had no real agenda except for trying to get well.

Given that Gehrig's condition had gone undiagnosed for perhaps a year, what transpired at the Mayo Clinic was remarkable. The first physician who saw Gehrig was Harold Habein, an internist. As Habein later told the story, Gehrig minimized his symptoms, stating only that his left hand was clumsy. But this assertion represented the final moment of the collective denial in which Gehrig and his friends had engaged. According to his later statements, Habein quickly grasped the severity of Gehrig's condition, in part because he had an intimate connection to it. "The most serious observation was the telltale twitchings or fibrillary tremors of numerous muscle groups," he wrote. "I was shocked because I knew what these signs meant—amyotrophic lateral sclerosis. My mother had died of the same disease a few years before."[15]

Beyond the coincidence of ALS in Gehrig and in Habein's mother, how could the Mayo doctors have reached such a dramatically different conclusion than those Gehrig had seen in New York? Donald Mulder, a neurologist who joined the Mayo Clinic staff in the 1940s and knew Habein, says that making the diagnosis of as distinctive a disease as ALS would not have been difficult for a well-trained neurologist of the era. It seems that the earlier doctors had simply missed the boat. But it was not uncommon for ALS to remain undiagnosed for a year or more as doctors confronted sometimes subtle symptoms. In Gehrig's case, his dual status as an athlete and a VIP probably further blinded the physicians. Also, in an era before television, the number of doctors who had actually witnessed Gehrig's difficulties on the ball field at close range was probably quite small.[16]

As Gehrig prepared to leave the Mayo Clinic, he had to deal not only with the ramifications of his diagnosis but also with whether or not to reveal it. By this point, with the press actively following the story, deception would have been difficult. Gehrig ultimately decided to first tell the Yankees—specifically Barrow and manager Joe McCarthy—and then let the Mayo Clinic issue a press release. Barrow read Habein's statement to the public on June 21, 1939:

TO WHOM IT MAY CONCERN:

This is to certify that Mr. Lou Gehrig has been under examination at the Mayo Clinic from June 13 to June 19, 1939, inclusive.

After a careful and complete examination, it was found that he is suffering from amyotrophic lateral sclerosis. This type of illness involves the motor pathways and cells of the central nervous system and in lay terms is known as a form of chronic poliomyelitis (infantile paralysis).

The nature of this trouble makes it such that Mr. Gehrig will be unable to continue his active participation as a baseball player inasmuch as it is advisable that he conserve his muscular energy. He could, however, continue in some executive capacity.

Harold C. Habein, M.D.[17]

Habein's words were reprinted on the front page of newspapers nationwide. As discussed below, the media would have a difficult time in processing this information, in part because the ALS was wrongly characterized as a type of polio. In reality, it was a disease of the spinal cord and lower brain that caused progressive weakness of the extremities and the trunk, culminating in an inability to swallow and then breathe. But Gehrig's illness and prognosis had definitely become the public's business.

Even though Lou and Eleanor Gehrig and others had begun to suspect, before the Mayo visit, that Gehrig had a medical problem, the diagnosis of ALS was still a bombshell. "What my physical examination revealed came as a distinct shock to Mrs. Gehrig and myself," Gehrig stated on June 22. "What the tests showed was the one thing I never suspected." "I knew something was wrong with him," said Gehrig's roommate Bill Dickey, "but I had no idea it was as bad as this." "None of us ever expected anything so dreadful," said Clara Kauff, a Yankees fan from the Bronx.[18]

Although Gehrig pursued a definitive medical diagnosis at a leisurely pace, a sense of urgency would characterize his treatment. Immediately upon leaving Mayo, he began taking a series of vitamins, including vitamin C and niacin, part of the vitamin B family. Later, Gehrig would also be given vitamin B_1 (thiamine) pills.

There was no known therapy for ALS. But given the recent advances in treating diabetes and bacterial infections, there was tremendous optimism about what research could accomplish for diseases like ALS. "We do hold hope, though," Habein had stated, "that soon medical research workers here and elsewhere may uncover the means of keeping the ailment static or retarding its progress." Indeed, doctors predicted that Gehrig's very public bout with ALS would promote these medical advances and the larger research agenda in the United States.[19]

The choice of vitamin therapy for ALS reflected recent developments within medicine. Researchers had uncovered a series of diseases caused by vitamin deficiencies. Some of these conditions, such as pellagra, which is due to an insufficiency of niacin in the diet, caused neurological damage. In all of these cases, prompt administration of vitamin therapy led to recovery. For his part, Gehrig participated willingly, traveling to Mayo for periodic assessments.

Gehrig received an estimated thirty thousand letters. As in the case of Franklin Roosevelt, Jr., these came from well-wishers, alternative healers, and people with a similar affliction—ALS or other neurological diseases—seeking information. In contrast to Roosevelt, whose illness was self-limited, Gehrig's chronic condition truly made him a touchstone for fellow sufferers. Gehrig and Eleanor diligently answered these letters, evidently being careful not to raise false hopes. In one surviving letter, dated October 1, 1939, Eleanor declined to describe the exact nature of Gehrig's yet unproven treatment. To do so, she wrote, "would be unfair and possibly harmful."[20]

How was Gehrig doing? In truth, it is hard to know. After Gehrig went to the Mayo Clinic for a checkup in August 1939, Harold Habein issued a statement saying that "the general condition of Lou Gehrig is definitely improved." Habein added that there had been no progression of the disease. After his next Mayo checkup in January 1940, Gehrig reported that he was definitely holding his own.[21]

Another cause for optimism was a series of medical studies apparently showing that vitamin B_1 therapy was effective for ALS and other neurological diseases. In November 1939, Toronto physician W. J. McCormick reported vast improvement or complete recovery for fifteen patients treated with the vitamin. One of the patients had ALS. Newspapers picked up the story, reminding readers that Gehrig had ALS and was also on B_1 therapy.[22]

But the big story broke on March 13, 1940. "Remedy Is Found for 'Gehrig Disease,'" announced the New York Times, both giving ALS a new name and providing a major dose of optimism. The physician making this claim was Israel S. Wechsler, chief neurologist at New York's Mount Sinai Hospital, a Renaissance man whose friends included Sigmund Freud and Albert Einstein. In an experimental protocol, Wechsler had treated nine ALS patients with vitamin E pills and injections. Three showed no benefit, four showed improvement, and two, he claimed, had completely recovered—the first two such instances in history. "The results of treatment have been so spectacular thus far," he later wrote in the *Journal of the American Medical Association*, "that I am constrained to make this preliminary report."[23]

In one case, a 52-year-old insurance agent had come to Wechsler complaining of loss of power in the left hand. After a few weeks of vitamin E, the patient was once again able to button his coat and tie his tie. Symptoms returned when the vitamin E was stopped and again disappeared when therapy was resumed. The second case was a 36-year-old housewife who had developed difficulty walking and swallowing. After several weeks of vitamin E therapy, both of these symptoms considerably improved.

Wechsler generated even more momentous news at the June 6, 1940, meeting of the American Neurological Association. He presented additional data, now involving twenty ALS patients taking vitamin E. Nine of the patients were the same or worse, but eleven "showed varying degree of improvement": two had recovered, four had marked improvement, and five had moderate improvement.

What was particularly interesting about Wechsler's data was patient number four, described as "L.G., male, age 36." This was, of course, Gehrig. With the approval of his Mayo doctors, he had entered Wechsler's experimental study in February 1940, receiving vitamin E pills and injections. As of June, Wechsler reported, L.G. was walking better, his muscles had stopped fibrillating (spasming), and his thumbs had gained power. In the case of L.G., Wechsler announced, the condition "may be regarded as definitely arrested and somewhat improved."[24]

It is not known how many physicians at the meeting or readers of the *American Journal of the Medical Sciences*, which published the data later in 1940, figured out that Wechsler was treating Gehrig. But for Gehrig, the news had to be reassuring, despite the fact that his overall condition still remained poor. For his part, Wechsler truly believed that patient L.G. was improving.[25]

There is an old joke about what doctors tell fellow physicians about an exciting new treatment: "Rush back to your office and order it for your patients before it stops working." In the case of vitamin E and ALS, a series of studies would be published as early as 1943 calling Wechsler's findings into question. One study, conducted at the Mayo Clinic, reported on eleven cases (not including Gehrig). One patient had remained stable but the rest had worsened or died. "We have found no conclusive evidence," the authors wrote, "that Vitamin E alone or in combination with Vitamin B6 and other vitamins is of benefit in amyotrophic lateral sclerosis."[26]

How could Wechsler's findings be squared with these negative results, which have been corroborated over subsequent decades? Did Lou Gehrig truly improve between February and June 1940? And, if so, how?

These questions strike at the very basis of how one obtains proof in medicine. In some instances, proof can be reasonably straightforward. For example, if patients are treated for blood in their urine or stool, objective tests exist to determine whether the therapy has prevented further bleeding. The success of medications that treat high cholesterol can be determined by checking blood cholesterol levels.[27]

But in the case of ALS, where the outcomes of treatment are much more difficult to assess, it is considerably harder to generate accurate data. That is, measurement of muscle fibrillations, arm and leg strength, walking ability, and swallowing is, by definition, subjective. Even though scales can make such assessments more scientific, a human is still recording the information.

Moreover, Wechsler's study was uncontrolled: there was no comparison group not receiving vitamin E. As a result, what Wechsler might have been observing in the case of Gehrig and the other patients was the placebo effect, in which as many as one-third of patients improve simply as a result of receiving any treatment whatsoever. In addition, the promise of a new experimental therapy might have lifted the spirits of Gehrig and his fellow sufferers, thereby getting them to try harder both at home and at the doctor's office.[28]

One other important criterion to consider is the variability of diseases such as ALS. The same disease progresses at different rates in different people. There may also be periods during which the disease process slows down or perhaps reverses. If this occurs while a person is undergoing a new treatment, the intervention may seem to be responsible. But this may or may not be the case. It is all of these types of observational biases that randomized controlled trials seek to avoid.

So it is impossible to know whether Gehrig actually improved for a time. If he did, this likely had nothing to do with the vitamin E. But the connection between the therapy and recovery was a powerful one for Lou and

Eleanor Gehrig. The vitamins symbolized the commitment of Gehrig's physicians and, by extension, medical science to try whatever was available to thwart the ALS. Indeed, Gehrig continued to receive vitamin injections even when he dramatically deteriorated in the spring of 1941. While the vitamins clearly were not having any effect by that point, it was still possible to say that something was being tried.

Wechsler must have been profoundly disappointed when he attended the annual meeting of the American Medical Association in Cleveland on June 5, 1941. His experimental subject, Lou Gehrig, had died three days earlier. During a session on nervous and mental diseases, Russell M. DeJong, a Michigan neurologist, presented data that showed "no outstanding response" to the use of vitamin E in 19 ALS patients. By this time, Wechsler, too, was having less success in his vitamin E experiments. But, noting his earlier results, he raised a crucial issue after DeJong's talk. "The more important question," he stated, "is whether in even a single case an invariably progressive and fatal disease has shown improvement [due to vitamin E]." Although this question was perhaps no longer justified by the scientific data, it was nevertheless one that patients and their families still wanted asked.[29]

If Gehrig was optimistic about vitamin treatment, at least initially, what, exactly, did he expect it to accomplish? Another way to phrase this question is, Did Lou Gehrig know that he was dying, and, if so, when? Speculations about Gehrig's prognosis began as soon as he received his diagnosis from the Mayo Clinic. Yet, while the scientific literature was unambiguously gloomy about ALS, different people nevertheless chose to "know" different information. Thus, what Gehrig actually believed may be less interesting than how he—and those around him—chose to rationalize his quite certain death.

In trying to understand Gehrig's conception of his illness, we first have to ask where he would have received his information. The first source, of course, was the medical staff at the Mayo Clinic. As is revealed in a letter to Eleanor, Gehrig seems to have been given similar information to that contained in Habein's press release. "The bad news is 'lateral sclerosis,'" he wrote, "in our language chronic infantile paralysis."[30]

The next phrase in Gehrig's account of his discussion with his doctors is the most interesting. "There isn't any cure," he informed Eleanor. "The best they can hope is to check it at the point it is now and there is a 50–50 chance for that." This 50–50 statistic would appear frequently in subsequent journalistic accounts of Gehrig's ALS. Given that ALS was always progressive and fatal, such a statement by a doctor would have been outright deception. "It seems unlikely," journalist David Noonan wrote in 1988, "that the Mayo Clinic doctors would have told an ALS patient any such thing."[31]

In Noonan's scenario, Gehrig probably made up the 50–50 number, to protect both Eleanor and the American public from the grim truth. And, as Mayo physicians never corrected Gehrig, at least in public, it would have meant they had silently chosen to go along with his decision.

This series of events is plausible, but unlikely. Deception was widespread in medicine during the 1930s and 1940s. Patients with cancer, for example, were routinely lied to about their diagnoses, being told of "growths," "tumors," or "inflammation." One such patient would be Babe Ruth, whose wife and doctors concealed his diagnosis of throat cancer, even when the dying Bambino was admitted to Memorial Hospital, a renowned cancer facility in New York City, in 1948. Physicians justified this practice by arguing that it preserved hope, encouraged patients to participate in available treatments, and, at times, prevented suicides. Family members, who were generally told the truth, willingly participated in the secrecy.[32]

Thus, while Gehrig was told the actual name of his disease, it is reasonable to assume that, at least initially, the Mayo physicians fudged the issue of his prognosis. The "50–50" chance of recovery left open the very real possibility that Gehrig would worsen and possibly die, but also held out hope that he could stabilize at his current level of disability.

Statements Gehrig gave to the press in June 1939 seem to corroborate the idea that he saw his future as either uncertain or reasonably hopeful. The *New York Herald-Tribune*'s Rud Rennie listened in on a conversation that Gehrig had with his teammates on June 21, 1939, the day that Gehrig's illness was announced. When one Yankee asked him whether his condition was curable, he replied, "I don't know." Jimmy Powers of the *New York Daily News* reported that Gehrig "believes the disease can be checked and that it will not get any worse."[33]

Some sportswriters interviewed physicians about Gehrig's prognosis, and, in certain cases, ominous details appeared in newspapers. But most journalists who learned that ALS was fatal kept quiet. Rather, press accounts were upbeat, even going beyond Gehrig's cautious optimism.

"Gehrig Sure He'll Beat Illness," announced a front-page headline in the June 22, 1939, *New York Journal American*. "In a broader sense," wrote Joe Williams, "the tragedy is softened by the promise that Gehrig will ultimately win out in his fight for complete health." That the public believed this story is suggested by the thousands of empty seats on July 4, 1939, when Gehrig gave his famous "luckiest man" speech. Had Gehrig's remarks really been his "farewell speech," as it was later dubbed, Yankee Stadium surely would have been packed.[34]

There are several reasons why the press told this hopeful story. Even though tabloid newspapers had made celebrity illnesses fair game to some degree, much secrecy still existed. In addition, the rare nature of Gehrig's disease, and the irony of its attacking such a strong and decent man, probably led to a degree of denial among reporters. This was not cancer in a 70-year-old. Thus, when Gehrig dangled the 50–50 statistic, the press latched onto it, interpreting it as positively as possible.

In doing so, however, these optimistic reports created a type of feedback loop. Once the press announced enough times that Gehrig's condition would remain stable or improve and that he could look forward to decades of productive life, it became hard not to believe it. Gehrig himself may have taken some solace in the optimistic pronouncements that appeared in the newspapers.

There was another reason that the press slanted its coverage of Gehrig's illness. Besides Bill Dickey, Gehrig's other best friends were the reporters who traveled with the Yankees—Richards Vidmer, Joe Williams, Grantland Rice, and John Kieran. Train trips between American League stadiums meant endless poker games for Gehrig and these writers. The New York press, therefore, was covering the fatal illness not simply of a beloved athlete but of a friend. To the degree that these reporters knew the truth, telling it to the public was not an option.[35]

Only after Gehrig died, in June 1941, did the reporters admit that their coverage had been incomplete. Gehrig's impending death "was not a story that anybody on the sports page would have written," wrote Bill Corum, a *New York Journal American* writer and a friend of Gehrig's since high school. Corum's editor, Max Kase, agreed. "Lou Gehrig could still read papers and did—and you couldn't, not even in ink, end the hopes of one of the greatest gamesters you had ever met in sports."[36]

Another person telling Gehrig what he wanted to hear was his wife,

Eleanor; after his death, she began to tell her version of her husband's illness. Throughout these accounts, Eleanor portrayed herself as having successfully kept the truth from Lou. She stated, for example, that she secretly researched ALS at the New York Academy of Medicine and frankly spoke to her husband's doctors, most notably Mayo Clinic physician Paul O'Leary, without his knowledge. "He never knew he was doomed," Eleanor said shortly after Gehrig's death. "He thought, right up to the last few days, that he would get well." In her 1976 book, Eleanor said the same.[37]

But what did Lou Gehrig himself know or think? Some commentators believed that he absolutely knew his fate. On the day after Gehrig died, *New York Sun* sportswriter Frank Graham wrote a column entitled "He Knew It All the Time." Graham related two stories to back his claim. One incident, which occurred in 1939, involved a sportswriter, later identified as Rud Rennie. Rennie had been walking with Gehrig when a group of Boy Scouts had wished the Yankee good luck. "They're wishing me luck," Gehrig supposedly told Rennie, "and I'm dying." In another instance, on Lou Gehrig Day in July 1939, Gehrig had reportedly told another sportswriter: "It is going to be very hard to leave all this." Most of Gehrig's biographers have dutifully repeated these quotations. Gehrig, wrote journalist Ray Robinson in *Iron Horse*, "gave out hints, from time to time, that he realized his chances for survival were slim."[38]

One other account of Gehrig's life suggested that he knew he was dying. In the 1942 Hollywood movie *Pride of the Yankees*, Gary Cooper, playing Gehrig, directly confronts the physician giving him his dread diagnosis. "Tell it to me straight, Doc," Gehrig importunes. "Is it three strikes?" The doctor nods, sadly, in reply.

At times, historical questions are impossible to answer because of inadequate documentation. For decades, it seemed that it would be difficult to ever know what the deteriorating Lou Gehrig was thinking. But recently discovered correspondence between Paul O'Leary and both Lou and Eleanor Gehrig provides some answers. In researching his 2005 biography of Gehrig, *Luckiest Man*, journalist Jonathan Eig received permission to quote from the letters, which went into great detail about Gehrig's ALS and his treatments. Eig discovered that Gehrig repeatedly asked O'Leary for the truth. "Paul," he wrote to the doctor, who had also become a friend, "I feel you can appreciate how I despise the dark, but also despise equally as much false illusions." On another occasion, Gehrig, after describing worsening symptoms, wrote: "What is your conclusion? And honestly, please."[39]

O'Leary, albeit regretfully and thoughtfully, deceived his patient. As late as January 1940, he gave Gehrig a 45 percent chance of making some sort of recovery. And when Gehrig met a musician, Al Reiser, who told Gehrig that he had recovered from ALS, O'Leary did not tell his patient that Reiser had actually been suffering from another, less severe, form of sclerosis. "I have always disliked to tell falsehoods," O'Leary wrote to Eleanor Gehrig, "but I feel that with Lou we must keep his morale up, not only for the benefit and help it may be to him, but also in order to save him the shock that accompanies such discussions."[40]

Thus, Eleanor Gehrig's account of her husband's last two years were essentially accurate. Consistent with the paternalism of the times, she, O'Leary, and the other doctors had largely kept Gehrig in the dark, despite his suspicions they were doing so. As the twentieth century progressed and patients' rights became a rallying cry, such deception would become much more difficult to carry out. Yet, as we shall see, Gehrig's ability to maintain hope and confidence in the face of almost certain death—in other words, simultaneously believing conflicting versions of his fate—would become the standard approach for severely ill patients in a society increasingly familiar with the concept of medical miracles.

Just as the press had misgivings about discussing Gehrig's terminal illness, so, too, did it gingerly cover his impending death in the spring of 1941. At the end of 1939, Gehrig had accepted an offer from New York mayor Fiorello LaGuardia to become a city parole commissioner, deciding the fates of various criminals. Each day, Eleanor drove Gehrig to work from his new home in the Bronx to downtown Manhattan. At some point, Gehrig could no longer hold a pencil. But he dutifully continued to work until early 1941, when Eleanor was forced to submit a letter of resignation to LaGuardia in his behalf. Gehrig now remained home, listening to Eleanor read aloud and playing with his dog, Yankee.[41]

To New Yorkers who happened to see Gehrig at work, his deteriorating state would have been evident. In this sense, his impending death was quite public. In addition, a steady stream of friends visited Gehrig at his home, even when he had become essentially bed-bound by May 1941. These included Bill Dickey, Ed Barrow and other Yankees, the comedian Pitzy Katz, and the actress Tallulah Bankhead. Gehrig looked gravely ill.

"I was shocked at how he looked," New York Giants' manager Bill Terry later stated. "It made me want to cry. He must have lost eighty or ninety pounds."[42]

Other frequent visitors were Gehrig's good friends, the New York sportswriters. One was John Kieran of the *New York Times*, whose son, James Kieran, remembers what his father reported about those visits. The elder Kieran spent many mornings playing cards with Gehrig and entertained him with an accordion. Meanwhile, Eleanor Gehrig had pulled Kieran aside to ask for help with the upcoming funeral arrangements.[43]

None of this, however, made its way into the newspapers. The *World Telegram*'s Joe Williams later explained why: "But all of us, or rather most of us, in the newspaper game, had decided we'd let Gehrig die in peace. There were two reasons: one was Lou, the other Eleanor, and nobody ever had a finer girl." Thus it was respect and privacy—not some type of taboo against discussing death—that kept the reporters quiet. After all, in the case of Thomas Edison a decade earlier, reporters had maintained the equivalent of a death watch.[44]

Gehrig's death was an old-fashioned one. Until the early twentieth century, death almost always occurred at home. Death was a ritual: dying individuals and their families often choreographed the final days and weeks, inviting over relatives and friends to say their last good-byes. Physicians largely helped nature take its course. With the rise of the modern, technologically advanced hospital, however, more people found themselves dying as inpatients. In the hospital, individuals were surrounded not by their loved ones but by strangers. Probably because physicians had nothing more to offer him, Gehrig bucked this trend, dying quietly at home on the evening of June 2, 1941. It was exactly sixteen years to the day since he had taken over at first base for the Yankees. He was 37 years old.[45]

What were Gehrig's actual dying weeks like? Here again, there are many competing stories. A few accounts provided fairly graphic details of both Gehrig's death and the toll it took on his family. An interview conducted by journalist Harold Weissman with Gehrig's New York physician, Caldwell B. Esselstyn, was particularly revealing. The last six weeks were "nightmarish" for Eleanor and her mother, Nell, who subsisted on three hours of sleep per night. At the end, Esselstyn said, Gehrig died of "Dreaded Bulbar Paralysis," which "clogged his respiratory organs."[46]

In *My Luke and I*, Eleanor Gehrig detailed what she termed ALS's "grim progression." Her husband's hands and arms, she wrote, "grew increasingly useless, then his legs could hardly support him; later, speech and even swallowing were impaired." The period between Gehrig's diagnosis and death, she concluded, was "two years of ruin."[47]

But the predominant version of Gehrig's final weeks and months emphasized the positive. His death had been a peaceful one in which he remained optimistic and interacted meaningfully until almost the last moment. These accounts emerged immediately following his death and have persisted ever since. For example, the *New York Journal American*'s Max Kase termed Gehrig a "champ to the end," reporting that, as he died, his lips had formed the name "Eleanor." In his 1941 biography of Gehrig, journalist Richard G. Hubler reported that Gehrig, just before dying, opened his eyes to acknowledge Eleanor and his parents. He then supposedly tightened his grip on Eleanor's hand (something that would have been physically impossible by that time), smiled, and then passed away. In her own book, Eleanor Gehrig wrote that at the moment of death, a "most beatified expression instantly spread over Lou's face."[48]

A positive spin also characterized accounts of Gehrig's last two years. In a 1948 article in *Sport* magazine, journalist Jack Sher concluded that Gehrig's last two years were "supremely happy," as Gehrig enjoyed the admiration and sympathy of baseball fans everywhere. When, toward the end, he could no longer hold a book, Gehrig "was humorous and sheepish about it. There was almost no self-pity." Gehrig, wrote sportswriter Earle W. Moss, "pursued his work to the very end without a word of bitterness or complaint."[49]

There is probably some truth in these accounts. Patients with ALS do generally die quietly by simply stopping breathing, although there may be a period in which they gasp for air. In addition, given Gehrig's generous nature and good-humored approach to life, he almost surely complained less about his fate than others might have.

But the descriptions of Gehrig's death ultimately had as much to do with how people wanted to imagine it as with the actual events. As a baseball player, Gehrig was associated with competition and winning, as were the other athletes and politicians who dominated celebrity life in the mid-twentieth century. Thus, a ballplayer as indestructible as Gehrig surely had to have fought his disease tooth and nail. This version of events was promulgated by his friend, sportswriter Max Kase, in a June 3, 1941, column:

"Lou Fought Game Battle with Death." Kase praised Gehrig's determination to beat his illness, even at the end, making it "his creed to carry on." While admirable in and of itself, Gehrig's grit served an even broader purpose, making him a "symbol of hope" for fellow sufferers of ALS. "Paralysis victims, thousandfold," Kase waxed poetically, "were looking to him for the spiritual strength to help them shed their shackles."[50]

Biographer Hubler, in his zeal to show how Gehrig had ably fought his disease despite dying, wrote that no man "had ever outlived [Gehrig's] disease, chronic polio, for more than two years." But Gehrig, he said, had beaten that record by a month. Not only did Hubler once again confuse ALS with polio, but he also exaggerated Gehrig's achievement. Yes, Gehrig had set the record for most consecutive baseball games, but many others had lived longer with ALS.[51]

Hubler also wrote about a journalist named Quentin Reynolds who had recently learned the story of a heroic English soldier. This soldier had single-handedly dug up and safely disabled a time bomb planted by the Nazis. When the storyteller was through, someone had commented to Reynolds: "You, I'll wager, have never seen anything approaching such courage." Reynolds disagreed. "Yes, I have," he said. "I knew Lou Gehrig."[52]

The connection of Gehrig to World War II would become even more pronounced after the United States entered the war in December 1941. In July 1942, RKO released *Pride of the Yankees*, based on Gehrig's life. The film opened with a statement by the noted writer Damon Runyon: "He faced death with that same valor and fortitude that has been displayed by thousands of Americans on far-flung fields of battle. He left behind him a memory of courage and devotion that will ever be an inspiration to all men. This is the story of Lou Gehrig." The analogy of Gehrig to the heroic soldier was thus complete. Even though Gehrig had simply been the unfortunate victim of a disease, it was as if he had given his life for his country. Fighting disease had become the moral equivalent of fighting war.[53]

A few reviews chided *Pride of the Yankees* for its unabashed romanticism and sentimentality, with one even suggesting that it was exploitative. But critics generally praised the movie, which was based on a book by sportswriter Paul Gallico. One critic, for example, said that it "will renew your faith in and love for the American way of life."[54]

The film's account of Gehrig's illness and death was greatly simplified, revealing even less than had New York's sportswriters. Gehrig, played by Hollywood legend Gary Cooper, is depicted having trouble on the baseball diamond, choosing to end his streak, and then going to "Metropolitan Clinic," where he receives his diagnosis. Aside from the "three strikes" line, which alludes to his fate, there is no mention of either dying or death. The scene then shifts to Yankee Stadium, where Cooper delivers Gehrig's famous, moving speech.

Then, amidst a swell of romantic music, Cooper quietly trudges into the Yankees' locker room and the film ends. The reality of Gehrig's subsequent physical deterioration and death is subsumed by the symbolic image of a dignified man accepting his unlucky fate. Edwin Schallert of the *Los Angeles Times* praised the decision to end the movie with the speech, which "compels with its glowing courage." The *New York Times* critic Bosley Crowther wrote that Cooper, as Gehrig, "accepts with silent courage his seemingly merciless fate."[55]

Although most Americans were familiar with the outlines of Gehrig's story, it was not until *Pride of the Yankees* that they actually saw the tragedy played out. The movie was quite successful, grossing more than $3 million and earning eleven Academy Award nominations. Director Sam Wood deliberately blurred fact and fiction by casting several Yankees, including Babe Ruth, to play themselves. In choosing Gary Cooper to play Gehrig, director Sam Wood selected an actor who was known for playing characters that fit Gehrig's persona: strong, silent, and stoic. *Variety* approved of Wood's strategy, praising the film as having "consummately fused" reality and art. "Gary Cooper is Lou Gehrig," enthused the reviewer.[56]

But it might be more reasonable to state that Lou Gehrig had become Gary Cooper. By telling Gehrig's story as one of unabashed heroism and sacrifice in the face of illness, *Pride of the Yankees* both validated earlier myths about his life and influenced future accounts. Later recollections about Gehrig's illness were as likely to refer back to the Hollywood film as to any first-hand written accounts, which, as we have seen, themselves downplayed unpleasant aspects of his last weeks and months.

So powerful was the Gehrig legacy that in 1995, when Baltimore Orioles infielder Cal Ripken, Jr., seemed poised to break the consecutive games record, there was resentment. Someone calling himself "Lou Gehrig, Jr." phoned in a death threat to Ripken. The broadcaster Larry

King urged Ripken to stop his streak after tying Gehrig at 2,130 games, enabling the two players to become "a twin example of the best in us." Gehrig, King wrote in *USA Today*, "walks with the angels."[57]

With Ripken chasing Gehrig, it could not have been easy to criticize the Yankee great. But an essayist, Florence King, did. In an op-ed piece in the *New York Times*, she raised doubts about Gehrig's streak, pointing out that he had left many games in the late innings, and pitied Eleanor Gehrig for her decades-long service as keeper of her husband's flame. "Frankly," she wrote, "I am tired of Saint Lou Gehrig." But almost no one else was.[58]

In the decades after he died, Lou Gehrig's death became transformed into a paradigmatic good death—a tragedy, to be sure, but one to be admired. First, Gehrig had fought nobly, willingly undergoing experimental therapy just as America had begun to champion clinical research. Not only did this treatment hold out the possibility—however remote—of saving him, but it also provided hope to his fellow sufferers. After her husband's death, Eleanor Gehrig kept this upbeat message alive, tirelessly raising money to fund research into another neurological disease, muscular dystrophy, and even pondering a "Gehrig Foundation" to further this cause.[59]

Second, once the experimental treatment failed, Gehrig ultimately accepted his fate in a dignified, courageous manner. "Gee, there was no pity coming out of him at all," recalled Yankee teammate Tommy Henrich about his final visit to Gehrig's home. "Whatever it was that was eating him up, he was taking it as he always did." "He certainly was given a bad break," wrote Richard Bak, "but he never expressed regrets because he truly had none."[60]

Today, it has become customary to describe a death in terms of a good fight followed by gradual acceptance. But it is worth remembering how Gehrig and *Pride of the Yankees* helped to idealize this model of death and, more importantly, to ensure that this is how survivors would remember such deaths. It was, after all, a comforting script.

Roughly a decade after Lou Gehrig died, another baseball player became ill in plain view of the press and the public. Jimmy Piersall's problem was not neurological but psychiatric—he had severe mental illness. Piersall proved to be far more forthcoming than Gehrig had been, providing several detailed accounts of his illness. Although Piersall, like other famous patients of the post–World War II era, never really challenged the system, the concept of the celebrity as disease activist was emerging.

Chapter 2

Crazy or Just High-Strung?

Jimmy Piersall's Mental Illness

.

The subjective nature of the illness narrative might best be exemplified by the story of baseball star Jimmy Piersall. In 1955, Piersall wrote an autobiographical account of his manic depression (now known as bipolar illness) for the *Saturday Evening Post;* this was later expanded into a book, *Fear Strikes Out.*

Piersall's decision to go public was remarkable. Popular understandings of mental illness in the 1950s were as diverse as the labels given to Piersall. He was variously described as "crazy," "berserk," "being eaten alive," a "mixed-up kid," and as having had a "nervous breakdown." Some believed that Piersall was truly sick, while others viewed his eccentric behaviors as opportunistic. By the time of the 1957 movie, also called *Fear Strikes Out,* the focus had shifted to the supposed cause of Piersall's mental problems; the blame was pinned on his father, John Piersall. The story of what happened to Jimmy Piersall had less to do with the actual events than with who was doing the telling.

In contrast to Lou Gehrig, Jimmy Piersall recovered from his public illness and has lived for another fifty years, allowing not only journalists but also Piersall to revisit his story. As time went on, Piersall rejected many of the assumptions of the psychiatric profession that had ostensibly "cured" him. The tellings and retellings of what happened to an energetic 22-year-old baseball player, beginning in 1952, demonstrate how stories of celebrity illness can simultaneously enlighten and mislead the public.

Some facts about Piersall's story are not in dispute. He was born in

Waterbury, Connecticut, in 1929, the son of a house painter, John, and his wife. John Piersall was a former semipro baseball player who remained frustrated at his own lack of success in the sport. As soon as Jimmy Piersall was old enough to play baseball, his father began grooming him for the career that he himself had never had.

Meanwhile, Piersall's mother was troubled. During much of her son's childhood, she was in and out of institutions. Piersall never learned his mother's actual diagnosis, except that it was a "mental condition."[1]

John Piersall's efforts paid off. By the time Jimmy entered high school, he was not only an excellent baseball player but also talented at football and basketball. Baseball scouts had already begun to make inquiries about him. The plan, however, was for Piersall to gain a baseball scholarship at Duke University.

But problems had already begun. Jimmy Piersall had an extremely high energy level, what we might now label "hyperactive." He was highly animated, especially on the baseball field, where he chattered and screamed constantly. Piersall also developed headaches, but told no one.

Piersall's plans to attend Duke changed in March 1947 when his father suffered a heart attack. John Piersall had to stop working, and the family decided that it was time for Jimmy to become the breadwinner. Jimmy initially took a job loading freight cars but soon thereafter signed a contract with his favorite team, the Boston Red Sox.

Piersall spent 1948 playing for a minor league affiliate of the Red Sox in Scranton, Pennsylvania. There he met a nurse, Mary Teevan, whom he would marry in October 1949. In 1951, Piersall hit .346 for another minor league team, the Birmingham Barons. He also was a spectacular center fielder, routinely making catches that amazed both teammates and fans. There was talk that Piersall would start in the outfield for the Red Sox in 1952.

His minor league years, however, had been troubled ones. Piersall remained very high-strung and, it seemed, incapable of relaxation. He worried not only about his performance on the baseball field but also about his family's finances. He and Mary had their first child, Eileen, in 1951, and a second was due in early 1952. Piersall was also still supporting his aging parents.

It was in the winter of 1951–52, when Piersall's mental condition began to worsen, that his story becomes trickier to tell. The most definitive description of this period comes from Piersall's own writings—the two articles published in the *Saturday Evening Post* and his book *Fear Strikes Out*, all co-written with Boston sportswriter Al Hirshberg. But, because these accounts were autobiographical, they presented Piersall's worsening state of mind and eventual breakdown quite subjectively.[2]

With this caveat, here is Piersall's version of what occurred. In December 1951 he was reading the baseball "bible," the *Sporting News*, when the following words "seemed to leap up from the printed page and crack me right across the face":

> One planned move [by the Red Sox] is the converting of Jimmy Piersall, minor-league outfielding sensation with Birmingham last season, into a shortstop. Piersall will be the chief target of the Red Sox brass at the special training camp which opens in Sarasota January 15.

Writing in 1955, Piersall described his reaction: "It was impossible! I wasn't a shortstop. I was an outfielder . . . Why, it could ruin me. Ruin me? Maybe that's what they intended." He concluded that the Red Sox were trying to get rid of him.[3]

Piersall's wife, Mary, told him that he was mistaken, but he refused to be convinced: "As the days went by and the inner turmoil increased in intensity, I drew further and further from reality. I couldn't face people. I was a pariah."[4]

Piersall acted strangely the rest of the winter, going to movies by himself and roaming the streets of Scranton, where he still lived. When Piersall announced that he was not going to the Red Sox training camp in Florida, Mary called his father, who convinced him to go.

On the plane to Tampa in January 1952, Piersall reported, he grew even more anxious. He was especially worried about supporting Mary, Eileen, and the baby to come. By the time he arrived at the team's hotel, his heart was "beating a frantic tattoo" on his ribs, his head was "bursting," and his eyes were "smarting."[5]

Piersall entered the hotel lobby. That, he told readers, was the last thing he remembered until he woke up seven months later in the "violent room" of Westborough State Hospital.

Piersall's amnesia, which his physicians would attribute to a combination of his illness and the electroshock treatments he received, meant that he had to reconstruct what had occurred between January and August 1952.

He did this through a combination of discussions with Mary and supportive teammates and by reviewing a series of scrapbooks that John Piersall had kept.

He had begun the 1952 season at shortstop, Piersall reported in the *Saturday Evening Post* and in his book. In May he got into a fight with Billy Martin, the Yankees' shortstop, and with one of his own teammates, Maurice McDermott. Sensing that Piersall was too stressed, Red Sox manager Lou Boudreau shifted him to the outfield. During games, Piersall began to stage a one-man show. He made elaborate gestures after catching balls, did calisthenics, and clowned with the fans. He also made fun of other players.[6]

Then, on June 12, 1952, after reaching first base, Piersall mocked the pitcher, the legendary Satchel Paige, by "jumping up and down and making noises like a pig as I gestured." A few days later, at Chicago's Comiskey Park, Piersall did a "hula-hula" dance in the outfield.[7]

Finally, on June 28, the Red Sox had had enough, sending Piersall back down to Birmingham. But things only got worse. He climbed into the stands to lead cheers for himself, heckled umpires, ran around wearing only an athletic supporter, and, on July 17, sprayed home plate with a water pistol when an umpire called him out. The next day, Piersall agreed to be evaluated at a private sanitarium in Boston. After becoming violent there, doctors transferred him to Westborough State Hospital.[8]

Piersall's account of his breakdown was a thoughtful one, based on what information he could acquire. But as with most retrospective narratives of illness, his version contained a sense of inevitability and fate that was not present at the time. Thus, his breakdown was portrayed as a more or less linear story in which a volatile individual was given bad news—that he would be moved to shortstop—which precipitated a progressive and perhaps inevitable decline. The sudden demotion to Birmingham then fanned the flames. Eventually, Piersall's antics became more and more severe, until the Red Sox concluded that he needed professional help.[9]

But in reality, Piersall's story was more complicated. Well into the 1952 season, he was seen not as undergoing a mental deterioration but as someone who was outlandish and trying to attract attention to himself. Bernie Sherwill, his childhood friend, was "shocked" by Piersall's breakdown. A lot of players, teammate George Kell recalled, even encouraged Piersall to do wild things. "I couldn't really see his breakdown coming," Kell stated.

Nor did Red Sox third baseman Fred Hatfield. No one thought about sending Piersall to see a psychiatrist, according to Hatfield: "We just thought he was nuts."[10]

A useful source of information about Piersall's condition is contemporaneous newspaper coverage. As was the case with Lou Gehrig, whose neurological illness was characterized as a hitting slump, so, too, was Piersall portrayed not as sick but as an eccentric and entertaining ballplayer. Among the adjectives sportswriters used to describe him were "prankish," "bouncy," "impish," and "zany." Even when Piersall was sent to Birmingham, the *Boston Globe* termed him the "Clown Prince of Rookies." Lou Boudreau had demoted Piersall, wrote Arthur Daley of the *New York Times*, to "settle down his ebullient problem child."[11]

Even the sportswriters who suspected something might be wrong were far from sure. "Was Piersall serious or was it an act?" asked Harold Kaese in a June 30, 1952, column in the *Globe*. Piersall had been sent to Birmingham for "clowning, boasting and making disparaging remarks," Kaese stated. But, he asked his readers, didn't such charges seem too light for demotion to the minor leagues?[12]

One journalist, although unsure that any organic problem existed, nevertheless pushed the issue further than did his peers. What worried Austen Lake of the *Boston American* was Piersall's "immediate and frenzied flood of real tears when benched or scolded." His angers, Lake continued, "are violent and sudden, flaming into challenges and fist-slugging." Lake, in retrospect, was a good clinician. Others who had witnessed the crying had teased Piersall, nicknaming him "Johnnie Ray," after the emotional crooner of the 1950s.[13]

One reason for the confusion was that the vast majority of these journalists—perhaps all of them—had never witnessed a professional athlete's breakdown. There were moody ballplayers, of course, such as Boston slugger Ted Williams, but such individuals basically kept it together. Without a frame of reference, it makes sense that the journalists were as surprised as anyone when Piersall was eventually committed.

This ignorance about mental illness helps to explain the vast range of terminology used to describe Piersall's condition. The *Boston American* diagnosed him with "nervous exhaustion," while the *Boston Globe* chose "mental exhaustion." A 1953 article by Al Hirshberg in *Sport* magazine stated that Piersall had experienced a nervous breakdown. Piersall's *Satur-*

day Evening Post pieces were entitled "They Called Me Crazy—and I Was!" "He wound up berserk in a mental hospital," read a tag line introducing the first of the two articles. Nor did the book *Fear Strikes Out* provide readers with any type of definitive diagnosis. What he had experienced, Piersall wrote, was a "mental collapse."[14]

Reporters did not pursue more definitive information about Piersall's diagnosis or prognosis. If it had become acceptable to pry for details about Rudolph Valentino's intestinal rupture and possibly Lou Gehrig's ALS, mental illness continued to be off limits. Still often treated in locked institutions with lobotomies, straitjackets, and other seemingly barbaric techniques, mental patients and their lives remained secret and shameful. The sportswriters evidently did not even interview expert psychiatrists to get generic details about such breakdowns.[15]

Had these reporters pursued the story, they might have learned Piersall's actual diagnosis. According to materials contained in Al Hirshberg's papers at Boston University, Piersall had experienced a "manic depressive reaction, manic type." Manic depression, in which a person alternates between periods of great euphoria and sadness, was named by the renowned German physician Emil Kraepelin in 1899. A physician at Westborough State Hospital wrote that Piersall often showed "push of speech," now known as pressured speech. In addition, he was "overactive, facetious [and] euphoric." In later years, Piersall revealed his diagnosis of manic depression.[16]

Piersall was discharged from Westborough on September 9, 1952, after a one-and-one-half-month hospitalization. His treatment included sessions with a Mexican-born psychiatrist, Guillermo Brown, and electroshock therapy. At the time of discharge, he was termed "recovered." By early 1953, Piersall was back at the Red Sox spring training camp in Sarasota. When the season opened in April, he was the team's starting right fielder.

One person who took special notice of Piersall's saga was Don Slovin, a Chicago man who had recovered from mental illness. Slovin had founded an organization called Fight Against Fears, named after the 1951 Lucy Freeman book of the same title, which was a support group for people with various mental illnesses. In 1954 Slovin convinced Piersall to tell his story on a popular Chicago television talk show, hosted by newspaper columnist Irv Kupcinet.

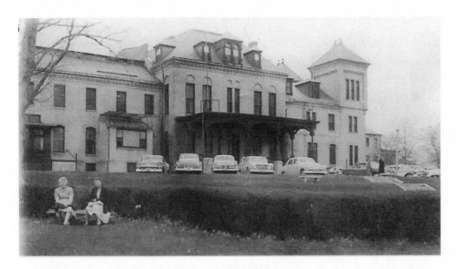

Westborough State Hospital, where Jimmy Piersall was hospitalized after his breakdown in 1952. Photograph of main building, taken in 1958. Courtesy of the Massachusetts Department of Mental Health.

Although newspapers had covered Piersall's story, the Kupcinet appearance was really his "coming out." Television, which would eventually become a common vehicle for sick celebrities to go public, made stories of illness seem more intimate and personal. Piersall frankly told Kupcinet's audience about his breakdown, his institutionalization, and his subsequent recovery. "I pointed out the need for coming into the open," Piersall later wrote, "and letting the world know that there were thousands like me, who could be cured if people would try to understand them."[17]

The response was highly positive. Piersall received more than a hundred letters from Chicago residents, most of whom had experienced some type of mental illness. Piersall, and through him Fight Against Fears, represented a real opportunity for interested people to obtain information. One Chicago woman wrote, "I've had this for about 8 years. I got better for awhile but had a setback about 5 years ago. I haven't been more than a block from the house in that time unless I have a few beers ahead of time but I've come to the conclusion [that] that is not fighting it the right way. I know it is all mental but I can't do anything about it. The minute I know I'm going some place I start worrying maybe I'll get this spell and by the time I'm ready to go I'm a wreck. I feel as if every nerve in my body is tight and that I'll pass out. People think it's so easy to get over something like this but I can't." She concluded her letter with a request for books that could help her.[18]

An East Chicago woman praised Piersall as having provided "a source of inspiration to anyone who has gone through an experience similar to yours." Piersall, she concluded, had "resolved a possible tragedy into this ultimate victory."[19]

Thanks to Piersall's efforts, membership of Fight Against Fears rose to five hundred people by the summer of 1954. Piersall generously donated his time to the group when he was in Chicago.

While Chicago had heard about Piersall's breakdown, the rest of the country still knew few details. Boston sportswriter Al Hirshberg saw this as an opportunity. Hirshberg had befriended Piersall in 1952 and had been writing a story on him for the *Saturday Evening Post* at the time of the outfielder's demotion to Birmingham. *Post* sports editor Harry T. Paxson had told Hirshberg to put the story on hold. But by mid-1953, with Piersall playing well and experiencing no apparent mental problems, Hirshberg broached the topic again. "A year ago," he told Paxson, "he was on his way to the nuthouse and there was a definite question as to whether or not he'd ever get out." But Piersall had shown no signs of "cracking" so far. The real story was his comeback, which was "one of the most unusual in the game's history."[20]

Paxson remained cautious, telling Hirshberg to wait until the end of the 1953 season. But Paxson was interested, realizing the newsworthiness of the potential article. "A Piersall story," he told Hirshberg, "should be primarily the case history of a guy who has gone through the grinder and come back—so far at least—both in the mental-health and playing-field departments." In February 1954, Paxson told Hirshberg to go ahead. "We would want his mental problem gone into as thoroughly as good taste permits," he stated.[21]

But problems remained. How could the *Saturday Evening Post* be sure that Piersall was telling the truth? After all, he had told Hirshberg that he had no recollection of what had occurred during much of 1952. And how would Hirshberg validate the claims about Piersall's mental illness? With Piersall's permission, Hirshberg solicited letters from Guillermo Brown and Morris L. Sharp, the superintendent of Westborough State Hospital; both basically corroborated what Piersall had said. Later, the *Post* sent a draft of the piece to an independent psychiatrist, who gave his approval. Paxson was now satisfied.[22]

Piersall, however, was not. He was now asking to be paid for the story. As always, Piersall, who would eventually have eight children with Mary, was concerned with supporting his family. Although the *Saturday Evening Post* did not pay people featured in its publication, it did pay authors. So Hirshberg came up with a clever idea. Piersall would be the author of the two pieces, which would be billed as "as told to Al Hirshberg." In this manner, Piersall could be paid. He ultimately received $3,500 for the two articles. Response to the *Post* articles, published on January 29 and February 5, 1955, was very positive. Piersall estimated receiving more than fifteen hundred letters, all of them supportive.[23]

Several months before these articles were published, Hirshberg was already planning to convert them into a book. In September 1954, he sent a pitch letter to Boston publisher Little, Brown. The book on Piersall, he stressed, would focus as much on mental health as on baseball. That Little, Brown proved interested is not surprising. As Nancy Reynolds, a friend of Hirshberg's in the publishing industry, told him: "All the ingredients of a best-seller are here—a nationally known figure, an unusual problem, a story of great courage and compassion." Reynolds was correct. As of 1961, six years after its publication, *Fear Strikes Out* would be in its thirteenth printing, having sold roughly three hundred thousand copies. The topic of mental illness in a famous person, formerly seen as taboo, had become compelling. As Mary Piersall later wrote, "It was the first time anyone in the public eye had ever openly identified himself as a former mental patient."[24]

Piersall and Hirshberg's book, *Fear Strikes Out*, was published in May 1955. Reviews were positive. "His case is more than substantial proof," wrote John N. Makris of the *Boston Herald*, "that mental illness, so frightening to many people, can be cured."[25]

The role played by "fear" in his experiences had taken center stage for Piersall. The word also appeared in the title of Lucy Freeman's book and in the name of Slovin's Chicago group. In addition, Guillermo Brown had stressed the issue of fear, according to Piersall. "You worried yourself into this place by being afraid of the future," he quoted Brown as saying. "You thought the whole world was against you." As such, the solution Brown had provided was clear-cut: "It's that fear which you have to avoid."[26]

This focus on fear, as opposed to the specific illness in question, fit well with the political climate of the United States, which was entrenched in the Cold War. In the mid-1950s Senator Joe McCarthy was at his height, playing on the fears of Americans as he detailed the supposed communist takeover of Hollywood and the government. Outing mental illness, like outing the Soviet threat, made sense.

The emphasis on fear was also related to trends in psychiatry during the 1950s. By the start of the twentieth century, many physicians viewed insanity and other mental illnesses as being caused by various biological abnormalities located in patients' brains. This construct led physicians to devise a series of so-called somatic treatments designed to fix these problems. These included the frontal lobotomy, which involved cutting nerve pathways within the brain, and two procedures designed to produce brain seizures: insulin shock therapy and electroshock therapy. Although doctors did not know exactly how such treatments worked, they believed that they often helped.[27]

Concurrently, however, there was growing interest in an alternative model—one that saw mental illness as primarily psychological, resulting from one's early life experiences. The main figure responsible for this development was Sigmund Freud, the Austrian-born psychiatrist who believed that unconscious motivations determined behavior. According to Freud, psychological problems, ranging from hysteria to neuroses, stemmed from repression of painful past experiences, particularly childhood events. The best strategy for such patients, therefore, was not changing the biology of the brain but psychoanalysis, in which a psychiatrist would help identify these painful memories. This knowledge, once exposed, would help patients return to normal mental health.

By 1910 Freud had gained an international following. Indeed, some psychiatrists had begun to advocate psychoanalysis or a less rigorous program of psychotherapy for patients with diseases that Freud had not emphasized—notably schizophrenia and manic depressive illness. The Freudian approach to psychiatric disease reached its peak in the United States in the years after World War II, thanks in part to the success of psychotherapy in treating soldiers suffering from stress disorders. By the 1950s, psychoanalysts dominated many medical school psychiatry departments and even state hospitals like Westborough.[28]

Given this climate, it is not surprising that Hollywood latched onto the themes of Piersall's fear and inner turmoil. In fact, in the decade before the opening of the film *Fear Strikes Out* in 1957, Hollywood released several other movies depicting people with psychiatric illnesses arising from earlier life crises. Most notable among these was *The Snake Pit*, a 1948 film in which the heroine's psychotic breakdown was revealed through flashbacks to earlier traumatic events. When *Fear Strikes Out* was released, *Time* magazine even joked about Hollywood's "Vienna lobby," a group of "psychiatric doctrinaires" who made movies based on the medical charts of psychiatrists.[29]

The Hollywood movie was actually not the first production of Piersall's life story. On August 18, 1955, the CBS television show *Climax!* presented an hour-long version of *Fear Strikes Out*, starring heartthrob Tab Hunter as Piersall. In this production, the cause of Piersall's breakdown was his "fear of failure." At the end of the film, Piersall himself appeared in a clip shot shortly after his recovery. In it, he expressed concern about his ability to return to the major leagues. Mary Piersall, sitting next to him, would have none of this. "Jimmy," she implored, "you can't live your life in fear."[30]

The Hollywood version of *Fear Strikes Out*, starring a young Anthony Perkins as Piersall, was released in February 1957 to generally strong reviews. "Paramount," wrote the *Hollywood Reporter*, "has what looks like a real winner." Interestingly, promotional material for the movie emphasized yet another societal concern of the 1950s: it characterized Piersall as a juvenile delinquent, an adolescent gone bad. "Here's the whole heart-story of today's mixed-up kids!" read one advertisement for *Fear Strikes Out*. A second advertisement showed Piersall being restrained by policemen. Piersall, according to the accompanying text, was not ready "for the savage thing inside that twists him toward the ragged edge of violence."[31]

The delinquency angle may have attracted audiences, but the Hollywood movie returned to the theme raised by Piersall's book and the *Climax!* film: the inner turmoil of one young man. Moreover, it told Piersall's story using an explicitly Freudian story line. Guillermo Brown's earliest efforts to try to help his patient are through psychotherapy, in which the two of them explore Piersall's upbringing. Piersall is uncooperative at first. "Jim has escaped into a world of his own and built a wall around it," Brown tells Mary. "Until we can break through that wall there's no way to reach him." At this point, Brown proposes trying electroshock therapy; after some trepidation, Mary consents. But even this treatment is characterized as a way to foster subsequent therapy sessions. Finally, after several shock treatments, Piersall becomes receptive to Brown's questioning and talks about his upbringing. The story that Piersall eventually tells is one of an overbearing father obsessed with making his son a major leaguer. Piersall's fears, which led to his breakdown, resulted from his father's relentless hounding.

To what degree was this aspect of Hollywood's version of *Fear Strikes Out* realistic? There is no doubt that John Piersall desperately wanted his son to become a major league baseball player. But while he appears as an importunate father in Piersall's book and in the *Climax!* presentation, he has become a monster in the Hollywood film. Indeed, the production, beginning with scenes of Piersall as a child, is framed around the father-son conflict.

As vividly portrayed by Karl Malden, John Piersall relentlessly badgers and insults his son for any perceived transgressions on or off the baseball field. In an early scene, John Piersall throws the baseball to his son with such force that the boy starts crying. The father does not notice. When Jimmy's high-school friends convince him to go ice-skating, the teenager returns home with a broken ankle. John Piersall is so upset that he collapses to the ground, almost suffering a heart attack. This event did not actually occur. Later in the film, when John Piersall visits his son in Scranton and learns that he is third in the league in batting, he can only criticize. "It isn't first," he says. With a father like this, the film strongly implies, it is no wonder that Jimmy Piersall had a breakdown.

Why was John Piersall transformed in this manner? As was the case with the Lou Gehrig story, *Pride of the Yankees*, film biographies strive less for the truth than a good story, and in the 1950s, a Freudian tale of childhood hardship was especially compelling. Thus, it made sense to overemphasize John Piersall's overbearing qualities and blame him for his son's breakdown.[32]

The degree to which the movie *Fear Strikes Out* reflected both the psychiatric theories of the day and the need to tell a good story can be gleaned from a memorandum written during revisions of the script in 1956. Piersall's mental illness was "non-organic," the unknown author stated, "the result of intra-personal conflict." Thus, "for our purposes of dramatic presentation," the conflict between John and Jimmy Piersall needed to be highlighted even more. The author recommended further development of

John Piersall's character as a way to explain why he put such pressure on his son. He went on to suggest two fictional events that would achieve these goals: that Piersall's father be even more vindictive after the broken ankle and that Jimmy drive himself even harder because of his guilt over John Piersall's near heart attack. It is not clear what, if any, changes were made based on these suggestions, but the final version of *Fear Strikes Out* surely simplified Jimmy Piersall's breakdown into a story of the damaging effects of an imperious father.[33]

Jimmy Piersall later strongly criticized Hollywood's version of *Fear Strikes Out* for this emphasis. (He also thought Anthony Perkins was terribly unathletic and "threw like a girl.") He believed that his father's behavior, and its supposed connection to his breakdown, had been exaggerated. "They made my father out to be a real bastard, one who was trying to drive me to a mental breakdown," Piersall later recalled. "Well, he wasn't."[34]

The decision to frame Piersall's story as a triumph over fear, beginning with his book and continuing through both films, had a paradoxical effect. It rendered invisible just what Piersall and others like him were being treated for: severe mental illness. Thus, those who corresponded with Piersall about the topic of mental illness often did not mention it by name. For example, Don Slovin wrote that fighting fears could "help these people who have temporarily lost confidence in themselves regain that new confidence and begin a new life with a new hope." A Chicago woman who had been hospitalized for a suicide attempt wrote, "Mr. Piersall, I most certainly agree with you that the most we have to fear is fear itself." Piersall himself would later state that "the reason for all breakdowns is a fear of failure—failure to succeed at work, failure to succeed as a husband, failure to succeed at anything."[35]

Also pushed to the background was the most probable cause of Piersall's recovery and what it signified. To his credit, Piersall was thoroughly open about the fact that he had received electroshock therapy, a treatment that in the 1950s conjured up associations of cruelty and even torture. First introduced in 1938, electroshock therapy caused seizures—tremendous shaking of the body—as it tried to "shock" the brain to normal. But psychiatric textbooks of the era agreed that electroshock, and not much else, was effective in treating manic depressive illness.[36]

Shock therapy, however, was most certainly a biological treatment, the success of which spoke to a formulation of mental illness that was primarily organic—not psychological—in nature. Nevertheless, given the atmosphere of the era, Piersall's recovery was largely configured as a Freudian success story of exposing and then overcoming one's emotional problems, with the role played by shock therapy greatly downplayed.

The emphasis on this particular story line becomes especially relevant when assessing Piersall's subsequent behaviors. By all accounts, Piersall had experienced a remarkable recovery. The man who had been confined against his will to a mental hospital in 1952 did indeed play right field for the Boston Red Sox in 1953. He stayed with the team until 1958, hitting serviceably and always amazing fans with his acrobatics in the outfield.

There were, to be sure, rocky patches during these years. For one thing, certain fans teased him mercilessly about his illness. There was no better example of why mental illness needed to be destigmatized than the taunts Piersall experienced. In Detroit, *Look* magazine reported in 1954, fans called him a "goony bird." Another common ploy was to make a siren noise and then announce the imminent arrival of men in white coats. Not only fans behaved this way. Dick Williams of the Baltimore Orioles sang "cuckoo, cuckoo, cuckoo" whenever Piersall was in earshot.[37]

One sign of Piersall's recovery was his ability to endure these taunts. He was still animated, of course, and caused his share of problems on and off the field. But the highly dramatic antics that had characterized his breakdown had ceased.

But things began to deteriorate in 1960. After the 1958 season, the Red Sox had traded Piersall to the Cleveland Indians. As someone who had grown up in Connecticut and achieved his lifelong goal of playing for Boston, Piersall was displeased. He made it through 1959 without any major incidents. In 1960, however, his behavior once again became erratic. Some of the problem stemmed from conflict with the Indians' manager, Joe Gordon, who took a dim view of Piersall's pranks.

What was Piersall doing? Many of his antics were reminiscent of 1952. Piersall constantly fought with the umpires, eventually being ejected from eight games. He sprayed bug repellent in the outfield to protect himself from insects. In Chicago on May 30, 1960, in response to being hit with an orange thrown from the stands, he rifled a baseball against the scoreboard. In Cleveland, Piersall came to the plate wearing an oversized batting helmet. Two innings later, he became dizzy and asked to be taken out of the game. In the locker room he burst into tears and took tranquilizers.[38]

Things came to a head late in June at a Sunday doubleheader with the New York Yankees in Cleveland. During the second game, Piersall argued a call with the umpire and was thrown out of the game. The Indians had a day off on Monday and Piersall wanted to see his family, who still lived in Boston. He left the ball park early to catch the six o'clock flight, the last one of the day.

What happened next is a matter of controversy, but a rumor spread that the outfielder had deliberately gotten himself ejected to make the last plane. Moreover, a reporter had apparently convinced Joe Gordon and Frank Lane, the Indians' general manager, that Piersall needed to see a psychiatrist. Regardless of the exact chain of events, by the time Piersall arrived in Boston, Mary Piersall had received a phone call from Donald Kelly, the Indians' team physician. "Jim's not to report back to the ball club until we send for him—or until he sees a doctor there," Kelly told her. Piersall consented to see a Boston psychiatrist who, according to Piersall, gave him a clean bill of health.[39]

Piersall was back in the outfield within a week, but his misbehavior continued. During a pitching change in Yankee Stadium, he sat down behind a group of monuments dedicated to old Yankee stars. Later in the game, he stood behind second base when Yankee pitcher Ryne Duren, a poor hitter, came to bat. Things did not settle down until August, when Frank Lane made a surprise move, trading his manager, Joe Gordon, for the Detroit Tigers' manager, Jimmy Dykes. Dykes was much more supportive of Piersall than Gordon had been.

Throughout 1960, Piersall remained a favorite of the fans, who appreciated his attempts to animate slow-moving games on hot summer afternoons. Many sportswriters also defended him to the hilt, either because they genuinely liked him or because they knew he could always be relied upon for a pointed quote. But those within baseball, including some of his teammates, often tired of his constant showboating.

Just what was going on with Piersall in 1960? One sportswriter who believed that Piersall had relapsed suggested that the ballplayer pen a sequel to his book, entitled "Fear Doubles to Left." An article by journalist Dave Anderson posed (but did not answer) the key question. Its headline read, "Putting on an Act—Or Really Sick?" It depended whom one asked, reported Ed Linn in *Sport* magazine. One colleague believed that Piersall "could stop it completely any time he wanted to." Another said, "It's not an act; it's a compulsion."[40]

This confusion largely stemmed from the vague way that Piersall and the media continued to describe his illness. Although members of the press wrote numerous articles connecting Piersall's recent behavior with his 1952 breakdown, they provided few medical details. Manic depression was again unmentioned. Reporters did not revisit Piersall's earlier treatments, such as psychotherapy and electroshock therapy, or ask if they needed to be resumed. While it is possible that journalists tried to raise these issues and were thwarted by Piersall or by a mum medical profession, there is no suggestion that such an attempt was made. As such, most of the opinions rendered about Piersall in 1960 were just that—opinions.

For his part, Piersall vehemently denied that 1960 equaled 1952. Guillermo Brown, Piersall had written in *Fear Strikes Out*, had pronounced him "cured." "It's all over now," he had quoted Brown as saying. "You're starting from scratch." Piersall often referred to himself as a "former mental patient."[41]

This focus on cure, by both Piersall and his doctors, bespoke the reigning cultural model for understanding disease, which was that of acute infections. If someone developed pneumonia or a blood infection, as did Franklin Roosevelt, Jr., he either died or completely recovered. But with rates of infectious diseases declining in the 1950s, attention was turning to chronic conditions—heart disease and some types of cancer—that persisted but did not necessarily kill you. Most mental illnesses fell into this latter category, but it was hard for Piersall, or anyone else, to see anything but a complete cure as a realistic goal.[42]

Piersall did not affirmatively deny that mental illness could recur; he simply believed it was not happening in his particular case. His antics were not crazy but funny, he asserted, as when he had gotten into an argument with umpire Bill McKinley. "All I know is that they shot the wrong McKinley," Piersall had told him. Piersall also claimed, with good reason, that many of his transgressions had occurred in response to harassment from fans and opposing players. Mostly, though, Piersall argued that his pranks, by allowing him to relax, *prevented* a relapse of his illness. He admitted that he sometimes got "keyed up" during ballgames and did things that landed in the newspapers. "But," Piersall insisted, "this is all letting off steam."[43]

Well aware that his behavior was raising concerns, Piersall drew careful distinctions between his current problems and his earlier breakdown. "The last time I had headaches, and I blacked out, and I thought everyone was against me," he told his wife. "None of those things is true now. I'll be all right, Mary. You watch."[44]

But Mary Piersall was unsure. In March 1962, with the help of Al Hirshberg, she wrote an article for the *Saturday Evening Post* entitled "Why Do They Call My Husband Crazy?" An earlier draft of the article can be found in Hirshberg's papers. In this draft, Mary rejected claims that her husband had been mentally ill during the 1960 season. His battles with umpires and aggressive play, she wrote, "might have made him different, but it certainly didn't make him crazy." She had known that Piersall was sick in 1952, Mary added, but knew he was not in 1960.[45]

But a second draft of the article, which was nearly identical to the printed version, told a different story. Nineteen sixty had become a "nightmare season," Mary Piersall stated, as her husband "exploded in a series of antics that reminded me of the year I wanted to forget." Piersall, she wrote, "was in a fight—a battle far greater than he might have had with an umpire." Mary then told a story of how Piersall had been waving his arms and dancing around at a game that she attended with two of her children. When umpire Ed Hurley approached Piersall, the outfielder charged him. As would be expected, Piersall was ejected from the game. "For a moment I sat in silence," Mary recalled, "then realized I just had to go somewhere and hide. I told the others to wait for me, and fled to the ladies' room."[46]

Despite all of this, Mary Piersall concluded, her husband was clearly not as bad as he had been in 1952. For example, his behavior at home, which had been erratic eight years earlier, was "calm and sensible." In contrast to 1952, Piersall had the ability "to leave his pressures on the field and in the locker room."[47]

Even though Mary Piersall ultimately assured readers of the *Saturday Evening Post* that her husband had not been crazy in 1960, her own ambivalence about the events spoke volumes. The question was not really whether Piersall was crazy but whether he had become crazier, and he surely had. Medical textbooks of the era described manic depression as a relapsing illness, one that often returned in a more or less severe form.

The media, while covering the story, still held back. Perhaps because they liked him or respected his candor, sportswriters generally acceded to

Piersall's version of the story: he was not crazy, merely trying to deal with the constant scrutiny he received because he had once been crazy. "Free expression on the field of his turbulent emotions," wrote Murray Robinson of the *New York Journal American*, "has acted as his safety valve." But Robinson had drawn this conclusion by speaking not with a psychiatrist but with "Dr." James Piersall.[48]

In hindsight, it is reasonable to conclude that Piersall's exploits in 1960 probably were due to a flare of manic depression, albeit a milder case than had earlier landed him in the hospital. Perhaps the best diagnostician was Piersall's teammate and friend Vic Power. "He said he wasn't crazy anymore," Power later recalled, "but he still was sick."[49]

Incidents continued to occur through the rest of Piersall's playing career. In 1961, Piersall punched and kicked two fans who had leapt onto the field at Yankee Stadium and accosted him. In 1963, by then with the New York Mets, he ran around the bases backward after hitting his one-hundredth home run. Piersall finished his career with the California Angels in 1967, having played major league baseball for sixteen years.

Piersall has had an eventful professional and personal life since then. He divorced Mary, remarried, got divorced again, and then married his current wife, Jan. Piersall has held a series of jobs, including running ticket sales for the Oakland Athletics, broadcasting Chicago White Sox games on radio, and hosting a sports talk show in Chicago. In many of these positions, issues about Piersall's mental health have arisen. For example, after a dispute with Oakland owner Charles Finley in 1972, Piersall became depressed and checked himself into a rehabilitation center. He was given psychotherapy and medications, and he eventually improved.[50]

In 1974, Piersall was hired by the Texas Rangers on the condition that he see a psychiatrist. This physician recommended that Piersall begin to take lithium, recently approved as the first medication specifically for manic depression. After a month on lithium, Piersall later wrote, "I could see that it was working." The drug modified the "extremes" in his feelings, providing him with "the proper chemical balance" in his system. Such a response, of course, belied the frequent claim that Piersall's manic depression had been "cured" in 1952.[51]

But even after Piersall began to take lithium, he was still prone to mood swings and outbursts. One of the most infamous of these events occurred in 1980. As a radio broadcaster for the Chicago White Sox, Piersall prided himself on his honesty. (His second autobiography, published in 1984, was called *The Truth Hurts.*) During games, Piersall pointedly questioned decisions made by White Sox manager Tony LaRussa and team owner Bill Veeck. When Piersall called Veeck's wife, Mary, a "colossal bore," antagonism toward Piersall increased. Eventually, LaRussa conducted an informal poll of the players to see whether they thought Piersall should be fired.[52]

On July 2, 1980, Bob Gallas, a reporter from a local paper, was interviewing White Sox players about LaRussa's poll. Piersall confronted him and things escalated. Accounts of the brawl differ, but some witnesses claimed that Piersall had tried to choke Gallas, which Piersall later denied. On the same day, Mike Veeck, son of Bill and Mary, got into a shouting match with Piersall, which also led to a physical altercation. Afterward, suffering from pains in his chest and "mental upset," Piersall was taken to Illinois Masonic Hospital, where he stayed for a week.[53]

"I did need a rest," Piersall later wrote. "I did need to get away from the pressures." To his surprise, he was not fired but given a leave of absence. Once again, his biggest supporters were the fans, who hung banners at Chicago's Comiskey Park urging his return. Piersall came back, but again found himself in hot water for calling the wives of baseball players "horny broads." "Controversy follows him the way May follows April," wrote one Chicago journalist.[54]

Although Piersall has spoken forthrightly about mental illness for almost fifty years, his case underscores the ways in which this type of disease still remains hidden and poorly understood. Were Piersall's outbursts the result of his illness or his underlying personality, which was intense, effervescent, and confrontational? The line between being distinctive and pathological is often a fine one. Piersall himself has pointed this out, arguing that his behavior, which would merely be seen as eccentric in others, has reflexively been seen as disease in his case.[55]

Over time, Piersall has consistently obscured aspects of his own disease and treatment. For example, he has often analogized mental illness to breaking a limb—an easily definable medical problem that can easily be fixed by pursuing appropriate treatment. But mental illness has always represented a major challenge, due to its complexity. Piersall, the sportswriter Bill Madden perceptively noted in 1980, had spent half of his lifetime "simultaneously proving and disproving he had licked his affliction."

In contrast to Piersall, Kay Redfield Jamison, professor of psychiatry at the Johns Hopkins School of Medicine and a successfully treated manic-depressive, has come to terms with the unpredictability of her disease: "I long ago abandoned the notion of a life without storms."[56]

Despite his evident admiration for Guillermo Brown in his book *Fear Strikes Out*, Piersall has also displayed a dim regard for mental health professionals. "Psychiatry isn't the answer," he said in 1976. "It's just a crutch. Psychiatrists don't really tell you anything constructive." He reiterated this point when interviewed for a 2001 ESPN documentary. All psychiatrists do, he said, "is ask you what do you think." Psychologists did not fare any better in Piersall's eyes: "They talk too much and they do nothing."[57]

As an alternative, Piersall has increasingly emphasized the value of self-help, arguing that individual effort—as opposed to shock treatment or psychotherapy—was the key to managing and overcoming his disease. "Someone who is emotionally disturbed has lost control of the ways of conducting himself," he said in a UPI interview. "He is someone who needs to be loved by his parents, who needs someone to relate to, someone to assure him that all is well." Mental illness, he told ESPN, is like any other sickness. "You can cure it, or you can lick it, if you want to." Without discounting the virtues of self-help, the vast majority of modern mental health professionals would never suggest that it serve as the primary intervention for manic depression.[58]

Well before it became fashionable to do so, Jimmy Piersall went public with his mental illness in magazines, in books, on television, and in a Hollywood film. Yet, rather than a coherent account of one man's manic depression, we are left with a series of stories. Depending on the version at hand, Piersall's breakdown was due to the Red Sox decision to play him at shortstop, his overbearing father, or a severe biological illness. He has been alternatively described as cured, recovered, or still nuts. His ability to overcome his mental illness has been attributed to Freudian psychiatry, shock therapy, lithium, or personal initiative. In other words, different audiences have placed their own spin on Piersall's story.

Such a conclusion can be frustrating for a historian who seeks to definitively document "what happened." Yet, as we saw in the case of Lou Gehrig, illness narratives are not only about the "truth." Rather, they derive their power and, ironically, their validity from the meanings and lessons that people draw from them. When the movie *Fear Strikes Out* was released, a perceptive reporter from *Life* magazine actually thought to ask Jimmy Piersall's father, John, what he thought of the film. After all, the elder Piersall had been depicted as cruel and the cause of his son's breakdown. But John Piersall said that he approved of the film, explaining that it might help others in trouble.[59] In his mind, this honorable goal apparently outweighed any concerns about accuracy.

It is reasonable to assume that, as a prominent figure, Jimmy Piersall has had excellent medical care. But, perhaps due to his ambiguous feelings about psychiatry, he never has actively sought out the "best" or most cutting-edge treatments. The renowned photojournalist Margaret Bourke-White did. When she developed the early signs of Parkinson's disease in the 1950s, she underwent a controversial new operation and then told her story to the public. Bourke-White believed that the procedure had helped her. But proving this—to the medical profession, others with Parkinson's, and, eventually, even herself—would be a difficult challenge.

Chapter 3

Picturing Illness

Margaret Bourke-White Publicizes Parkinson's Disease

As with a brain surgeon who develops brain cancer, Margaret Bourke-White's illness was ironic. A jet-setting photographer for *Life* magazine and other publications, Bourke-White relied on dexterity, quick reflexes, and being in the right place at the right time. Among the first symptoms of her Parkinson's disease was difficulty snapping photographs.

Bourke-White, as a journalist, had access to individuals who knew about the latest developments in Parkinson's. She became an ardent consumer of such information, particularly that concerning a controversial new brain operation, which she underwent in 1959. Bourke-White then told her story in a 1959 article in *Life*, in a unique 1960 television broadcast, and in her 1963 autobiography; her neurologist later stated that she had provided "the most vivid and clear neurological description of the early, subtle signs of this disorder."[1]

Like Jimmy Piersall, Bourke-White corresponded with fellow suffer-ers—other people with Parkinson's. But these individuals saw her not only as a courageous figure who gave them hope and alerted the public about their disease but as someone who knew a great deal about both the prog-nosis of Parkinson's and new therapies coming down the pike. Bourke-White's decision to assume this role made her a forerunner of celebrity disease activists who would emerge in subsequent decades. But she and her compatriots had to contend with an unfortunate reality. The highly touted new interventions for Parkinson's that Bourke-White advocated in print, notably the operation that she underwent, were not panaceas. Being an advocate for treatments of limited value proved to be a complicated task.

Bourke-White excelled from an early age. She was born in the Bronx in 1904 and moved to New Jersey at age 4. In high school, she was president of the drama club and editor of the school's newspaper and yearbook. At Columbia University she took a class in photography, leading her to abandon a potential career in zoology. A transfer to the University of Michigan followed, as well as a short marriage. Finally, having earned her bachelor's degree from Cornell University, Bourke-White was free to pursue her new career: photojournalism.[2]

In 1927 she moved to Cleveland and opened a photography studio. Among her subjects was an area of the city known as The Flats, which housed steel and other industries. Bourke-White ventured onto the factory floors, snapping pictures that made the machinery look like works of art. Her industrial photographs gained her local renown, although some were skeptical that a woman had taken them.

One person who saw Bourke-White's photographs was Henry Luce, the publisher of *Time* magazine. In 1929 Luce hired her to work on a new magazine, *Fortune*, which featured business and industry. Bourke-White traveled across the country, photographing workers and factories at places as varied as the Campbell Soup Company and the Chrysler Corporation. Later, working with the writer Erskine Caldwell, she photographed poor families in the South; a book, *You Have Seen Their Faces*, resulted.

In 1936 Bourke-White moved to another new Luce publication, *Life* magazine. It was for *Life* that she would take her most famous and memorable pictures, "telling of people and their bravery in the face of sufferings." Her subjects included President Franklin D. Roosevelt and his family, Soviet leader Joseph Stalin, and the Buchenwald concentration camp at the end of World War II. After the war, Bourke-White went to India, chronicling Mohandas Gandhi's rise to power; South Africa, documenting the imposition of apartheid; and Korea, covering her second war. It is no exaggeration to state that Bourke-White was the most accomplished woman photographer of her era.[3]

It was in Korea that she felt what, in retrospect, would be the first stirrings of her Parkinson's disease: "a dull ache in my left leg, which I noticed when I walked upstairs." The first formal description of the disease had been by an English physician, James Parkinson, in 1817, but it had existed since Biblical times, when it was termed the "shaking palsy." Individuals with Parkinson's develop rigidity of their muscles, difficulty in moving, and, at times, tremors of their arms or legs. They also suffer from a "masked" face, due to immobility of the facial muscles. Physicians now know that the disease results from damage to brain cells that produce dopamine, a compound that facilitates movement of the body.[4]

Bourke-White initially downplayed her symptoms. She was, after all, "Maggie the Indestructible," someone who had fearlessly traversed the world in pursuit of remarkable images. Upon returning from Korea she consulted a series of physicians, but, in a situation that Lou Gehrig or Jimmy Piersall would have recognized, none of them figured out her problem.[5]

Finally, in January 1954, after twenty months of symptoms, Bourke-White wrote to Howard Rusk, an acquaintance and well-known specialist in the rehabilitation of polio patients. She was 49 years old. At this time she complained that her left hand was stiff, preventing her from typing, and that her left leg "has a slight drag . . . I seem to slap my foot a bit instead of walking evenly." Rusk referred her to his colleague Morton Marks, a neurologist. Yet when Marks made the diagnosis of Parkinson's, he kept it secret from his patient. "I am not going to give it a name," he told Bourke-White, "because someday you may see a very advanced case and that might discourage you." Marks, like Gehrig's physician Paul O'Leary, was a paternalist, taking upon himself the burden of Bourke-White's diagnosis and treatment.[6]

The photographer, urbane as she was, evidently did not press for details. Although Bourke-White eventually urged people with Parkinson's to learn as much as possible about the disease, we should not project back in time an initial inclination to challenge her physicians, something she may not even have perceived as an option. At the start of her illness, at least, she was quite comfortable assuming the passive "sick role," a theoretical model then being described by the sociologist Talcott Parsons, in which patients were expected to cooperate with medical practitioners who were laboring to make them well.[7]

Marks prescribed rehabilitation, referring Bourke-White to a therapist named Jack Hofkosh. After some initial skepticism, Bourke-White actively embraced Hofkosh's exercise regimen, which included crumpling newspapers into balls and squeezing out wet clothes. She also tried to walk four miles a day, even when on assignment in remote areas or confronted by bad weather. Throughout her illness, Bourke-White remained a staunch devotee of exercise, constantly urging reluctant fellow sufferers to persevere.[8]

By June 1955 she reported some improvement, particularly in her left hand. Successfully typing the early chapters of her autobiography, *Portrait of Myself,* which would be published in 1963, she told one of her doctors that "there is no doubt that the fingers have improved considerably." Her left leg, unfortunately, still ached and lacked strength. She still had no tremors of her arms or legs. Bourke-White's Parkinson's was the akinetic form of the disease, in which muscle stiffness interferes with movements, such as walking, turning, and writing. In 1957 she underwent three weeks of intensive physical therapy at Howard Rusk's Institute of Physical Medicine, located in New York City.[9]

Throughout these years Bourke-White kept working, traveling across the United States and abroad. She initially did not tell her editors at *Life* about her impairment. But colleagues gradually deduced that something was wrong. One story Bourke-White covered in the mid-1950s was the construction of the New York State Thruway, which required her and another *Life* journalist, Richard Stolley, to charter a small plane. As she prepared to lean out of the plane to take pictures of the enlarging highway, she bragged to Stolley that she had never dropped anything on her many flying excursions. Almost immediately thereafter, Bourke-White dropped her lens cap. "I still vividly recall the look of anguish on her face," Stolley said in a recent interview.[10]

It is not exactly clear when Bourke-White learned her actual diagnosis—probably 1955 or 1956. Her biographer, Vicki Goldberg, says that the revelation occurred when she saw "Parkinson's disease" written on an insurance form. Bourke-White was grateful for the knowledge, quickly discovering that the disease affected roughly one million Americans, including many notable people: the photographer Edward Weston, Australian nurse and polio expert Sister Elizabeth Kenny, and the playwright Eugene O'Neill, to name just three. Bourke-White soon became a vocal advocate for full disclosure. "If I could give only one message after sifting down this experience," she would later write in *Portrait of Myself,* "it would be to urge others to banish the secrecy."[11]

Passivity was never really an option for Bourke-White; she naturally became a student of her disease. Perhaps due to an inherent inquisitiveness or because Parkinson's so directly threatened her passion and livelihood, photography, she became immersed in cataloguing her limitations and her efforts to surmount them.

Typical was a section of her book that described her problems with balance. "Balance is a mysterious and highly personal thing," she wrote, noting that even her cat brushing against her legs could make her topple over. Bourke-White described her body as a "Tower of Pisa" that leaned different ways on different days. But there were strategies she could use. For example, quickly throwing one arm up over her head could interrupt a fall. In addition, she always paid close attention to potential obstacles. "As I walked into a room," she wrote, "I surveyed it much like a pilot in a single-engine plane surveys the ground beneath to spot a little landing strip in case of emergency."[12]

Beyond physical therapy, a number of drugs were available for the treatment of Parkinson's at this time, including trihexyphenidyl (Artane). Unfortunately, none of them was especially effective. But the 1950s were also the heyday of aggressive surgery in the United States. Surgeons who had served in World War II, performing risky and novel operations, had returned with a great confidence about what they could accomplish. At this time, for example, surgeons removed the ribs and limbs of many patients with metastatic cancer, with the hope of eliminating all remaining cancer cells. While Parkinson's was very different from cancer, the prospect of surgical intervention generated a similar optimism.[13]

The surgeon offering hope with his scalpel was Irving S. Cooper, an assistant professor at the New York University School of Medicine. Cooper had devised his new brain operation in 1952, during a mishap involving a Parkinson's patient. The surgeon, then 30 years old, had been performing another procedure, which involved cutting certain nerves in the brain. This latter operation was only used for patients with severe tremors and worked, unfortunately, by partially paralyzing certain muscles in the body. During one such procedure, Cooper evidently tore a blood vessel in the brain known as the anterior choroidal artery. Although Cooper aborted the operation, the patient's tremor markedly decreased, leading the doctor to hypothesize that his mistake—by depriving a certain part of the brain of oxygen—was actually therapeutic. Cooper convinced another Parkinson's patient to allow him to tie off the same artery on purpose. This patient also had relief of his tremor without paralysis.[14]

Cooper was sitting on a possible medical bombshell. But he did what physicians in the 1950s usually did with this sort of information. He quietly recruited a series of patients and offered them the operation, thereby accumulating what is known as a case series. Then Cooper presented his data to his fellow physicians.

But such results, even if preliminary, did not stay within the confines of the medical profession. During the 1950s, the public became increasingly exposed to medical topics, due to publicity efforts by the American Medical Association as well as growing coverage of scientific advances by the press. A few reporters had begun to specialize in science and medicine. Some, like Walter C. Alvarez, formerly of the Mayo Clinic, were retired physicians with good writing skills. Others were formally trained reporters. Like any journalists, they sought out big stories and thus kept close tabs on major medical journals and the meetings of prominent medical societies. When the findings suggested a breakthrough, it was time to alert the public.[15]

And so when Cooper published early data on thirty patients in the journal *Surgery, Gynecology and Obstetrics*, reporters noticed. "A surgeon can now go into a brain and destroy a particular artery and therby [*sic*] do something big against Parkinsonism," announced Delos Smith of United Press International. Given the novelty of the procedure, Cooper had operated only on patients with very severe symptoms of Parkinson's. But this is what made his findings so striking. As Smith reported, three of Cooper's patients, who had been "utterly helpless" for seven to twenty-five years, now "walk, talk, dress and feed themselves." Many others had also improved. When Cooper presented data on fifty patients at a November 1954 conference, similar press coverage ensued. Thirty-five of the fifty, reported *New York Herald-Tribune* science editor Earl Ubell, had experienced reduction or elimination of their rigidity and tremors.[16]

The media coverage of Cooper's procedure, it should be noted, was muted. The headline of Smith's article merely read "Parkinsonism Aid Found." And reporters noted the major drawback of the procedure: a mortality rate of 10 to 13 percent. That is, one out of every eight to ten of Cooper's patients had died during or shortly after the surgery, which, after all, required burring a dime-size hole in the skull and manipulating the brain. Still, the potential import of Cooper's work was apparent, certainly to any physicians or patients who were familiar with the frightening sensation of being trapped within one's own body. The apparent improvement experienced by some of Cooper's patients, Walter Alvarez allowed, was "miraculous."[17]

And Cooper, who moved to St. Barnabas Hospital in the Bronx in 1954, was busy refining his procedure. After treating his first fifty patients with anterior choroidal ligation, he now tried so-called chemosurgery. Cooper would again burr through the skull but would now inject small amounts of alcohol onto either the globus pallidus or the thalamus. He termed these operations "chemopallidectómy" and "chemothalamectomy," respectively. In a 1955 article in the journal *Science*, Cooper reported moderate to dramatic benefit among Parkinson's patients.[18]

Bourke-White seems to have first learned about Cooper's new operation from a 1957 newspaper clipping. She initially concluded that the procedure was not for her. She was busy pursuing physical therapy, for one thing, and her condition was not nearly as severe as that of the patients being treated by Cooper.

But the possibility of the operation helped Bourke-White begin to shed the customary sick role. She was miffed when staff members at the Rusk Institute dismissed her inquiries about the procedure. "Instead of getting a quiet reply," she wrote to a friend, "I would get a minor oration on why this should not be considered by me." And, she added, she knew that Parkinson's was a progressive disease: "I cannot close my eyes to the knowledge that my malady marches relentlessly along no matter, leaving me a little worse each year." Her response to this state of affairs was to increase her knowledge. "I want to learn as much as I can about any developments in Dr. Cooper's work," she said, "or that of others which touch my field."[19]

By November 1958, Bourke-White had decided to forge ahead with the operation, which Cooper eventually performed on the right side of her brain (to relieve her left-sided symptoms) in January 1959. Her description of her rationale provides fascinating insights into why she—and many other Parkinson's patients—proved willing to submit to a new, invasive, and fairly risky procedure. Bourke-White made clear one potential factor that had *not* played a major role in her case. Although she had "combed the field of clippings" from newspapers describing Cooper's operation, her choice, she told Cooper, was not based on "sheer arithmetic." That is, the numerical odds that she would benefit rather than suffer had not turned the tables for her.[20]

Rather, Bourke-White told Cooper and her friends, it was her faith in modern medicine that made her go ahead. The operation, she would later write, was a "gift of science." Bourke-White had seen frequent coverage in her own *Life* magazine of medical "miracles": not only penicillin, but also the first curative antibiotics for tuberculosis and the polio vaccine. Familiar with historical reasoning from her coverage of World War II and other major events, Bourke-White the patient came to see herself as a historical actor in a specific era. "I am very glad," she told Cooper, "I was born into the right century and the right decade to get the benefit of advancing medical science at the time I needed it the most." Writing to a friend, she analogized her photography, which relied on being in the right place at the right time, to the fact that she had developed Parkinson's just as Cooper had developed his operation. Finding Cooper, she wrote excitedly, was like a journalistic "scoop."[21]

Yet, why go ahead with surgery at this particular time? Cooper had done close to a thousand operations as of late 1958, reporting improvement in 80 percent, which impressed Bourke-White. But the majority had been performed on persons with much more advanced Parkinson's, who were nearly frozen on one side or were experiencing incapacitating tremors. As with her faith in medical science, Bourke-White's decision to proceed stemmed from a personal belief. "Well-meaning people frequently advise that you must learn to accept your illness," she later explained. "My conviction was just the opposite. Try to take a realistic approach, yes. But accept an illness, never."[22]

In the case of Parkinson's, this philosophy meant not waiting until the disease was so far advanced that "anything will be an improvement." Rather, one should undergo Cooper's operation from a position of strength. "Don't wait passively on the sidelines for a shambling old age," she implored fellow Parkinson's sufferers. "Go into it as young as possible. Bring all the assets you have, and play to win!"[23]

This stance is remarkable for a number of reasons. While Bourke-White saw Cooper's operation as exemplifying the best that medicine could offer, she was not willing to wait for more definitive scientific data about the actual value of the procedure in less advanced cases such as her own. In this manner, she was simultaneously embracing and rejecting medical science, basing her decision to proceed on a mixture of scientific knowledge and sheer hope.

Bourke-White's sports metaphors also bear scrutiny. Much has been written about the ways in which metaphors, particularly military metaphors, may be used by powerful groups—such as physicians, pharmaceutical companies, and activist groups—to oversell medical interventions to vulnerable patients. It is also worth noting how one patient chose to incorporate the optimistic and vigorous language of sports into her individual medical calculus. Is such a strategy self-deceiving and ill-advised in the face of real disease and risky treatment? Or is it a viable way to arrive at decisions that are intensely personal?[24]

Notably, patients who later wrote to Bourke-White made decisions in a similar way, using science as only a guidepost for more instinctive choices. One woman, a clerk from St. Louis, described how her physician had candidly told her that an operation might greatly improve her tremor but might also leave her partially paralyzed and unable to talk. "I said yes," the woman wrote, "because I wanted it more than anything I had ever wanted in my life." She, like Bourke-White, simply had a good feeling about what would happen: "The fact is I was so sure I was going to come thru the operation O.K." Another patient, one of Cooper's first candidates, told Bourke-White that "I took the big risk," although Cooper had warned him that the procedure was experimental and had major downsides. By the time of the operation, the man perceptively admitted, "I had forgotten the prediction of possible death or even complete paralysis."[25]

Bourke-White and her correspondents were also fond of using the term "guinea pig." Given that Cooper had done so many operations before hers, the photographer did not really consider herself a guinea pig, but told a friend that she would have been one if it had been necessary. One does not know for sure whether Bourke-White was serious, but she clearly had respect for those willing to take a risk. A California woman hoping for surgery told Bourke-White that she would consent to be a guinea pig "in the interest of trying to help get a cure for this disease." Noting how the disease was going to progress, she said she was determined not to reach a point where she could not keep her body clean. "If I lose," she poignantly asked Bourke-White, "so *what?*"[26]

These letter-writers had learned about Bourke-White's case because she went public with the details of her operation. There was a recent precedent for a famous woman to openly discuss her illness: the athlete Babe Didrikson Zaharias had disclosed her diagnosis of colon cancer in

1953. The idea to chronicle her own illness and operation for *Life* had ger-
minated when Bourke-White was at the Rusk Institute postoperatively. A
frequent visitor was her dear friend and *Life* colleague, the photographer
Alfred Eisenstaedt ("Eisie" to Bourke-White). When at Rusk, Eisenstaedt
did what came naturally: he took photographs of Bourke-White as she underwent rehabilitation. What began as a "personal record" of his friend's
recovery grew into a collaborative article for *Life* in which Bourke-White
wrote text to accompany Eisenstaedt's pictures. Bourke-White had not
intended to be a celebrity patient, but she recognized a good story, even
though it involved highly personal revelations.[27]

The *Life* piece, entitled "Famous Lady's Indomitable Fight," was published in the June 22, 1959, issue of the magazine. The authors included
photographs of Cooper performing a chemothalamectomy, the same
operation Bourke-White had undergone, on an unnamed man. In another
photograph, Bourke-White, wearing a surgical mask, observed the operation. "I watched fascinated," she wrote. "I stood in the small room where,
a few weeks before, my future had been given back to me, and I watched
the hands of the surgeon, then the trembling hands of the patient."[28]

In describing her own surgery, Bourke-White explained that she was
conscious throughout, even when Cooper drilled a hole into her skull. This
enabled her to participate in the operation. As they worked on her brain,
the doctors had peppered Bourke-White with requests—that she clench
her fist, move her wrist, or raise her arm. As the procedure continued, she
was "suddenly aware of an extraordinary feeling," Bourke-White reported.
"I just knew the doctors were doing the right thing. I could tell by a kind
of inner harmony, almost an ecstasy." The procedure, she concluded, had
been a "gift."[29]

To her credit, Bourke-White was careful to warn readers that such surgery might not benefit—and might harm—some Parkinson's patients.
"Much of it is new," she wrote, "and much is hedged with qualifications so
that it cannot guarantee improvement." And she wrote about a series of
unpleasant sensations, such as heaviness of her arms, that occurred in the
days after surgery. Still, her passionate advocacy of the surgery was palpa-
ble. Writing of the man whose operation she observed, Bourke-White
stated that he would soon be up and around, relieved of his tremors. "I
never met the man, or heard his name," she stated, "but I shared with him
a miracle."[30]

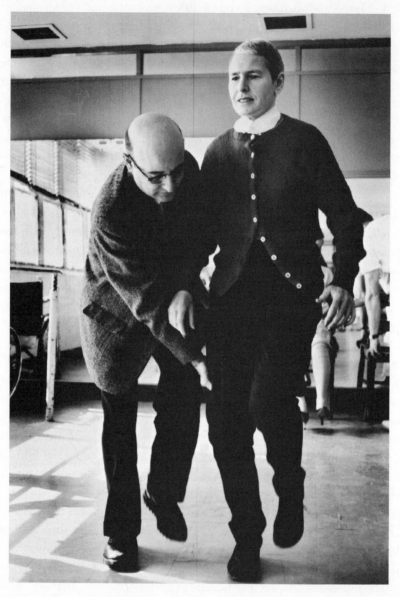

Margaret Bourke-White undergoing rehabilitation with therapist Jack Hofkosh at Howard Rusk's Institute of Physical Medicine in 1959. Photograph
from the Margaret Bourke-White papers, Special Collections Research Center, Syracuse University Library, Getty Image. Printed courtesy of Time-Life.

It is worth underscoring that this account of Bourke-White's operation was written by her. The press never independently researched the story, before or after she went public, and subsequent accounts of Bourke-White's illness and surgery essentially repeated her own version. The first of these was a play, *The Margaret Bourke-White Story*, based on the *Life* article and televised on NBC's *Sunday Showcase* on January 3, 1960. Teresa Wright, who had played Eleanor Gehrig in *Pride of the Yankees*, starred in a production that sought to "present in meticulous clinical detail the medical problem of a celebrated patient." Bourke-White was omnipresent on the set, working closely with the director and actors and communicating her story with what Wright later termed a "ferocious intensity." A complimentary review in the *New York Times* noted how the play's last act, featuring Bourke-White's operation, "illustrated how personal courage, medical skill and good fortune enabled her to survive seemingly hopeless odds." Bourke-White's later description of her surgery in *Portrait of Myself* was nearly identical to her *Life* account. Finally, Bourke-White's biographer, Vicki Goldberg, relied almost entirely on her subject's take on events in describing what happened in the operating room.[31]

The point of this recitation is not to question Bourke-White's accuracy or the editorial judgment of *Life* or NBC. She seems to have provided as truthful an account as possible of her experiences. But the constant repetition of the same story in multiple settings could not help but validate its two basic messages: that Cooper's operation demonstrated how medical science was triumphing over disease and that patients should seek out physicians (like Cooper) who took chances. Bourke-White had never disguised her adulation of Cooper. His blond hair and impressive height made him look "a little like a Greek God," she wrote. She also referred to the years before her operation as "B.C.—before Cooper," insinuating that her doctor, like Jesus Christ, was a savior. For these reasons, Bourke-White's version of her surgery read almost like an advertisement.[32]

Not surprisingly, many letters received by Bourke-White after the *Life* article and the television play told similarly positive stories about brain operations performed by Cooper or other surgeons. A Brooklyn man operated on by Dr. Robert M. Sengstaken reported that his left side was free of rigidity and his tremors greatly reduced: "The results were beyond anything I had anticipated." Another man stated that his operation had been "simply amazing," fixing his poor walking, leg tremor, foot and hand rigidity, and his "Parkinsonian face."[33]

But there also were dozens of letters describing problems resulting from operations. In many cases, they described initial improvement followed by deterioration. In other instances, there was little benefit at all—and sometimes worsening of the Parkinson's. While Cooper and other physicians seem to have regularly warned patients about these possibilities, such bad outcomes were nevertheless devastating.

The operation, wrote a woman from Brazil, had paralyzed her right side for several days. Eight months later, she reported, she still had problems with speech, walking, and writing, as well as difficulty concentrating. An Oregon bookkeeper who had undergone surgery in April 1957 had first experienced such improvement that he had appeared in front of the county medical association. But his symptoms returned, leading to a second operation in November 1958. It did not produce the same successful results, he told Bourke-White. "It seems to have weakened my legs some," he wrote, "and I am walking with a cane, which isn't too much of a draw back as I am already a cripple." His typed letter also mentioned that he could no longer write.[34]

Most upsetting to Bourke-White were a series of letters she received from her "sorority sisters," a group of women who had undergone Cooper's operation at St. Barnabas around the same time she had. One, a Michigan woman, told Bourke-White that Cooper had operated on her four times and that she had had to relearn to walk each time. "I find my re'cooper'a-tion is very slow," she quipped. A New York City woman wrote of "days when none of my limbs want to function properly and I get so discouraged again."[35]

Another woman from New York also had bad news. "I tense so much that one would think rigor mortis was setting in," she told Bourke-White in September 1959. "My greatest difficulty is when I handle small objects, cleaning my teeth, and when I am rushed." By early 1961 things had worsened. She told Bourke-White of trying to find her words "through the wilderness of this disease." In later years, the woman's husband had to continue the correspondence as his wife deteriorated further. "It sure does take a lot of grit to keep going," he told Bourke-White.[36]

Bourke-White dutifully replied to most letters, providing either advice or commiseration, depending on the situation. One reason was her empathy. She later wrote how her illness had "brought me closer to other human beings in a way I cannot put into words." But another reason was her continual desire to gain more knowledge about Parkinson's disease. Bourke-White asked her correspondents numerous probing questions about surgery, rehabilitation, and, as the 1960s progressed, the growing number of pharmaceutical agents for treating the disease. "I am so much interested in this subject," she told a Maine woman, "that I would like to have you drop me a line if you get any more information."[37]

Another reason that Bourke-White asked these questions was her growing interest in ascertaining just what Cooper's operation accomplished—both for her and others. Even though her *Life* article had made her the lay "expert" on Parkinson's, Bourke-White asked her fellow patients for information. "Do you have any idea how long good effects are supposed to last . . . if one has just one operation?" she asked one of her St. Barnabas roommates.[38]

Gradually, Bourke-White developed a more sophisticated view of her surgery that was at odds with her earlier assessment of it as a miracle. Rather, it had provided genuine relief, but only with strenuous physical therapy could she and other patients expect to retain such benefits. As a result of this thinking, Bourke-White became even more invested in exercise in the months after her operation. The piece in *Life* placed great emphasis on rehabilitation and contained several photographs of Bourke-White at the Rusk Institute, exercising, playing catch, and doing the tango. Her therapy, it seems, became a way not only to maintain her health but also to validate her decision to have undergone surgery.[39]

Vigorous therapy became a sort of talisman for Bourke-White—her way of trying to stave off the inevitable decline of Parkinson's disease. Physical therapy was "almost a religion" to her, she confessed. That is, if she just worked hard enough at rehabilitation, she could avoid a second operation or giving up work. "I cannot see how it would be possible for me to have a recurrence with all the exercises I am doing," she wrote to the woman from Maine. As Bourke-White got sicker over the next several years, she insisted on running and dancing even if they caused her to fall. "I do not want to live cautiously," she told her friend Myrle Morgan. "I believe just the opposite." As was the case with Lou Gehrig, the therapeutic value of "fighting" one's disease was taken as a given, requiring no validation.[40]

Yet, as one woman, the daughter of a Parkinson's patient, warned

Bourke-White, this type of reasoning was potentially problematic. The *Life* article, the woman stated, had been "too optimistic and will therefore cause much unhappiness to people later on." She went on to say that her mother had been a "strong-willed" person "who refused to believe that she was ill and that any illness could stop her from doing the things she wanted." But, she continued, her mother worsened nonetheless and was now "hopelessly imprisoned forever and a day" in her own body. "Please don't give people the impression that this can be conquered by one's own will, or that the operation is the answer," the woman entreated. "It is not so for all of us." In so writing, Bourke-White's correspondent likely became one of the first people to criticize a famous patient for overgeneralizing from a personal experience. In the coming decades, as sick celebrities became bolder in their claims, such criticisms would mount.[41]

For most of her correspondents, however, Bourke-White had gotten it just right. She had alerted them to a new combination of surgery and physical therapy, which seemed to help in a significant proportion of cases. But beyond the actual improvement that these interventions produced, her story itself had intrinsic value both to those with Parkinson's and to Americans in general. In other words, Bourke-White's decision to go public with her story was deeply meaningful above and beyond the issue of clinical effectiveness.

Hearing how a celebrated and accomplished woman courageously fought the disease provided hope and inspiration to others. A Utah woman whose husband had Parkinson's told Bourke-White that the televised play depicting Cooper's operation had given her husband new hope. "We were so thrilled to see and hear you on TV we just cried," she wrote. "Chad didn't think I saw him, but he wiped his nose and eyes." Having seen the play, a Los Angeles woman whose son had Parkinson's told Bourke-White that she had been "born anew." Thanks to God and Bourke-White's story, she stated, "I've got a lot of new hope." "The doctors here say there is no cure," wrote a West Virginia woman, "but your story made me believe there is some help and hope." Finally, a Philadelphia man commended Bourke-White for having "rendered a fine human service in extending hope . . . to many who are not inclined to hang on, to those whose tendency are [*sic*] to despondency."[42]

A man from Michigan wrote about the impact of the *Life* article on his wife. "I hesitate to use so important a word as 'inspire' but it really did inspire her," he said. "Her courage returned and her balance and vision improved. The courage is the most important." Another writer was a Brooklyn man with Parkinson's who was soon to undergo surgery. Bourke-White's story, he wrote, "should be an inspiration to all, handicapped and able-bodied alike."[43]

That Bourke-White's act of public writing was as important as or more important than her take on the scientific value of chemothalamectomy was underscored by the letters received by *Life* in response to Bourke-White's article. Twenty percent of the writers, who either had Parkinson's or knew someone with the disease, emphasized Bourke-White's apparently successful outcome and requested information about Cooper or other resources. But the majority of the correspondents, 62 percent, simply praised *Life* and Bourke-White for going public. "We congratulate LIFE on its contribution toward bringing understanding about this dread disease," one writer stated. Another termed Bourke-White's story "one of the most dramatic and courageous things I have ever read." Bourke-White, wrote another correspondent, "epitomizes the spiritual equivalent of a human being with the temerity to throw a rock at an advancing tank."[44]

The fact that Bourke-White was a celebrity made her story even more powerful. A feeling of intimacy with such a person, even if imagined, was nevertheless a source of comfort during illness. "I am not given to writing letters to celebrities," the Brooklyn man told her, "but I felt that we had so much in common." Another correspondent who acknowledged the power of celebrity was Jeanne Levey, chairwoman of the board of the new National Parkinson Foundation. Levey was inviting Bourke-White to join her in "turning the first spade of earth" for a Parkinson's rehabilitation institute soon to be built. "Your extraordinary qualities of perseverance, stamina and courage," Levey wrote, "would give added hope to the many frustrated sufferers."[45]

In this manner, Levey was trying to establish a loop that would become altogether familiar in the coming decades. In order to attract attention to a serious disease, she hoped to recruit a well-known celebrity who had the condition or a personal connection to it. The attendant publicity would help to increase funding for research and the number of top-notch scientists working on the disease. Therapeutic advances, which might benefit both the celebrity and other sufferers, would ensue. Michael J. Fox has served this role for Parkinson's disease activism over the past decade.

The blurring of an emotionally satisfying "battle plan" with actual clinical improvement could not have been clearer than in Bourke-White's own case. That the 1959 operation initially helped her seems to be beyond doubt. Her stiff left arm became much more flexible, the tight muscles of her back relaxed, she "jumped in" to cars rather than needing assistance, and she once again "conquered" typing. Most gratifying was an improved ability to work her camera—loading the film, changing lenses, and snapping photographs.[46]

But, as had been the case with many of her correspondents, her operation was no cure-all. Bourke-White continued to require constant physical therapy. By late 1960, her Parkinson's had worsened, forcing her to permanently give up both photography and lecturing. By January 1961, two years after her surgery, Bourke-White reported that she was "getting stuck in chairs, in corners and against the wall." That same month, Cooper performed a second operation, this time on the left portion of the brain, to alleviate the worsening stiffness, rigidity, and tremor on her right side.[47]

As before, Bourke-White described the results of her surgery in glowing terms. It was a "wonderful success," she told her general physician, Robert McGrath. In the postscript to *Portrait of Myself*, most likely written in 1963, she termed the second operation "a triumph of surgery." Specifically, her tremor had disappeared and her right hand had become much stronger. When she walked, she told McGrath, "I just sail along." As determined as ever, she recruited some neighborhood children in the summer of 1961 to help her to jump rope. After initial failure, she could finally report the "magnificent total of 47 jumps without missing."[48]

But, as Bourke-White would write in 1967, she had ultimately "been disagreeably surprised by the unwelcome offshoots of the operation." Most notably, the surgery had done lasting damage to her speech, a potential complication, she claimed, that she had been unaware of. In later years she suffered from hypophonia, in which speaking is soft and difficult to initiate. Her neurologist in the 1960s, Robert S. Schwab, believed that the second operation was "not as successful" as the first one. Her akinetic symptoms gradually worsened during the decade, with deterioration of her handwriting and "freezing" of her arms and legs.[49]

Bourke-White tried a series of medications for Parkinson's, eventually remaining on amantadine for several years. Unfortunately, however, she did not tolerate most of them. This was the case with l-dopa, a new and often effective dopamine supplement that provided many patients with dramatically improved mobility for several years. She tried it several times but always experienced severe side effects. In the summer of 1971 Bourke-White fell, breaking several ribs and becoming confined to bed. This immobility led to a series of other medical complications, which ended her life on August 27, 1971. She was 67 years old.[50]

In retrospect, was the bold new brain surgery an effective therapy for Bourke-White's Parkinson's disease? This is a complicated historical question. On the one hand, there can be no doubt that she perceived both operations as effective, so in this sense they surely "helped." Even as Bourke-White deteriorated, she remained fiercely loyal to Cooper. Robert Schwab also believed that the surgeries, on balance, had been beneficial. "Had you not been operated on," he told Bourke-White in 1968, "you would be, if you were alive, a complete invalid at about 35 percent of normal in your performance, almost bedridden with stiffness on both sides." Her therapist, Jack Hofkosh, also believed that the surgery had helped to extend her life.[51]

But all of this, of course, is impossible to prove. Bourke-White was only one case of a disease that is notoriously variable in its progression. Modern research indicates that more sophisticated versions of Cooper's operations are viable options for a subset of Parkinson's patients. These data suggest that patients like Bourke-White may have benefited from their operations, but it is also likely that a placebo effect was at play, with patients overestimating what had actually been accomplished. Indeed, surgical intervention for Parkinson's disease remains controversial.[52]

By going public with the intimate details of a poorly understood and even embarrassing disease, Margaret Bourke-White did a huge service. Her status as a well-known person and a star photographer at *Life* gave her a logical pathway to generate publicity, and she took it. Because of Bourke-White, people confronting Parkinson's could obtain information about surgery and the latest treatments much more easily. "I am not asking you to make the decision [about an operation] for me," wrote a man from Los Angeles in 1964. "Just give me the facts that you have experienced." "In short," asked a woman from Columbus, Ohio, that same year, "was the end result worth what you had to go through to get them [*sic*]?"[53]

Still, Bourke-White's major contribution was less her ability to disseminate medical knowledge than her upbeat message to thousands of suffering people. One person who recognized this was Jean Bradfield, the executive vice president of the Chicago chapter of the National Parkinson Foundation. People like Bourke-White and Irving Cooper, she wrote, had "brought life, hope and encouragement as well as usefulness into the lives of otherwise 'forgotten people.'" Indeed, Bourke-White retained a remarkable optimism even as her disease made her almost a complete invalid. In December 1970, Robert Schwab gingerly raised with his patient, who could no longer dress or feed herself or go to the bathroom without assistance, the question of moving into a nursing home. Bourke-White demurred, noting that she had turned her sun porch into a gymnasium and was planning a trip to see an exhibition of her photographs in Boston. In rejecting her doctor's suggestion, she retained her usual magnanimity. "You are the kindest person I know," she wrote, "and I especially appreciate your taking the time to guide me."[54]

As disease activism evolved in the 1970s and 1980s, Bourke-White's reassuring message—that patients should place their faith in the scientific establishment and its seemingly imminent breakthroughs—would need rethinking. Activists such as Morris Abram, Elizabeth Glaser, and especially Augusto and Michaela Odone rejected the notion that science was necessarily acting in their best interests. Rather, they argued, patients and families needed to learn the science themselves if they wanted to save their own lives and the lives of their loved ones.

This message would not get disseminated, however, until the press began to play a larger, and more confrontational, role in its coverage of medicine. Despite all of its attention to Bourke-White's illness, the press never picked up on the story that was apparent from the course of her disease and was sitting right in her voluminous correspondence: for many people, heroic brain surgery for Parkinson's did relatively little to stave off the grim progression of the disease.

There were glimmers of this more aggressive role of the media as journalists covered the illness of John Foster Dulles, who was diagnosed with colon cancer in 1956 and died in 1959. As Walter Reed Hospital dutifully provided details of the secretary of state's illness, a few reporters quietly began to question the veracity of what they were being told. That Dulles was the nation's point man in its fight against the "cancer" of communism only further complicated how the story of his illness would be told.

Chapter 4

Politician as Patient

John Foster Dulles Battles Cancer

No one likes being sick. But John Foster Dulles *really* didn't like being sick. When first hospitalized in 1956, he was embroiled in a crisis regarding the Suez Canal. One of America's most recognizable secretaries of state, thanks to his tenure during the Cold War, Dulles was eager to return to work as soon as he recovered. But the 68-year-old diplomat was not through with his cancer of the colon (large intestine). Two years later he would again be treated, this time unsuccessfully.

The Dulles case demonstrates how celebrity illness was gradually being transformed in the middle to late 1950s. Abandoning some of the caution it had previously exhibited when covering the sicknesses of political figures, the press avidly reported on Dulles's condition, freely using the word *cancer* and explaining the disease to its readership. Although patients and families still often discussed cancer in hushed tones, it was a very public topic in the 1950s.

Dulles was both an extraordinary and an ordinary patient. On the one hand, some Americans assumed that someone who could so effectively fight the "cancer" of communism was especially capable of doing the same for the cancer in his body. On the other hand, other citizens deluged the "nation's most famous invalid" with letters of advice that described their own successful treatments. Their recommendations included faith in God, new chemotherapeutic agents, and controversial, unorthodox remedies. These writings—plus the media coverage of Dulles's illness—reveal the diverse ways in which the public attempted to come to terms with concepts such as prognosis and cure.[1]

Dulles was the son of a Presbyterian minister and had contemplated a career in the pulpit. Although he did become an elder of the Presbyterian Church, Dulles instead chose diplomacy, entering the foreign service after graduating from Princeton University. He served as a delegate to the United Nations from 1946 to 1948, helping to negotiate a series of treaties in the wake of World War II. As secretary of state under Dwight D. Eisenhower beginning in 1953, Dulles advocated an aggressive policy of "brinkmanship"—refusing to back down—as a way of intimidating the Soviet enemy.[2]

Early in November 1956, Dulles was dealing with an enormous crisis. Israel, fearing a Soviet-sponsored arms buildup in Egypt, had invaded its western neighbor and was heading toward the Suez Canal. Great Britain and France, without conferring with their ally, the United States, had lent military support to Israel. Even though Dulles announced his opposition to the military incursion, he was strongly criticized by the press for being blindsided. On the night of November 1, 1956, he addressed the General Assembly of the United Nations, calling for, among other things, an immediate cease-fire. And the Middle East crisis was not the only one worrying Dulles. The Soviets had just invaded Hungary and would soon take over the country.[3]

Dulles felt well when he went to bed the next night but awoke in the early morning of November 3 with shaking chills and severe abdominal pains. His wife, Janet, called the family physician, Alva D. Daughton, who immediately paid a house call. The diagnosis was unclear, but a decision was made to admit Dulles to Walter Reed Army Hospital. Logistically, this proved to be a nightmare as he was in too much pain to walk and the spiral staircase in his home prevented the ambulance workers from carrying his broad-shouldered, six-foot frame down the stairs. Dulles solved the problem by sitting and bumping down the steps one at a time. During the entire episode, he gave detailed instructions to his assistant, William Macomber, about work that needed to be done while he was sick. He insisted on speaking with several other colleagues before allowing physicians at Walter Reed to begin treating him.[4]

The provisional diagnosis, given Dulles's fever and excruciating belly pain, was appendicitis. But when Major General Leonard D. Heaton and his surgical colleagues opened up their patient's abdomen, they were shocked. Dulles's appendix was fine but he had a perforation (hole) in his large intestine. And the cause seemed to be a large cancer. Tissue sent to the laboratory confirmed the diagnosis. Having removed both the cancer and the damaged section of the intestine, the surgeons stitched together the healthy portions of the colon.

There were two decisions to be made. Would the physicians tell Dulles the truth? And what would the public be told? As Margaret Bourke-White learned, concealment of grave diagnoses from patients was still routine in the paternalistic 1950s. Cancer was a case in point. One study reported that 90 percent of doctors preferred not to tell cancer patients their actual diagnosis. But Dulles apparently insisted on candor, and his wife was amenable.[5]

Dulles's openness extended to the public, even if it made the Eisenhower administration politically vulnerable. The decision to announce the cancer diagnosis represented a marked departure from the deception that had surrounded the illnesses of presidents Woodrow Wilson and Franklin D. Roosevelt. Eisenhower himself had ushered in this new openness when he suffered a heart attack in 1955. After a period of confusion, the press and public were fully informed of what had happened. One of Eisenhower's cardiologists, Paul Dudley White, used the occasion to try to educate Americans about heart disease. Other public figures in the 1950s, including athlete Babe Didrikson Zaharias and Ohio senator Robert A. Taft, had revealed their cancer diagnoses. In this spirit, a front-page headline in the November 5, 1956, *New York Times* announced "Dulles' Surgery Removed Cancer." The word was out.[6]

At the time, Dulles received no additional treatment besides surgery. He did well for two years. But in November 1958 he began to experience severe abdominal pains and to grow thinner and more haggard. As before, this occurred during an international crisis, this time involving West Berlin. The Soviet premier, Nikita Khrushchev, had issued an ultimatum for the Western countries to leave the city, which they had occupied since the end of World War II.

On December 5, 1958, Dulles finally went to Walter Reed Hospital, where he was diagnosed with diverticulitis, an inflammation of a portion of the colon. Although the doctors were concerned that Dulles's cancer had returned, they found no evidence that it had. One week later, Dulles left Walter Reed against doctors' orders. He had insisted on going to Paris, where the allies were addressing the Berlin situation.[7]

Dulles made it to Paris, then traveled to Jamaica for a well-deserved two-week vacation. He returned to work at the beginning of January 1959, but had not regained his health. Dulles made his last diplomatic trip during the first week of February, flying to Great Britain, France, and West Germany to further discuss Berlin. Those encountering Dulles realized that something was terribly wrong. He was in evident pain and had difficulty eating. In a biography of Dulles, Deane and David Heller speculated that everyone knew it was the secretary's last diplomatic mission: "Everywhere, honors and courtesies were extended to the Secretary of State far in excess of the requirements of protocol."[8]

At the completion of the trip, Dulles again checked into Walter Reed. He had developed a hernia in his lower abdomen at the site of the pain. When Heaton operated on February 12, he found a large cancerous mass. Thus began the last few months of John Foster Dulles's life. He would receive radiation therapy and then radioactive gold at the site of the cancer. A period of improvement followed, allowing a trip to Florida on March 30, 1959. But while there, Dulles developed neck pain. He flew back to Walter Reed, where x-rays of the neck vertebrae revealed metastatic cancer.

Although this area of cancer would also be treated with radiation, there was no denying its significance. On April 15, 1959, Eisenhower announced that Dulles had resigned due to his health. The president had rebuffed an earlier effort by the secretary of state to resign after the first recurrence in February. Eisenhower named Dulles's assistant, Christian Herter, to fill the post, and named Dulles a special consultant to the president on foreign affairs. But this was a formality. Dulles continued to grow weaker, and died at Walter Reed on May 24, 1959.

This timeline of basic medical facts about Dulles's terminal illness follows, in retrospect, a familiar path: surprise diagnosis of cancer, apparent cure, recurrence of cancer, additional treatment, positive response, deterioration, and death. It also seems straightforward with respect to the issue of disclosure. Due to changing norms and Dulles's own wishes, his diagnosis of cancer was made public from the start. But as events were unfolding, there was actually a great deal of ambiguity as well as a series of difficult choices to be made. And even though there was no overt concealment, efforts to ascertain the medical and political significance of Dulles's cancer raised a complex series of questions.

What was Dulles's actual prognosis when he was first diagnosed with colon cancer in 1956? The medical profession's understanding of how colon cancer spread was undergoing major changes in the 1950s. For centuries, cancer was considered to be a slow-growing disease that remained localized for years at its site of origin. Gradually, cancers would spread to the nearby lymph nodes; they would become metastatic only late in their course, with cancer cells spreading first to the bloodstream and then throughout the body.[9]

One of the first classifications of colon cancer, the Dukes system, built on this reasoning. The Dukes method used the letters A through D, which were assigned based on the clinical and pathological findings: "A" cancers affected only the inside lining of the intestinal wall; "B" cancers had invaded partially into the muscular layer of the intestine; "C" cancers had gone all the way from the inside layer to the outside layer of the intestine; and "D" cancers had metastasized. The prognosis was directly related to these classifications. Five-year survival was as follows: "A" cancers, 80 to 90 percent; "B" cancers, 60 to 80 percent; "C" cancers, 30 to 50 percent; "D" cancers, less than 10 percent.[10]

The treatment of colon cancer also reflected its designation as a local disease. Surgeons performed extensive operations designed to encompass not just the cancer but a large portion of the intestine and the surrounding lymph nodes. This wide procedure allowed them not only to sample the nodes for cancer but also to try to remove any and all cancer cells in the region of the primary cancer. Doing so successfully was considered the best possible way to cure the disease.

Dulles's cancer was most likely a "Dukes C." Since it had caused perforation of the large intestine, it likely had already eroded through the bowel wall. Though the nearby lymph nodes were clear of cancer, as were his distant organs, the intestinal damage added a negative prognostic factor. "In the course of this perforation," Heaton later recalled, "cancer cells were naturally extruded into the abdominal cavity." Even though he and the other surgeons attempted to clean out the abdomen, it is overwhelmingly likely that some of the millions of cancer cells were left behind—something the surgeons surely knew. This would have raised the chance of a recurrence even higher than the 50 to 70 percent chance that the Dukes scale suggested.[11]

There was one other piece of bad news. A group of surgeons had recently begun to sample blood vessels in the region of colon cancers. They found, in contrast to standard teaching, that cancer cells were often present at these sites. By suggesting that colon cancers spread to the bloodstream early in their course, often invisibly, this finding helped to explain why perhaps a third of patients with supposedly curable "Dukes A" colon cancer died from recurrent disease. For Dulles, given all of these factors— a "Dukes C" cancer that had perforated and might have spread to the bloodstream—the odds of a recurrence would have been extremely high, perhaps 90 percent.[12]

Lacking Dulles's medical record and relevant correspondence from this time, it is hard to know exactly what Dulles's physicians thought about his prognosis or what they formally told him. But it seems that they were hedging their bets. A 1962 biography by military historian Richard Goold-Adams reported that Dulles's doctors had given him a time frame. If there was no recurrence of the cancer within eighteen months, he could consider himself cured. In a 1966 interview, Heaton recalled that Dulles regularly asked him about the possibility of recurrence. No one knows, Heaton would reply, "except the Lord of all of us."[13]

For his part, Dulles thought the operation had been successful. And the basic message to the public, which Dulles surely saw in the newspapers he read religiously, was optimistic. His surgeons, for example, were quoted as saying that "complete removal of the diseased tissue was accomplished." There was "no evidence whatsoever," they stated, "of extension of this lesion to any other organ."[14]

Since no cancer was seen at the end of the operation or in the excised lymph nodes, these statements were technically true. But it was commonplace for cancer surgeons, when they could, to announce they had "gotten it all," even though in most such cases the cancer would eventually recur. If pushed on the matter, most surgeons would probably have admitted that this statement was more of an optimistic ritual than a meaningful statement of prognosis. The language chosen thus obscured the unfortunate reality of the intestinal perforation, which rendered Dulles's prognosis quite poor.

The optimism persisted when Dulles was admitted for his bout of diverticulitis in December 1958. It was now two years since his original operation and six months past the magical eighteen-month mark given to him by the doctors. With hindsight, Dulles's cancer had surely recurred at that point. But routine testing revealed only the infection, and Dulles pressed his caregivers to release him from the hospital. So his doctors gave the situation a positive spin, confidently announcing that there was "no recurrence of the malignancy."[15]

In retrospect, one might be tempted to ask why no reporters challenged this story. The answer is that, from their perspective, there was no story. The Dulles situation, with its candid disclosures, seemed entirely opposite from the case of Woodrow Wilson. It was not until July 1959, two months after Dulles died, that Marguerite Higgins, an award-winning war correspondent with the *New York Herald-Tribune*, wrote a three-part series revisiting the secretary of state's illness. While most of the article was a laudatory account of how Dulles and his family dealt with his deterioration and death, she nevertheless connected the ruptured intestine in 1956 to his prognosis. "Sooner or later," she stated, "the escaped cancer cells would seed themselves on other parts of the body." The diagnosis of diverticulitis in 1958, Higgins concluded, was merely a "happy respite" from the upcoming diagnosis of cancer.[16]

Nevertheless, true investigative reporting about famous patients' illnesses lay in the future. Higgins did not accuse Dulles's doctors of either deception or undue optimism. Nor had reporters written about the diplomat's obviously grave condition during his last trip to Europe. Still, the article by Higgins signaled the beginnings of a sea change. Thus, when Dulles was readmitted to Walter Reed Hospital on February 10, 1959, first with a hernia and then recurrent cancer, his condition became fair game for reporters. Press conferences, held at Walter Reed and the State Department, resembled those that Dulles held on foreign policy matters. Just as journalists might probe military buildups or proposed treaties, here they asked doctors and hospital spokespeople detailed questions about the extent of the cancer, treatment options, and Dulles's potential recovery.

For example, when told that surgeons had found cancer cells in fluid adjacent to the cancer, a reporter asked whether that meant there was likely to be malignancy elsewhere in the body. "Is there any conclusion or tentative conclusion," asked another reporter on February 20, 1959, "about the chances of arresting it, or controlling it, or curing it?" The notion, fifteen years earlier, of reporters pressing President Franklin Roosevelt's physicians for details of his persistent cough (which turned out to be congestive heart failure) would have been unthinkable.[17]

These inquiries led to extensive and informative coverage. United Press International (UPI) and other wire services issued daily stories published in newspapers across the country. Based on interviews with physicians not connected with the case, a *Washington Post* reporter explained why Dulles's cancer was a "highly malignant type." Meanwhile, in *Newsweek*, readers learned considerable details about new technologies, such as the million-volt x-ray machine housed in a "concrete-shielded room behind a 1-ton door of lead" at Walter Reed, that they were unlikely to have previously encountered in the press.[18]

Based in part on the candid interchanges at the press conferences, early coverage of Dulles's cancer recurrence was quite gloomy. A front-page article in the February 15, 1959, *New York Times* quoted physicians as saying that the secretary of state's outlook was "grave." A headline in *Newsweek* was equally blunt: "Dulles—The Cruel Facts of His Future." Dulles, the magazine concluded, was "a victim of incurable cancer."[19]

Nor was there optimism about his treatments, such as the radiotherapy to his abdomen. The secretary of state was about to begin "massive" x-ray therapy, UPI reported on February 20, that would at best arrest—not cure—his disease. *Newsweek* stated that even though Dulles was going to receive radiotherapy, the cancer still "was likely to scatter through the lower abdomen." Benjamin Bradlee of *Newsweek* quoted experts as saying that adenocarcinoma of the colon did not respond particularly well to radiation.[20]

Although it was Dulles's position as a government official that had promoted disclosure, the resultant candor surrounding his cancer was still impressive, given its obvious political ramifications. In February 1959, two Democratic senators, Hubert H. Humphrey of Minnesota and Stuart Symington of Missouri, seized the opportunity to call for Dulles's resignation. Overseas newspapers, such as the *Parisien Libéré*, openly worried about the diplomatic effectiveness of a country with a chronically ill president and secretary of state.[21]

These political concerns led to the publication of some overly optimistic articles suggesting that all was well with the secretary of state. Not surprisingly, one such piece appeared in a military magazine, the *Stars and*

Stripes, earmarked for veterans and their families. "An impressive number of people believe John Foster Dulles will win his second bout with cancer," it stated. "This includes his own wife."[22]

But it was not only politics that caused some journalists to ignore the facts in favor of a hopeful assessment. Part of what drove this coverage was Dulles's apparent improvement at the beginning of his radiotherapy. At the end of February 1959, Dulles's doctors were "gratified" at his progress after eight radiation treatments. A month later, they were "impressed" by their patient's condition; results of the treatment were "promising." Amid the forest of gloom, physicians—and reporters—looked for one hopeful tree.[23]

The inclination to be upbeat was even more apparent among the thousands of letters Dulles received, both in 1956 and 1959. Media coverage of his illness caused an outpouring of concern from individuals—not only Republicans but also Democrats who opposed Dulles's politics. A small boy alerted Dulles to this phenomenon. "It seems when you were well, you were terrible," he explained, "but now that you are sick, you are wonderful." Dulles responded with a hearty laugh.[24]

A review of this correspondence provides excellent insight into public understandings of cancer in the 1950s. Although the veil of secrecy about the disease was seemingly being lifted for the first time, a very distinctive set of beliefs about cancer clearly already existed. And they suggested—at least among those who chose to write letters to famous victims—a striking optimism about curability. Specifically, four consistent themes emerged: (1) the importance of faith, (2) the relevance of previous ("n of 1") cases of colon cancer, (3) the value of unorthodox medical treatment, and (4) the unique ability of Dulles to fight his disease.

The most notable characteristic of these missives was their overtly religious sentiments. Dulles was a religious man. Not only had his father been a clergyman, but Dulles's son, Avery, a convert to Catholicism, was studying to become a priest. Writers frequently told Dulles they were praying to God for his recovery. Typical was a November 1956 letter from a couple in Waterford, Pennsylvania, who wrote, "May our Lord guide you and grant you a speedy return to good health and a long life." The letters often included religious imagery and artifacts.[25]

This correspondence underscores the primacy of religious thought in America in the 1950s. But many of the correspondents were not simply recommending prayer as advisable but emphatically argued that it would cure Dulles—or at least improve his chances. "You may be assured," wrote a New Hampshire woman in November 1956, "that we are praying for you that God will give you a normal recovery." A Virginia man wrote that Dulles's recovery to health would be permanent because man's fate was in God's hands.[26]

Many letters further invoked the role of religion in cure by referring to God or Jesus Christ as a doctor. "By knowing that God is the great physician," wrote a St. Louis man after Dulles's 1959 recurrence, "you will be back in the front ranks serving your God and country better than ever." God, a Michigan man wrote, was a "Great Physician who has never lost a case that we know of." Such letters, it should be noted, generally neither disavowed nor endorsed the medical treatments that Dulles was receiving. They simply advocated prayer as the most effective way to achieve physical recovery.[27]

But these faith-based assurances were not based on faith alone. Many of the letter-writers who invoked God supplied an "n of 1" anecdote offering supposed proof of divine healing. This was the second type of optimistic assertion that characterized the correspondence to Dulles. One man, also a Presbyterian elder, wrote that he had been diagnosed with cancer in 1928 and then cured because he had "such faith in God." A Minnesota woman wrote that she had been cured of cancer through prayer three different times. In the last instance, she wrote, she was on her deathbed with only a few days to live: "There is One to whom you can go and be sure of your deliverance, and that is Christ Jesus, our Lord."[28]

The letters were potentially even more powerful when the "n" in question was greater than one. A woman from Cohoes, New York, sent Dulles a Green Scapular of Our Lady, a Catholic artifact that had supposed healing powers. "Your son the Priest can explain it to you," she said, but told him that the scapular had cured her sister's cancer. The woman added that she had sent "over 598 Scapulars to sick people who were cured or relieved by it."[29]

Not all of the "n of 1" letters were of a religious nature. A Chicago man told Dulles how his father-in-law, operated on for colon cancer twenty-two years earlier, was very much alive at the age of 94. "I report this case," he wrote, "just to reassure you that modern medicine can completely eradicate that former bugaboo—carcinoma." A 73-year-old Delaware man told

Dulles in November 1956 that he had undergone the same surgery three years earlier and had never felt better in his life. "So I trust," he concluded, "that you will improve rapidly, steadily, and gradually resume the wonderful service that you have been rendering."[30]

Without more details, it is difficult to know why people felt compelled to send such "n of 1" stories, although some of the motivation was surely to cheer up a man who was greatly respected. Nor can one assess the validity of what they wrote. For example, the people telling their stories may not have had cancer. Or those who ostensibly recovered due to prayer might have recovered anyway. And, most notably, the fact that one person could be cured of colon cancer did not necessarily have any relevance to another case, as cancer experts were beginning to teach the public. But what is important is the sincere belief among certain members of the public that an earlier positive outcome in another person, achieved with or without prayer, offered some type of proof that Dulles was likely to recover—even when newspapers were quoting physicians as saying his prognosis was extremely poor. Famous patients in succeeding decades would routinely receive similar assurances.

The third category of optimistic letters were those advocating that Dulles and his doctors consider unorthodox cancer treatment. For centuries, healers had treated serious diseases in a variety of ways. In the early 1900s, the orthodox approach taught in mainstream medical schools competed with homeopathy, chiropractic, and osteopathy.[31]

By the mid-twentieth century, cancer had become a particular battleground. Orthodox medicine had asserted its authority through advocacy of radical surgery, based on the notion of cancer as a local disease. And it promoted radiotherapy as an adjunct treatment when surgery was inadequate. But in reality, the vast majority—perhaps 75 percent—of cancer patients eventually died from their disease. Once surgery and radiation had failed, there was little that orthodox physicians could do for cancer patients except prescribe opiates for their pain.

This situation inspired a series of alternative treatments. While there were surely major differences among these unorthodox practitioners, many were united by a similar philosophy. Cancer, they argued, was a systemic rather than a local disease. The aggressive use of localized surgery and radiation was not only unhelpful but perhaps even interfered with the body's ability to fight off the cancer. What was needed, rather, was an approach that treated the entire body, restoring the imbalance that had led to the cancer in the first place. Moreover, because different individuals had different types of imbalances, the exact type of therapy recommended would vary from case to case.

Among the major unorthodox cancer therapies touted during the 1950s were the Gerson treatment, a strict dietary regimen that supposedly cured cancer by restoring normal metabolism; Krebiozen, an injectable chemical advocated by the well-known physician-researcher Andrew C. Ivy; and the Harry Hoxsey botanical treatment, a mixture of roots and barks. Hoxsey supporters often blended their advocacy of his medication with an antipathy for government and non-Christians. Morris Fishbein, editor of the *Journal of the American Medical Association*, had no patience for the marketing of expensive elixirs and powders to a vulnerable public. "Of all the ghouls who feed on the dead and dying bodies," he wrote, "the cancer quacks are the most vicious and the most unprincipled."[32]

An additional issue in these debates was the language used by many alternative practitioners, who generally promised their patients a "cure." A cure, of course, was also what orthodox cancer doctors wished to achieve. However, because the nontraditional healers advertised this goal most loudly, the word *cure* acquired a negative connotation. Anyone who promised a cure, no matter what his or her approach, was suspect.

The letters sent to Dulles are full of testimonials to various alternative therapies—additional evidence that cancer was not a mystery to Americans in the 1950s. Dulles's family and staff sent these letters to his physicians, who generally dismissed them as coming from "crackpots." For example, one man wrote to urge Allen Dulles, the brother of John Foster Dulles and head of the Central Intelligence Agency, to advocate for Krebiozen. Ninety percent of doctors thought it was quackery, he admitted. "Nevertheless, I believe that if your brother could have the drug now the cancer would be arrested and perhaps completely eliminated." "In case of further cancer trouble," a California man urged after Dulles's first operation, "please go to the Hoxsey clinic at either Portage, Pa. or Dallas, Texas."[33]

Not surprisingly, these letters often recounted "n of 1" stories: someone the writer knew had been diagnosed with terminal cancer and had tried one of these remedies as a last resort. To his or her surprise and relief, they had worked. One woman told Isidor S. Ravdin, a consultant on Dulles's case, that she had been diagnosed with metastatic cancer in both 1953 and 1956. The second time she had received a medication called "Mucorchin" for six months. It was "like a miracle what it did for me and countless other doomed cancer victims," she wrote.[34]

Because well-known alternative practitioners gained a large clientele, the "n of 1" case potentially became a much larger—and convincing— number. A 13-year-old girl from New Mexico earnestly urged Dulles to try the Hoxsey treatment: "Would you *please* go to see Hoxsey and be cured before it is too late?" The Hoxsey clinic, she explained, had successfully cured a cancer on her mother's neck. But she also stressed how her mother was only one of many patients whose case histories served to legitimize this approach. "Mr. Hoxsey has cured thousands of people," she told the secretary of state, "and *he* has *proof.*"[35]

Many of the letter-writers bolstered their case by pointing out how little conventional medicine had to offer Dulles and other patients with recurrent cancer. One woman, having heard on television that doctors had "abandoned hope," wrote to Allen Dulles urging a trial of a "bio-chemo-therapy" developed by a Romanian-born physician, Emanuel Revici, then practicing in New York City. Revici, she explained, had cured several hopeless patients and was an upstanding member of the New York State Medical Society. "What's there to lose?" she asked.[36]

Some letters came from physicians, who stated their credentials to avoid being lumped with disreputable practitioners. One such letter was sent to Allen Dulles by Ernesta Barton, an old acquaintance. She reminded Dulles that her father had been president of Lehigh University, her brothers, Cecil and Philip Drinker, were scientific researchers at Harvard, and her sister, Catherine Drinker Bowen, was a reputable historian who checked her facts carefully. "I was born into a family," she stated, "who requires pretty substantial proof before believing."[37]

She then sang the praises of Revici, describing a series of cases in which he had produced remissions for supposedly terminal individuals, including patients with tongue and liver cancer. Barton also emphasized Revici's relatively modest claims: that his therapy did not always work and that his goal was arresting, not curing, cancer. Barton closed by urging Dulles to look into the Revici treatment for his brother. "Even if Ravici [*sic*] can't restore him to health," she wrote, "in all probability he will be able to spare him the physical pain attendant on such cases."[38]

When seemingly reputable clinicians were involved, Dulles's physicians paid closer attention. In one instance, a heart surgeon named Gorelik contacted Allen Dulles to alert him to intravenous medication known as peroxydases. Dulles had referred the matter to his assistant, Frank M. Chapin. Gorelik explained to Chapin that he had recently had a small number of patients with terminal cancer to whom he had administered the drug. The results, he said, were "absolutely amazing." And then, to prove his point, Gorelik put on the phone a patient, formerly with a large cancer, who told Chapin that he had been written off by doctors at the Bethesda Naval Hospital. Thanks to the peroxydases, the patient stated, his cancer had "disappeared" and his weight had increased from 143 to 180 pounds.[39]

Whatever anyone thought of an "n of 1" case and unorthodox treatments, hearing an oral report of possible cure from an actual patient had to raise hopes. Allen Dulles passed along the information to his brother's physicians, who declined to try the medication. Peroxydases, they explained, were "in the research area" and should not freely be used in the treatment of cancer.[40]

Dulles's physicians ultimately rejected all of the proposed unorthodox remedies. But an interesting tension was emerging. By the 1950s, orthodox medical researchers had begun testing the first chemotherapeutic drugs to treat cancer. The era of chemotherapy had been ushered in by the chance observation that soldiers exposed to nitrogen mustard suffered severe damage to their bone marrow. This led physicians to develop a series of related chemotherapeutic drugs, known as alkylating agents, to try to shrink cancers. Meanwhile, in Boston, Sidney Farber had successfully used an antagonist to the vitamin folate to treat certain childhood leukemias.[41]

Early agents were quite toxic, killing not only cancer cells but healthy cells and tissues throughout the body. Patients suffered nausea, vomiting, and hair loss. Because most of the medications suppressed the bone marrow, patients became highly susceptible to infections, which were potentially fatal. Still, researchers forged ahead, developing a series of multi-institutional clinical trials designed to formally assess the value of such treatments.

What made chemotherapy so novel was its ability to treat cancer systemically. That is, conventional treatments, surgery and radiotherapy, had sought to eliminate local pockets of disease, either when the cancer first appeared or when it recurred. Chemotherapy was based on the notion that medications, taken by mouth or vein, would enter the bloodstream and then kill cancer cells throughout the body.

This concept, however, was the same one that unorthodox healers had been promoting for decades. Now, too, orthodox physicians could begin to talk of cured patients whose cancer would never recur. All of a sudden, the goals of these cancer physicians had started to resemble those of the unorthodox practitioners they had so long reviled. There was a distinction, of course, between mysterious elixirs developed by unsavory practitioners and chemicals being tested at major medical centers. But to certain members of the public, unorthodox healers, and at least a few mainstream physicians, the line between these two approaches was blurred.[42]

Why was the orthodox medical profession now able to discuss chemotherapy and cures after it had warned against such language for decades? How clear was the distinction between treatments developed by outsiders versus insiders? The truth was that in the years after World War II, mainstream cancer physicians were increasingly in the "hope business," searching for possible lifesaving interventions—radical surgery, radiotherapy, and now chemotherapy—for cases previously deemed untreatable. "Cancer, Dulles and Hope" was the title of an article in the February 22, 1959, *New York Times*. Written by New York rehabilitation expert Howard Rusk, who had helped treat Margaret Bourke-White, the piece described exciting advances being made in cancer research.[43]

A few physicians not involved with Dulles's case had favored treating his recurrence not only with radiotherapy but also with one of the new experimental chemotherapy agents then being tested for colon cancer. According to Dulles's surgeon, Leonard Heaton, some had even told Janet Dulles that omitting such agents was a "horrible error." After considerable discussion, Dulles's physicians had chosen not to try any of these agents, which included 5-fluorouracil and thiotepa, due to their toxicity and lack of proven efficacy. As Isidor Ravdin wrote, Dulles "should not be used as a guinea pig," the role that Bourke-White said she would have chosen for herself if necessary.[44]

The fourth optimistic message conveyed to Dulles by letter-writers addressed his supposedly unique ability to fight the cancer. Though not, like Lou Gehrig before him or Brian Piccolo after him, a professional athlete, Dulles was a large and formidable presence. He also had acquired a reputation as an indefatigable public servant. There was surely a tendency, once Dulles got sick, to celebrate his past durability as a positive omen for his cancer. For example, one newspaper reported in late 1958 that, at age 10, he had apparently survived being hit by a bolt of lightning and being knocked unconscious.[45]

There is some validity to the claim that Dulles was a tough customer. Before becoming secretary of state, he had suffered from several painful medical problems, including a slipped disc and gout. His physician during those years, Arthur Peckham, found Dulles to be "almost oblivious to pain." He said that Dulles was his only patient who insisted on walking normally during a gouty attack. As secretary of state, according to Deane and David Heller, Dulles worked at a pace "that left aides twenty-five years his junior exhausted." He logged close to six hundred thousand air miles during his tenure, considerably more than any of his predecessors.[46]

And there was another type of strength that Dulles evinced as secretary of state—his insistence on standing up to the Soviets. The concept of brinkmanship connoted a daring bravado, a willingness to stand up to any threat.

It was this supposed inner strength that convinced some people that Dulles could overcome his cancer. "With his courage, determination and rugged constitution," wrote one man in February 1959, "I feel sure he is going to win out in this." A writer from Skokie, Illinois, cited Dulles's "superb courage" and "indomitable character" as hopeful reasons that he would "triumph over the difficulty." Even Democratic Senator Lyndon B. Johnson conveyed this sentiment just after Dulles's cancer recurrence, as published in the *Congressional Record:* "If tenacity, dedication, and resoluteness of purpose are allies of medicine, then the prognosis is certainly encouraging, for Mr. Dulles has never been lacking in these qualities."[47]

As with the "n of 1" letters, it is hard to know the exact meaning of such sentiments. Did the authors of these statements actually believe that Dulles was more likely to recover, or were they merely engaging in wishful thinking? It is worth noting that Dulles's family members also linked his willpower with his recovery. In 1957, Dulles's sister-in-law, Clover, told him that his recovery from the previous year's cancer operation could be attributed to his "intense and real interest" in "the state of the world." Even after learning the grim significance of his 1959 recurrence, relatives still saw him as somehow bucking the odds. "Foster has more than the normal power of self-discipline," his sister, diplomat Eleanor Lansing Dulles, told *Time* magazine, "and in his case it isn't wise to go on averages."[48]

In this manner, the Dulles family likely resembled most families of cancer patients, famous or not. When presented with poor odds, it is only natural to think your relative might prove the exception. The family still privately held out hope for a cure in the weeks after Dulles's recurrence. Doctors rarely make mistakes about cancer, Allen Dulles mused, "but sometimes they're wrong."[49]

But the new area of cancer discovered in Dulles's neck vertebrae in early April 1959 ended such thoughts, leading to his resignation on April 15. The secretary of state had incurable disease. There would be no miracles. He was a tenacious individual, but he would not beat his cancer. Indeed, his two-and-a-half-year survival after his original diagnosis was no more than average.

Once the story of Dulles defying his cancer was no longer tenable, members of the press and the public put forth a new version of his illness: he had died as a martyr to a "hideous plague," a "cancer of the spirit . . . called communism." That is, Dulles had given his life to cancer as he fought the other cancer invading the globe. "He really has sacrificed himself for his nation and his world," wrote one woman to Allen Dulles. A couple from Wisconsin agreed, comparing Dulles's death to one of a general on a battlefield. "He has literally given his life for his country," wrote a couple from Palm Beach, Florida.[50]

These sentiments were fostered by growing public knowledge of how sick Dulles had been during the last months of his service. Newspaper and magazine accounts described how a gravely ill Dulles had insisted on making his final diplomatic trip to Europe in early 1959. For example, UPI quoted Vice President Richard M. Nixon as stating that his colleague had been in constant pain and "unable to keep down a single meal." Marguerite Higgins wrote about how Dulles had avoided painkillers during the daily negotiations but had to take them to sleep. "The nights were terrible," Dulles later told her. Reporters also quoted a friend of Dulles who said that the secretary of state had suspected before the trip that he had recurrent cancer but decided to go anyway.[51]

Having followed John Foster Dulles's struggle with cancer through the media, Americans also learned about his impending death from the press.

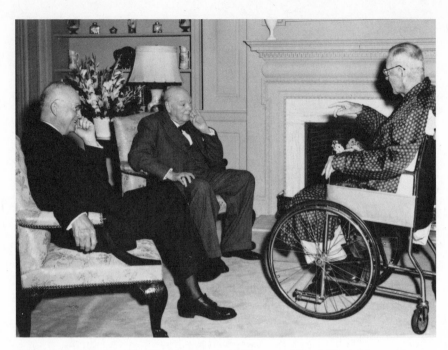

President Dwight D. Eisenhower and Winston Churchill visiting with a dying John Foster Dulles at Walter Reed Hospital in April 1959. Photograph from the John Foster Dulles papers, Seeley G. Mudd Library, Princeton University.

Reporters filed daily articles from Walter Reed, chronicling his gradual deterioration. Dulles, the public learned, spent his last weeks reading his beloved mystery novels, playing backgammon with his wife, and being briefed about world events. Among his many visitors were Eisenhower, Winston Churchill, and numerous members of Congress. Dulles's family, including sons John and Avery, visited frequently. Ironically, another former secretary of state, George Marshall, was dying of a stroke at Walter Reed at the same time.[52]

By the end, Higgins and others reported, Dulles surely knew he was dying. He stayed alert through May 20, 1959, refusing pain medications to do so. Shortly thereafter, however, Dulles developed pneumonia and his breathing became labored. At this point, doctors put him under "increasingly heavy sedation." His wife, sons, brother, and sister were present on May 24 when he finally stopped breathing.[53]

Despite the international attention to John Foster Dulles's colon cancer, including the sort of medical details not formerly released to the public, his case was ultimately an unremarkable one. He received standard surgery and, when that failed, standard radiotherapy. Neither his physicians nor Dulles himself chose to pursue any of a series of new therapies—orthodox or unorthodox—being touted for the disease.

But the thought that something more should have been done for Dulles continued to hover over the case, both before and after he died. When Ernesta Barton had written to Allen Dulles endorsing the Revici treatment, she included a story about Winston Churchill during World War I. During the German zeppelin raids over England, a man appeared at the war office claiming to have just the thing to stop them. Churchill's staff had dismissed him as a "crazy crank," but Churchill asked to speak with him. "That sort of crank is just what is needed," Churchill reportedly said. As a result of this encounter, Barton stated, the zeppelin raids ended. "The man," she told Dulles, "had invented the incendiary bullet."[54]

While the story may have been apocryphal, and the Revici treatment was soon consigned to history's dustbin, Barton's larger point was well-taken. Whether with alternative or mainstream therapy, the public was ready to support expanded efforts to develop cures for patients like Dulles. Within weeks of his death, the American Cancer Society and friends of the secretary of state proposed a "John Foster Dulles Memorial Cancer Drive." By June, the Senate's Health Appropriations subcommittee was considering raising the annual budget to the National Cancer Institute from $75 to $110 million. "Can money lick cancer?" asked *Newsweek*. If it could, "it would do so in the name of John Foster Dulles."[55]

Like the case of Dwight Eisenhower's heart attack, that of John Foster Dulles helped to establish a new standard: that the serious illnesses of politicians mandated media coverage. A few reporters had pushed further, gently questioning the information being provided to them. The widespread attention that resulted educated Americans about cancer, its treatments, and the issue of survival. And it would be cancer, as much as any disease, that remained in the public's eye as the practices of the medical profession increasingly came under attack in the 1960s and 1970s. Three cases that generated particular attention—those of Brian Piccolo, Morris Abram, and Steve McQueen—are explored in chapters 5 through 7.

Chapter 5

No Stone Unturned

The Fight to Save Brian Piccolo's Life

Like Lou Gehrig, Brian Piccolo was a famous athlete. And like John Foster Dulles, Piccolo developed terminal cancer. But Piccolo got sick not in 1939 or 1959 but in 1969, when medicine was on the verge of a series of transformations. Frank discussions of cancer were becoming much more frequent in the media. Patients were beginning to take a more prominent role in medical decision-making, challenging the existing model of the omnipotent and paternalistic physician. And, thanks to a series of technological innovations, doctors could significantly prolong the lives of critically ill people.

Piccolo's story is notable for another reason. Shortly after his death in June 1970, an extremely popular made-for-television movie dealt frankly and directly with his illness. But *Brian's Song* bore little resemblance to a contemporaneous account of Piccolo's saga, a candid book called *Brian Piccolo: A Short Season*, written by a friend of Piccolo with his cooperation. A comparison of these two very different versions of the same events illuminates how these new ideas about cancer, death, and the doctor-patient relationship were beginning to seep into public consciousness.

The story of Brian Piccolo was a milestone for another reason. After his death, Piccolo's family and his former team, the Chicago Bears, united to form a foundation to publicize and fund research into the disease that had killed him. Such activism, building on the illnesses of famous individuals, would later become commonplace. And, in a symbolic way, the Brian Piccolo Cancer Research Fund would ultimately accomplish what Brian Piccolo could not. It defeated disease.

As with Lou Gehrig, it has become hard to distinguish Brian Piccolo from the depiction of him in an enduring classic movie. But some facts are clear. He was born in Pittsfield, Massachusetts, on October 31, 1943, the youngest of three brothers. Piccolo's mother, Irene, was of German-Hungarian extraction and his father, Joseph, Italian. Brian was especially proud of his Italian heritage. When he was 3 years old, the Piccolo family moved to Fort Lauderdale, Florida, where his father first ran a driving school and then a restaurant. Brian Piccolo was a solid, if not spectacular, athlete, playing baseball, football, and basketball at Central Catholic High School. He originally played offensive tackle on the football team but became a successful halfback during his senior year, gaining hundreds of yards and scoring numerous touchdowns.[1]

Piccolo developed two striking characteristics during his high-school years—a rousing sense of humor and a strong sense of compassion. The humor was part of his gregarious nature. Whether at school, football practice, or the family restaurant, his friend Jeannie Morris later recalled, Piccolo struck up conversations with "pope and pauper" alike. Naturally irreverent, he poked fun at everyone, ranging from authority figures to himself. His compassionate side emerged through his interactions with Carol Murrath, who was the sister of his high-school girlfriend, Joy Murrath, and had cerebral palsy. Piccolo developed an independent friendship with Carol, taking her swimming or to sports events. "Brian was always so good to Carol," Herb Murrath, Carol and Joy's father, stated. "He was a big shot high school athlete, but he was never, never too busy." When Piccolo proposed to Joy in 1963, he bought rings for both sisters.[2]

Piccolo won a football scholarship to Wake Forest College, where he matriculated in 1960. The decision paid off. He became the team's star running back, and in his senior year, 1964, led the entire nation in rushing and scoring. But at six feet and 185 pounds, Piccolo was deemed too small and slow for professional football. So in the fall of 1964, the Atlantic Coast Conference's Most Valuable Player was not selected in the National Football League draft. Piccolo, who had fancied himself a first-round pick, was devastated. But there was good news. As Brian and Joy's wedding approached in December 1964, he was signed by the Chicago Bears as a free agent.[3]

Piccolo made the team and remained a Chicago Bear throughout his short career. Also joining the team in 1965 was an African American running back, Gale Sayers, whose friendship with Piccolo would be immortalized in *Brian's Song*. Sayers, who would eventually be inducted into the National Football League's Hall of Fame, quickly became the undisputed offensive star of the team. Piccolo plugged away over the next several years, often serving as Sayers's backup. Piccolo's best performances came in 1968, when Sayers suffered a severe knee injury. In one game, Piccolo rushed for 112 yards. By 1969, Sayers was back, but the Bears' fullback, Ronnie Bull, was injured in midseason. Piccolo took over the job, starting alongside his friend Sayers.[4]

Meanwhile, Joy and Brian Piccolo had begun a family. They had three daughters, Lori, born in October 1965, Traci, born in March 1967, and Kristi, born in December 1968. The Piccolos lived in Chicago.

When one examines the more complicated aspects of Brian Piccolo's life, it becomes harder to decipher fact from fiction. The idea for *Brian's Song* grew out of a chapter from Gale Sayers's autobiography, *I Am Third*, published in November 1970. The book did well, landing on the *New York Times* best-seller list. But it was the chapter on Brian Piccolo, in which Sayers described their interracial friendship and Piccolo's illness, that gave the book long life. The updated version of *I Am Third*, published in 2001, announced on the front cover that it was "the inspiration for *Brian's Song*."[5]

An understanding of how *Brian's Song* tackled the issue of race informs how it addressed Piccolo's illness. According to William Blinn's screenplay, the Bears management had decided that it was no longer appropriate to condone racial segregation on the team. In deciding that players should room together by position, the team had decided to make a test case of Piccolo and Sayers. The two had become increasingly friendly as the outgoing Piccolo persuaded the more quiet Sayers to emerge from his shell. Even more so than Piccolo's tragic illness, it was this friendship between a white man and a black man that was at the heart of the movie.[6]

Hollywood exaggerated some aspects of this relationship. For example, the two men, even after they became roommates, were never best friends. And, according to Sayers, the script overstated the magnitude of the Bears' decision to mix races. Aside from some initial apprehension, he wrote in *I Am Third*, "there was nothing to it." Some critics would later chide *Brian's*

Song as presenting a naive portrait of race relations at a time when American cities were being torn apart by racial strife. "It makes race relations look so simple and uncomplicated and so right that you wonder what the fuss is about," chided Don Page in the *Los Angeles Times*.[7]

Such criticisms, while valid, raise another question. If the issue of race in *Brian's Song* was handled simplistically, why did the film strike such an intense chord among Americans, becoming the fourth most-watched film in television history and winning several awards for promoting racial understanding? For one thing, the cohabitation of blacks and whites, whether as spouses or friends, was still a hot-button issue for many Americans in the mid-1960s. A letter sent to Piccolo underscored this point. "I read where you stay together with Sayers," it said. "I am a white man! Most of the people I know don't want anything to do with them. I just don't understand you." And the very fact that the two roommates, according to Sayers, spent a lot of time kidding each other about race (words like *spade* and *nigger* populate *Brian's Song*) suggests that they themselves were more self-conscious about the issue than Sayers claimed in his book.[8]

But perhaps the best explanation as to why the interracial relationship depicted in the movie proved so compelling was the exact reason that some critics had attacked it. Released only two years after the assassination of Martin Luther King, Jr., at a time when the Black Panther Party was at its peak, *Brian's Song* provided a reassuring representation of how the two races could and should get along. As media historian Douglas Gomery has argued, Sayers was a nonthreatening black, a "bashful hero" who "posed no problems."[9]

Despite its grisly reality, the depiction of Piccolo's illness and death in *Brian's Song* greatly resembled that of the friendship: it was well-ordered and somehow reassuring. As shown in the film, Piccolo's medical problems began in the fall of 1969, when he and Sayers were the starting running backs. In succession, Piccolo, as depicted by James Caan, loses weight, develops a cough, and then becomes extremely winded during a game. Next, the Bears' coach, George Halas, played by Jack Warden, decides that Piccolo needs to return to Chicago to see a doctor. Piccolo is furious but is comforted by his friend Sayers.[10]

The scene then switches to the locker room before the next week's game. Halas calls Sayers aside and tells him that he has just learned that Piccolo has cancer. An operation to remove part of Piccolo's lung is scheduled for the next day. At this point, Sayers decides that he wants to tell the team the news. In a powerful scene, Sayers asks his teammates to win the game for their ailing teammate and then present him with the game ball.[11]

In typical Hollywood fashion, the aforementioned scenes telegraph what is eventually going to occur. They are full of foreshadowing and ominous music. Even though the word *cancer* is used, an aura of secrecy and dread pervades this portion of the film. Disclosures about Piccolo's worsening condition occur during unwitnessed phone calls and in hushed conversations. Doctors are mentioned but never actually appear in the movie.

Aside from Piccolo, who cracks jokes about his condition and predicts his recovery, all other cast members are, pun intended, deadly serious. Sayers, for example, acts as if Piccolo has fatal cancer as soon as he first begins coughing. According to the stage notes for the movie, the character of Sayers was supposed to respond with "prayerful disbelief and awe" when Halas tells him Piccolo has cancer. Billie Dee Williams, as Sayers, follows this direction excellently. In the next scene, when Sayers addresses his teammates in the locker room, these rowdy football players are completely docile and almost reverent—even before they have any idea what he is going to speak about. A few shed tears.[12]

The scene next switches to the hospital, where Piccolo is recovering from his operation. His teammates are visiting and breaking the rules by drinking beer and eating pizza. As Sayers and Joy Piccolo, played by Shelley Fabares, leave, Brian Piccolo asks them to visit a girl he has met who underwent surgery the same day he did. When they reach the children's ward and ask for the girl, a nurse tells them that she died that morning. Joy Piccolo looks stunned. The implication of this scene is that the girl had the same disease as Brian Piccolo and did not make it. In reality, the girl that Piccolo met had suffered a broken neck. Although she did not survive, her death occurred weeks later. Once again, Piccolo's fate is being telegraphed. The Hollywood version of his story is marked with guideposts placed after the fact.[13]

As the movie proceeds, Sayers receives an urgent message from Joy Piccolo to come to her house. Sayers does so, with his wife, Linda. Joy tells them that the cancer has returned and additional surgery is necessary. She cries, but this scene typifies the "stiff-upper-lip" approach to cancer that existed before the 1970s. There is no anger and no questioning of either the doctors or fate. Even though it is 3:30 a.m., all three characters look well-groomed. Joy, despite her misery, has prepared a tray with coffee.[14]

The scene shifts back to the hospital, where an official interrupts a board football game that Piccolo and Sayers are playing. Piccolo does not yet know he needs additional surgery, as Joy was too frightened to tell him. When the official produces a consent form for the operation, he quickly realizes that Piccolo does not know about it. Sayers is then forced to come clean. "The tests show," he states, "there's more of the tumor than they thought, Pic. They have to operate again." The official pushes for a signature, but Sayers asks him to leave, for the time being.[15]

To our modern eye, this scene seems to be an indictment of the uncaring and even dangerous health care institution that would be immortalized in the 1971 George C. Scott film *The Hospital*. But circa 1969, this was the impersonal (and uninformative) manner in which operative consents were obtained. The confusion about the surgery is simply one more indignity that the dying Piccolo must stoically endure.

Piccolo's deathbed scene in *Brian's Song* suggests that the end was not pleasant. He has difficulty speaking and a spasm of pain. Joy Piccolo is depicted as distraught. But James Caan's face looks no different than it did at the beginning of the movie. He still has a full head of curly hair. The dialogue contains little anger or bewilderment but rather a clichéd discussion between Piccolo and Sayers in which they chronicle the highlights of their friendship. Piccolo describes his dire situation with a sports metaphor: "It's fourth and eight, man—but they won't let me punt." Sayers responds by saying, "Go for it, then," which might be seen as giving his friend permission to die.[16]

Joy Piccolo then takes Sayers's place at the bedside for one last interaction with her dying husband. He smiles and asks her, "Who'd believe it, Joy—who'd ever believe it . . . ?" After thus acknowledging his fate, Piccolo quietly dies.[17]

Brian's Song was probably no more or less accurate than most Hollywood dramas based on "true" events. Although written and filmed in cooperation with the Chicago Bears, neither Blinn nor director Buzz Kulik actively involved Joy Piccolo or other family members in the process. But Joy, her family, and friends did tell their version of the story at the time. And while no account is ever objective, this one had something in its favor.

It was based on a series of audiotapes made by an ailing Piccolo that were to have formed the basis of his autobiography. When he died, his collaborator, Jeannie Morris, did not plan to continue the project. But Joy Piccolo asked her to "finish Brian's book." Morris did so, she later wrote, to tell his story to the three daughters he barely got to know.[18]

Jeannie Morris was married to Johnny Morris, a wide receiver and teammate of Piccolo. Although the Morrises were several years older than the Piccolos, they became close friends—"family," as Jeannie Morris wrote in *A Short Season*. That Jeannie Morris became Piccolo's amanuensis is not a coincidence. Morris was at the time writing a column for the *Chicago Sun-Times* on the life of a football player's wife. Her column frankly suggested that all was not fun and games. Among the issues she discussed was the questionable role of team physicians in returning players to the lineup prematurely. To the degree that *A Short Season* had any agenda at all, Morris later recalled, it was to call into question aspects of Piccolo's early medical treatment.[19]

Whereas the book's title underscored its emphasis on Brian Piccolo's truncated football career and life, Morris strove to capture her subject's personality. She wrote of Piccolo's devotion to his family, stressing his unique relationship with his sister-in-law, Carol. And she made sure to highlight Piccolo's relentlessly upbeat personality and sense of humor. Morris often printed his words verbatim. For example, he had asked the nurses at Illinois Masonic Hospital, where he was first admitted in November 1969, "How do you expect a good Italian to take a crap if you don't give him any tomato sauce, for crissake?" When his teammates came to visit him at the hospital and his boyhood friend, Morey Colleta, a funeral home director, appeared, Piccolo announced, "Gentlemen, I would like you to meet my personal undertaker."[20]

Using, among other sources, Piccolo's actual medical chart from Memorial Sloan-Kettering Cancer Center, Morris documented his illness and death. The book is no indictment of the care that Piccolo received or of the medical profession. But Morris's narrative subtly raised a series of questions, which would burst forth in the 1970s and 1980s, about what patients with cancer should be told, how they should be treated, and who should be in charge of making decisions.

A Short Season begins with a story resembling that of Lou Gehrig: the delayed diagnosis of a famous patient. Piccolo had been coughing for several weeks as of mid-November 1969. Then he had become short of breath when running. The team trainer had treated him for bronchitis, but Piccolo only worsened. Finally, Piccolo went on his own initiative to Illinois Masonic, where the team physician, L. L. Braun, practiced. Braun was not in his office, so Piccolo went to get a chest x-ray. The technician then appeared and told him they needed another film; this was the "first inkling," Piccolo told Morris, that something was wrong. Piccolo then brought both films to Louis Kolb, one of the Bears' orthopedists. Kolb was hesitant to show concern, according to Piccolo, but the football player was alarmed at a shadow he saw: "I'm no expert, Doctor, but that's not supposed to be there."[21]

Piccolo was all too correct. The x-ray led to a cascade of tests, which culminated in a biopsy of his mediastinum, an area of tissue behind the breastbone and between the lungs. "They found it was a malignancy called embryonal cell carcinoma," Piccolo later informed Morris. "Christ, but they didn't tell me. Friday they told Joy. When she came up to see me, her eyes were about as big as they could be and very moist. So I assumed that whatever she knew wasn't very good." As in the cases of Lou Gehrig and Margaret Bourke-White, the inclination of the physicians was to keep secrets from Piccolo, something he did not appreciate. "I wanted to know everything," he later said.[22]

The cancer was a rare one, arising from cells that had not fully developed when Piccolo's body was being formed (hence the term *embryonal*). Eventually, the doctors discovered that these embryonal cells were part of a larger tumor, known as a teratoma. Teratomas are large masses that contain a variety of tissues from the body that should not be present at that location. They can be benign or malignant. Piccolo's was malignant, containing several types of rare cancers in addition to embryonal cancer: sarcoma, seminoma, squamous carcinoma, and possible choriocarcinoma.[23]

The doctors at Illinois Masonic all agreed that the entire cancer needed to be removed, but given the nature and location of the tumor, it would be a highly uncommon operation. Piccolo spoke to several people, including his friend Dick Corzatt, a physician. Eventually, Piccolo chose to be operated on at New York's Memorial Sloan-Kettering Cancer Center.

Piccolo's decision to go to Sloan-Kettering was important for two reasons. First, the hospital, founded as the New York Cancer Hospital in 1884, was the most renowned cancer facility in the United States. As would be the case with many other celebrity patients over the next decades, finding the "best" care available was an important objective for Piccolo and the Bears. "Ordinary" patients, especially those with rare diseases, would increasingly embrace such a philosophy as well, if they had the wherewithal to pursue such an option and the means and connections to gain access. In Piccolo's case, Chicago Bears' owner George Halas generously picked up the tab.

Second, the choice of institution signified that Piccolo would receive highly aggressive treatment. One did not go to Sloan-Kettering for conservative measures. Doctors there had pioneered operations, including those removing ribs and limbs, aimed at removing every last cancer cell. Radiation therapy was used liberally to kill any possible cells that the scalpel had missed. Finally, Sloan-Kettering was on the cutting edge of cancer chemotherapy, the new drug treatment that John Foster Dulles's doctors had declined to try. Indeed, there had been a brief discussion of sending the secretary of state to Sloan-Kettering had chemotherapy been approved.

The gung-ho spirit of Sloan-Kettering was well embodied by Edward J. (Ted) Beattie, chairman of the hospital's department of surgery. Beattie was warm, charming, and invariably upbeat, focusing all of his energy on one goal: beating cancer. And, moreover, he was a football man. Beattie had played defensive guard at Princeton University, which he thought was good training for his future job. "Football players make good surgeons," he told Jeannie Morris. "Surgeons are aggressive hard-charging guys."[24]

Piccolo bonded immediately with Beattie. At their first meeting they discussed football extensively. Beattie was even a Bears' fan, having worked in Chicago for eleven years. Piccolo remarked, admiringly, that Beattie was "the kind who knows the game." This connection helped Piccolo come to terms with his impending operation. "I felt like I was putting my life in his hands—and I guess my destiny—and I felt good about it," he stated. "He gave me confidence." The fact that Piccolo had succeeded in the National Football League against the odds may have made him seem to be an excellent candidate to battle cancer, both from his perspective and that of Beattie.[25]

Beattie performed the operation on November 28, 1969. It lasted four-and-one-half hours. Beattie had to split Piccolo's breastbone in order to remove the tumor, which was as large as a grapefruit. It was also necessary to remove a portion of Piccolo's left lung, which also contained cancer, as well as part of the pericardium, a thin tissue that surrounds the heart.

When Beattie met with Joy Piccolo immediately after the operation, he was very optimistic. He termed the surgery a success and told her that all visible tumor, plus some "insurance tissue," had been removed. Beattie later informed Joy that one of the nearby lymph nodes had contained cancer. The doctors decided to give Piccolo two types of chemotherapy, chlorambucil and actinomycin-D, initially at Sloan-Kettering and then back in Chicago after his discharge. Piccolo understood that the medications were intended to "work against any cancer cells that Beattie might have missed."[26]

What did it mean that all *visible* tumor had been removed? What was the significance of the positive lymph node? How successful was the chemotherapy likely to be? Nobody was asking or answering these questions, at least not openly. Perhaps the best summary of the situation appeared in Piccolo's discharge summary from Sloan-Kettering. "It is hoped," wrote the author in the passive voice, "that in this young man with complete surgical excision and with long range chemotherapy the prognosis will be good." Like the Piccolos, the doctors were hoping, too.[27]

Despite the ambiguities of Brian Piccolo's condition, by January 1970 he was telling Jeannie Morris and other friends that he had "been blessed and was cured of cancer." He had just been invited to Phoenix to play in a golf tournament for professional athletes; despite his recent surgery, he was eager to try to play. His partner was to be legendary Chicago Cubs shortstop Ernie Banks, which thrilled Piccolo. But his delight was cruelly interrupted during his second night in Phoenix. While fingering the operative scar, Piccolo felt a lump. Joy Piccolo noticed and asked, "What's that?" Piccolo replied, "What the hell do you think it is?"[28]

Piccolo returned to Sloan-Kettering and had a biopsy on February 16, 1970. The cancer had returned. This time, the doctors decided not to try surgery immediately but rather additional chemotherapy—a four-drug regimen. These drugs, never really discussed in *Brian's Song*, became the mainstay of his treatment for the time being. And Piccolo, who seemed especially susceptible to their side effects, hated them. "Brian," Jeannie Morris wrote, "loathed being sick with the degrading illness caused by chemotherapy." Morris had also learned what the latest news signified re-

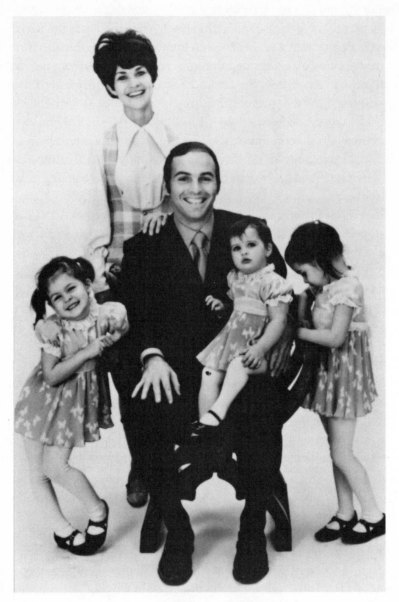

Brian Piccolo and his family in a photograph taken in December 1969, just after his first surgery. Piccolo looks remarkably healthy, but his body surely still contained extensive cancer. Courtesy of Joy Piccolo O'Connell.

garding Piccolo's prognosis. "In spite of their outward cheer," she wrote, "the doctors knew that now, with the recurrence, the odds on Brian's survival were short."[29]

Aside from a short trip to Chicago for his daughter Traci's third birthday on March 16, 1970, Piccolo remained hospitalized. Unfortunately, the chemotherapy did not have its desired effect. The tumor on Piccolo's chest, which was located in his left pectoral (chest wall) muscles, had increased in size and was uncomfortable. As a result, the doctors decided to perform a radical mastectomy, removing their patient's pectoral muscles and dissecting the lymph nodes under his arm.

This operation would prove especially difficult for Piccolo, both physically and emotionally. Not only were Beattie and his colleagues removing an enormous amount of muscular tissue from a professional athlete, but they were performing the operation used to treat women with breast cancer. Her husband, Joy Piccolo recalled, felt "very frustrated" and "extremely mutilated" due to the emasculating surgery. Even the fearsome Bears' linebacker Dick Butkus was taken aback when Piccolo later showed him the scar. The operation was performed on March 24, 1970.[30]

Although the cancer was now gone from Piccolo's chest wall, the doctors knew it had also returned to the left lung. Tests had shown no evidence of cancer in the liver or elsewhere in the body, leading Beattie to hope that it was confined to the lung and thus could be removed. When the surgeon told Piccolo about the need for yet more surgery, he informed his patient that he would never be able to play football again as a result. This statement underscores just how little Beattie had discussed the issue of prognosis up until this point. The notion of Piccolo playing football after a radical mastectomy for widely spread cancer was preposterous. The removal of the lung was just confirmation of this fact. And one cannot help but think that Beattie's admission, between two men who loved football, may have been his way of telling Brian Piccolo he was dying. Such euphemisms, which sent mixed signals, remained acceptable in the early 1970s.

Beattie performed the lung removal, known as a pneumonectomy, on April 9, 1970. The information obtained during the operation was even more discouraging. The operative note revealed that the surgeons had discovered tumor invading the left rib cage, the tissue surrounding the top of Piccolo's aorta, and even the mesh used to repair Piccolo's pericardium during the first operation. The cancer was everywhere. During the surgery, a radiotherapist, Basil Hilaris, placed radioactive iodine seeds wherever there was residual cancer. After the operation, Hilaris began administering a course of cobalt radiotherapy to this same area.[31]

By this time, Brian Piccolo was physically decimated. He had been through two major operations in a few weeks, still had cancer present, and was receiving radiation, which itself causes severe fatigue. Piccolo detailed these treatments for Morris: "The room, when it's finally your turn, is totally dominated by the Machine. And somebody with a rotten sense of humor, or I guess, maybe a futile desire to please, has covered one wall with a huge mural . . . Anyhow, I know the position well now: Flat on my back so the machine has a good shot at what's left of my left breast and shoulder. Hell, the Machine scares me, and the picture makes me mad, so I guess I just glaze my eyes and try not to see anything."[32]

During the radiation treatment, he and Joy stayed in an apartment near the hospital. Despite her urgings, Piccolo left the apartment infrequently. Often, Morris wrote, "he was simply drained—of everything." A particularly difficult problem was constant facial pain, resulting from infiltration of the cancer into his jaw and teeth. Even Piccolo's legendary humor was sometimes replaced by bitterness, both when speaking with Joy and with the many visitors he received. The cobalt treatment was completed on May 14, 1970, and Piccolo went home to Chicago on May 23.[33]

It was during this visit that a famous scene, depicted—largely accurately—in *Brian's Song* took place. The Professional Football Writers Association had awarded Gale Sayers the George S. Halas award as the most courageous player in football due to his successful return from knee surgery. On receiving the award, Sayers told the audience that it had been given to the wrong man.

> He has the heart of a giant and that rare form of courage that allows him
> to kid himself and his opponent—cancer. He has the mental attitude that
> makes me proud to have a friend who spells out the word "courage"
> twenty-four hours a day of his life. You flatter me by giving me this award,
> but I tell you that I accept it for Brian Piccolo. It is mine tonight, it is
> Brian Piccolo's tomorrow . . . I love Brian Piccolo, and I'd like all of you to
> love him too. Tonight, when you hit your knees, please ask God to love
> him.[34]

Sayers's words, like those uttered by Lou Gehrig in 1939 and those that would be spoken by Arthur Ashe in 1992, served as a type of pre-death eulogy for a doomed athlete.

On May 31, 1970, the Piccolos flew from Chicago to Atlanta to see their three girls, who had been living with Joy's parents, the Murraths. Brian visited with his family and many old friends, including Carol, who was graduating from a school for young adults with cerebral palsy. Morris wrote that he teased Carol about having received perfume and a nightgown from a boy in her class. But Piccolo was far too sick to horse around with his daughters. His cough had become "unbearable." Joy called Beattie, who told them to return immediately to New York. Before they left, however, Brian arranged for Monsignor Regan, the priest who had married him and Joy, to give him Holy Communion. A small altar was set up in the bedroom and the three children and Brian's in-laws sat down for the short service. Perhaps, as Gale Sayers later speculated, Piccolo knew by this point that he was dying, even as he kept a strong front for his family.[35]

According to Jeannie Morris, Piccolo's last hospital admission, which began on June 4, 1970, was "torture," consisting of "hours out of his bed, being wheeled, poked, turned, punctured, manipulated." Among the unpleasant things that Piccolo and others experienced in the last few days was a terrible smell. His body was literally rotting away. As was customary, nobody volunteered information to Piccolo about what was being done. Morris believed that Piccolo was too afraid to ask.[36]

The Sloan-Kettering staff tried to treat Piccolo's pain and cough but it was not easy. On Thursday, June 11, Joy found her husband on his hands and knees, pounding his head on the bed due to the pain. He received relief with more medication. But the next day, Beattie's colleague, Michael Small, had worse news: Piccolo was in shock due to low blood pressure. "I don't think Brian is going to live very long," he told the family.[37]

Joy Piccolo finds it hard to remember just when she knew her husband was not going to survive. Jeannie Morris, who was with her during the last days and interviewed her afterward, believes she had held out some slim hope until Small's words. "And *that* was the moment—no sooner—that Joy finally realized Brian was going to die," Morris wrote. Joy called the immediate family to come to New York as soon as possible to say goodbye.[38]

On Saturday, June 13, Piccolo received a blood transfusion from a New Jersey man who had been cured of embryonal cell carcinoma six years before. Even though the immunotherapist told Joy that it would not benefit her husband, she consented because there was possible value to both science and other patients. Such goals would increasingly interest Joy Piccolo in the coming years.

Sedated, Brian Piccolo remained silent most of the time, but continued to recognize visitors and make periodic comments. On Monday, June 15, he became more alert and interactive. He told Joy he loved her several times. But he was also seemingly still fighting, saying, "I'm going to lick this. I'm going to get out of here." Finally, he sat bolt upright and screamed, "Can you believe it, Joy? Can you believe this shit?" (The expletive was omitted from this sentence in *Brian's Song*, thus concealing Piccolo's fury.)[39]

At this point, Joy Piccolo decided, with Beattie's agreement, that more aggressive sedation was needed. Over the next several hours, Joy Piccolo later told Morris, her husband's breathing became more difficult: "There would be a breath, a huge gasp, and then a sigh." At 2 a.m. on June 16, 1970, Piccolo finally died.[40]

The account of Brian Piccolo's last months in *A Short Season* quietly raised questions about Piccolo's original prognosis and the treatments he received. The decision to send Piccolo to Sloan-Kettering reflected not only the atypical nature of his cancer but its gravity. Shortly after Piccolo's cancer was diagnosed, Morris reported, his high-school friend Dan Arnold shared the information with a pathologist he knew. The pathologist had flatly stated that the disease carried a six-month prognosis.[41]

If one looks at the medical literature from 1970, survival from an embryonal cell carcinoma was, in fact, quite poor. Less than 5 percent of patients lived five years. And because Piccolo's cancer was part of a teratoma, with other malignant tissues, his prognosis was even worse, something the Sloan-Kettering doctors surely knew. They, like other doctors of this era, were content to act optimistically, hoping for a miracle, even as they knew that death was surely inevitable.

Morris did an excellent job of capturing this mindset in her descriptions of Ted Beattie. On the one hand, she—like Brian Piccolo—was charmed by his sincere concern for his patients, his evident intelligence, and his great energy. But Morris also termed him a "salesman–politician–fund raiser," indicating how his job as physician was intimately tied up with his inclination to promote the virtues of Sloan-Kettering. Beattie described his approach as "aggressive optimism," the philosophy that one should never give up "until the last whistle." In Brian and Joy Piccolo, Morris remarked, Beattie had found two people who "played it his way." When the Piccolos, still reeling from the radical mastectomy, were told about the need for lung removal, Beattie had told them reassuringly: "We've removed lungs before." And he cited another famous cancer patient, John Wayne, who had survived such surgery and done well. Such optimism was infectious, according to Joy Piccolo. "You would listen to Dr. Beattie and you would go ahead and do."[42]

After having liberally used sports and war metaphors to rally the Piccolos, Beattie was especially devastated at his patient's continued deterioration. He held a family meeting on the Sunday before Piccolo's death, outlining how everything had been tried but to no avail. "We have failed," he said, with his voice breaking.[43]

But despite her great appreciation for Beattie and his colleagues, Joy Piccolo could not help but question this mindset after her husband died. Other individuals were doing the same at this historical moment. In 1967, Cicely Saunders, an English physician, had founded St. Christopher's, a hospice that emphasized dying as a natural part of life. Two years later, Swiss-born psychiatrist Elisabeth Kübler-Ross published her landmark book *On Death and Dying*, based in large part on her candid discussions with dying patients. Joy Piccolo later remarked that she wished she had been told more about Brian's actual condition, either by Beattie or by the competent but taciturn oncologist, Robert B. Golbey, who "probably knew" her husband was dying. Of course, she admitted, neither Brian nor she had ever told the doctors to pull back. "You didn't question it because you didn't know any better," she stated.[44]

Today, in retrospect, Joy Piccolo wonders whether she and Brian should—or could—have done anything differently. "If I'd known, I really wouldn't have put him through it," she states. "At the time it was a zero percent rate of cure. There was just no way in heaven he was gonna be able to survive this." But she remains realistic as well. Brian Piccolo was young and healthy and had three daughters. They would have pulled back, Joy Piccolo admits, only if they had been absolutely positive that all of the treatment would be of no value. "We just believed that tomorrow it would get better, that something would stop it."[45]

In *Shooting Kennedy*, his book on the imagery surrounding the assassination of John F. Kennedy, art historian David M. Lubin argues that we respond to catastrophes "with a prescribed set of physical and emotional responses." It is true that, thanks to the work of Saunders and Kübler-Ross and the improvements in physician-patient dialogue since 1970, patients like Piccolo today receive more realistic assessments of their prognosis. But when you are a 26-year-old professional football player with three daughters—then or now—you do what everybody else does. You "fight" your cancer. And the same usually goes for people who are not football players, people without children, and people much older than Brian Piccolo.[46]

When Dan Arnold was interviewed for a 2001 ESPN documentary on the life of his friend Brian Piccolo, he provided this epitaph: "Brian Piccolo was the living testimony [of] don't ever, ever give up. No matter what happens don't give up. Things can be worked out. You never know what the future holds." Of course, one can derive an entirely opposite message from Piccolo's story. That is, Piccolo never gave up but he died anyway. Arnold's recollection is reminiscent of a line uttered by a journalist at the end of the 1962 film *The Man Who Shot Liberty Valance:* "When the legend becomes the fact, print the legend."[47]

Why have Arnold and so many others embraced the inspirational version of Piccolo's life as depicted in *Brian's Song*? Although Jeannie Morris's book was a more accurate account of what actually happened to Piccolo, *A Short Season* posed a series of uncomfortable questions about medicine that American society was on the verge of confronting. In contrast, *Brian's Song* told not only a moving tale of a friendship between a black man and a white man but a simple and straightforward account of Piccolo's demise. A truly nice guy gets a very bad break at a young age. With the assistance of loving family and friends, he fights the cancer until the very end. He receives the best medical care imaginable. At the end, he dies, but as a hero. On the verge of a revolution in medicine—one that would challenge the credibility of physicians, urge patients to become active decision-makers, and question the reflexive use of heroic, death-defying technologies— *Brian's Song* was a reassuring paean to a disappearing era. Some will say that the movie was corny, said one viewer, President Richard M. Nixon. But, he insisted, "it was one of the great motion pictures I have seen."[48]

Other factors help to explain the movie's phenomenal success. The two young actors in the starring roles, Caan and Williams, were highly talented performers who would go on to illustrious careers in Hollywood. The affecting score by Michel Legrand, particularly the theme music, provided the compelling combination of sadness and hope that Piccolo's story embodied. And the film crossed gender lines. The fact that the dying cancer victim was not a brainy young woman, as depicted by Ali MacGraw in the contemporaneous *Love Story*, but a macho football player ensured viewership among a young, male population not normally apt to watch such a tearjerker.

Indeed, *Brian's Song* has the reputation of being the one movie at which men are "allowed" to cry. The entire Chicago Bears team did so when the film was first screened for them, according to Jeannie Morris, as did the technical staff at ABC-TV that produced it. On a 1994 episode of the television show *Frasier*, the fictional Martin Crane, the hard-boiled father of psychiatrist Frasier Crane, breaks down during a viewing of the movie.

Joy Piccolo continues to get mail from fans of Brian Piccolo, just as she and her husband did during his illness. Members of the Piccolo family, including Brian's daughters and his brother Joe, still get stopped on the street and asked whether they are related to Brian. When they answer yes, hearty handshakes ensue. More than once, according to Kristi Piccolo, who strongly resembles her father, strangers have asked to hug her. Hundreds of people have told Gale Sayers that they have named their children either Gale or Brian. *Brian's Song* may not have scored points for its veracity, but its story of perseverance proved meaningful for men—and women.[49]

There is an additional explanation for the lasting legacy of the movie. Although Piccolo died, there is a happy ending to his story. After his death, family and friends began the Brian Piccolo Cancer Research Fund, which has helped to raise more than $5 million to fund cancer research and education. The heart and soul of the fund has been Joy Piccolo, who, according to daughter Traci, is a "spitfire." Joy, presaging what hundreds of spouses, parents, and children would do in the coming decades, met with people across the country, forging a connection between a tragic death, needed research, and hope. For years, the fund sponsored two annual fundraisers, a golf tournament and a run. Television reruns of *Brian's Song* invariably bring a new wave of donations. Receipts also come from fines collected by the National Football League when its players commit infractions on the field. Traci Piccolo has quipped that she roots for players to misbehave in order to generate more money for the foundation.[50]

Initially, funds were earmarked to support the research of Robert Golbey, Piccolo's oncologist at Memorial Sloan-Kettering, who was studying
the treatment of both embryonal and testicular cancers. By the early 1990s,
the Piccolo fund had shifted its focus to breast cancer research. This transition made sense given Piccolo's traumatic experience with a radical mastectomy. The fund, headquartered at Chicago's Rush University Medical
Center, received a major shot in the arm when a made-for-television remake of *Brian's Song* aired in 2001.[51]

By this time, there was good news. The cure rate for embryonal cell
cancer, which had killed Piccolo, was going up. Forty to 50 percent of its
victims were living five years, and some were being cured. But the real success story was for a related disease, testicular cancer, which is what afflicted
Lance Armstrong. (Embryonal cancers originate in testicular cells that
have mistakenly migrated to the chest or other parts of the body.) As of
2004, up to 95 percent of men with testicular cancer experience long-term
survival.[52]

These improved survival and cure rates, particularly for testicular cancer, have provided a remarkably powerful last chapter to the Brian Piccolo
saga. Survivors and others writing about testicular cancer often emotionally—but inaccurately—cite Piccolo as someone who died from the disease
before there was effective treatment. "Most people think Piccolo died of
lung cancer," Armstrong wrote in his first book, "but it started as testicular cancer, and they couldn't save him." "If Brian Piccolo of the Chicago
Bears had gotten testicular cancer a few years later, instead of 1969," Arthur
Allen wrote at salon.com, "'Brian's Song' might have had a happy ending."
Piccolo is listed in the "Testicular Cancer Hall of Fame" of the Testicular
Cancer Resource Center.[53]

Some of the confusion about Piccolo's actual diagnosis likely stemmed
from the fact that the Piccolo fund did, in part, support research into testicular cancer. But more than this, the notion that the dreaded disease
that had killed Piccolo was now curable—thanks to the fund started in his
name—was simply too good a story not to tell. Piccolo, according to this
narrative, had not died in vain. Lance Armstrong, to name only one survivor, was living proof. As one anonymous fan wrote on an Internet memorial to Piccolo, "Your death has changed the world and saved many lives.
Not many people can say that. God bless." Or, as Piccolo's brother Joe has
stated, Brian's two greatest accomplishments were "finding a cure for this

cancer" and "saving a whole lot of other lives." That neither of these claims is strictly true matters little.[54]

Another cancer victim, however, would come to believe that he achieved both of these goals, and during his lifetime. This person was Morris Abram, a noted civil rights lawyer who developed acute myelocytic leukemia in 1973 and then went public with his story. Abram did what Brian and Joy Piccolo had been unable to do. He became a walking encyclopedia on his disease and challenged his physicians at every step. The era of the activist patient was dawning, and sick celebrities like Abram were leading by example. But whether Abram, who survived his leukemia against all odds, had actually helped to engineer his cure was a much trickier question.

Chapter 6

Persistent Patient

Morris Abram as Experimental Subject

Morris Abram had spent much of his life challenging the status quo, both as a Jewish boy experiencing anti-Semitism in Georgia and as a lawyer attacking segregation in the South. He developed leukemia at the age of 55, in 1973—at a time when critics had begun to take on medicine, arguing that hospitals were cold, uncaring institutions and that doctors were paternalistic and often arrogant. Abram became a very active participant in his medical care, closely monitoring hospital staff and pushing his physicians to consider new treatment options.

Although his doctors believed he was doomed, Abram refused to agree. He identified a series of experimental treatments for his leukemia and almost bullied his physicians into enrolling him into trials of these agents. It was almost inevitable, perhaps, that he attributed his subsequent recovery to his role as a proactive patient. Yet, while Abram may have survived in part because he sought out cutting-edge treatment, it would be hard not to acknowledge another factor: good luck. And if Abram simply got lucky, what lessons should another patient—or the public—draw from such a case? The question as to whether proactive patients could really influence the course of their illnesses received considerable attention in an August 15, 1977, front-page *New York Times* article that announced Abram's "cure." Abram would later formally struggle with the issues of experimental treatment and informed consent as chairman of the President's Commission for the Study of Ethical Problems in Medicine and Behavioral Research.

Abram was born to Jewish parents, Sam and Irene Abram, in predominantly Protestant southern Georgia in 1918. His father was a harness maker. Among the childhood memories that Morris Abram would later detail was anti-Semitism—being called, among other things, a "Christ-killer." Getting out of the rural South became a priority. Eventually he moved to Chicago, graduating from the University of Chicago Law School in 1940. His very evident intelligence was rewarded with a Rhodes Scholarship at Oxford University.[1]

With the outbreak of World War II, Abram did not go to Oxford but did public relations for the Army Air Corps. After the war, now at Oxford, he assisted the prosecution during the Nuremberg trials of Nazi war criminals. Abram then became an Atlanta lawyer, turning his attention to a problem he well knew from his childhood: the persistence of Jim Crow laws that denied African Americans their civil rights. For more than a decade he struggled to get the courts to disband Georgia's county unit system, a scheme that functionally erased African American votes. Finally, on March 18, 1963, with Attorney General Robert F. Kennedy arguing the case in front of the U.S. Supreme Court, Abram won the day, enshrining the "one person, one vote" rule. Among Abram's other accomplishments during these years was helping Martin Luther King, Jr., fight legal battles stemming from civil rights protests.[2]

Abram's successes earned him a series of prestigious positions: national president of the American Jewish Committee, U.S. representative to the United Nations Commission on Human Rights, president of Brandeis University, and president of the United Negro College Fund. It was his years at Brandeis, from 1968 to 1970, that cast a shadow over his career-long progressivism. His decision to oppose and punish student antiwar protestors during the Vietnam War not only led to his resignation but called into question his reputation as a crusader for change. Indeed, by the 1980s, Abram's political compass would shift far to the right.[3]

As of 1973, Abram was practicing law at a Manhattan law firm, Paul, Weiss, Rifkind, Wharton and Garrison. He had been married for twenty-nine years to Jane Maguire. The Abrams had five successful children, three sons and two daughters.

But all was not well. In early May, Abram left his wife. Six weeks later he received dreadful news. On June 19, 1973, his fifty-fifth birthday, Abram visited his internist, Hyman Ashman, for a routine checkup. When blood tests revealed an anemia, Ashman referred his patient to a hematologist, who removed a specimen from Abram's bone marrow, the internal portion of the bones where red and white blood cells are made. The examination revealed acute myelocytic leukemia (AML), a severe blood cancer. Physicians told Abram he would most likely be dead within six months.[4]

Yet this did not mean there was nothing to be done. By mid-September 1973, after a short period of watching and waiting, Abram had embarked on a course of aggressive chemotherapy at New York's Mount Sinai Hospital. Over the next several months, he experienced many complications: low blood counts, corrected by transfusions of red blood cells and platelets; severe infections requiring hospitalization; and hepatitis from a contaminated transfusion. But he remained alive. And the results of his bone marrow aspirations were improving. Abram went into remission, signifying the absence of leukemic cells in his bone marrow, within a month of beginning chemotherapy. The date of his predicted death came and went.[5]

By June 1974, Abram's chemotherapy was being supplemented by two novel experimental immunological treatments that he had helped to arrange. He did so well over the next several years that his doctors were not quite sure when to discontinue his various treatments. They did so gradually, giving him his last round of immunotherapy in 1979. The leukemia never returned.

As with the other illness narratives in this book, this skeletal account of what happened to Morris Abram, while essentially accurate, conceals as much as it reveals. Not only were the events surrounding Abram's illness and treatment much more complicated, but the story varied based on who was telling it. Crafting a definitive explanation of why Abram "triumphed" over his cancer would prove nearly as difficult as the toxic experimental protocol that seemed—at first blush—to have cured him.

To understand how Abram approached his illness, we need to know more about his personality and background. Growing up in a poor Jewish family, Abram saw himself as an underdog from an early age, determined that his upbringing should not circumscribe his life. His stellar legal career confirmed for him how action and determination, coupled with intelligence, paid dividends. For Morris Abram, it was what one achieved, not who one was, that mattered. In this sense, he was an optimistic person who relished challenging the system. Before his death in 2000, Abram said that he wanted his greatest accomplishment—"one person, one vote"—inscribed on his gravestone.[6]

But his achievements came with a cost. Abram had a "healthy narcissism" and no tolerance for incompetence, whether due to laziness or ineptness. His forthright, often brusque nature could be offensive, even to his friends. One, Joseph Letkoff, who had practiced law with him in Atlanta in the 1960s, once reminded Abram that he had been "the most ambitious and arrogant individual on Peachtree Street." When Abram published his autobiography, *The Day Is Short*, in 1982, one critic wrote that if the day is short, "the humility is even shorter."[7]

Before 1973, Abram had not applied his skills to the world of medicine. He was rarely sick, usually seeing his internist only for an annual check. But when Abram received his diagnosis of leukemia, his basic nature kicked into gear. Confronted with a highly serious, likely fatal, condition, Abram was not about to ride off into the sunset. Rather, he wanted the best doctors at the best hospital—the best hope, he believed, for saving his life.

Abram's insistence on the very best likely reflected the growing societal concerns about the competency of physicians. Critics had begun to chip away at the lofty pedestal that had supported the medical profession during the 1950s and 1960s. Many of the early charges were leveled by women, who challenged the arrogance and paternalism of male physicians. In 1969, for example, feminist author Barbara Seaman charged that physicians were concealing information about the side effects of birth control pills. Three years later, Babette Rosmond wrote a scathing account of how surgeons tried to force her into getting a radical breast operation. That same year, newspapers across the country reported on the Tuskegee scandal, in which, from 1932 to 1972, poor southern African American men with syphilis were deliberately left untreated by U.S. Public Health Service researchers. By the mid-1970s, social critics such as Ivan Illich would be publishing angry books arguing that American medicine did more harm than good.[8]

It helped Abram's mission that he lived in New York City, home to a number of top-notch medical institutions, one of which was Mount Sinai Hospital. Abram took an immediate liking to his Mount Sinai hematologist, Louis Wasserman, whom he described as "cagey" and "intuitive," someone who "smells his way from the labyrinth." When Wasserman announced that "the treatment of leukemia is an art as well as a science," it gave Abram confidence. Abram also liked that Wasserman referred him to another hematologist, James F. Holland. Holland, who had just moved to Mount Sinai from Buffalo's Roswell Park Cancer Institute, was internationally renowned, having won the prestigious Lasker Award in 1972 for his research in cancer chemotherapy.[9]

Holland practiced cutting-edge medicine. In the case of AML, he and a Roswell Park colleague, George Bekesi, had begun an experimental immunological treatment, which involved the injection of leukemic cells obtained from another leukemia patient. Before injection, the donated cells were treated with an enzyme, neuraminidase. The goal of this intervention was to stimulate the immune system of leukemia patients to better fight their disease. Abram would later receive this therapy. Abram also liked that Holland was in communication with a "network of specialists" across the world who were studying leukemia.[10]

Why did Abram have such faith in experimental medicine? The former Brandeis president later explained that he was "somewhat devoted to the academic world" and thus assumed that academic medicine was better than nonacademic medicine. But surely another source of appeal had to be the idea that those pursuing experimental treatments seemed to be fighters, just as Abram had always been. In his writings, he approvingly referred to the intense and strong-willed Holland as "the most aggressive cancer fighter" and someone who "attacked my illness as if it were a personal enemy, as if the mere existence of leukemia were an affront to his power."[11]

Abram always carefully underscored that he was no faddist. He was entirely uninterested in trying alternative treatments such as Krebiozen or laetrile, no matter how desperate he was. Chemotherapy and immunotherapy, in contrast, had a strong theoretical basis. And he believed that others with leukemia deserved to know this, especially once his treatment seemed to be going well. "I knew that in the hinterlands and indeed in the metropolis," he wrote, "the advanced treatment which seemed to be working for me was not merely unavailable but unheard of."[12]

But if Abram respected the prestige and science found at teaching hospitals, he questioned the day-to-day care they provided. Even though he liked Wasserman, Abram was uncomfortable with what he saw as the hematologist's paternalistic and secretive tendencies. In August 1973, Abram later wrote, Wasserman had been less than forthcoming, telling his patient not to draw "any negative inferences" if and when he eventually decided to treat—rather than continue to watch—the leukemia. Later during that visit, after getting Abram's blood test results, Wasserman abruptly told him to lie down for a bone marrow examination. Abram was "startled by the suddenness of this entirely unexpected procedure." In a draft of *The Day Is Short*, written in 1977, Abram asked: "What was he telling me without telling me? Whose body was mine; whose illness and whose life was this?" One can feel Abram's anger mounting at this interaction. The last thing he would tolerate was bullshit.[13]

Here the differences between the cases of Brian Piccolo and Morris Abram begin to emerge. True, Piccolo wound up at America's premier cancer hospital and underwent state-of-the-art treatment. But at no point in his illness did Piccolo or his wife, Joy, think to question the decisions of the physicians. Piccolo liked that Sloan-Kettering physician Edward Beattie was a football player and that he used sports metaphors to discuss medical issues. Such familiar touches, in contrast, meant little to Abram and, over time, even worried him. To some degree, these different responses reflected the divergent worldviews of Piccolo, a young, carefree football player, and the much older Abram, a savvy and seasoned veteran of legal and political battles. But more than this, Abram's unwillingness to simply accede to his physicians' wishes was very much a part of the nascent patients' rights movement that was forcing dramatic changes in medical practice.

When Abram entered the hospital, his frustration only grew. While Mount Sinai may have been "a wonder of modern science," it was "bureaucracy at its worst." Abram was stunned when a technician performing blood tests unsuccessfully jabbed his arm several times, even though his veins were clearly visible. He was left with a very large bruise. This was especially annoying, Abram wrote, because he "would need every site on every vein" for the blood tests and medications he was to receive.[14]

To make matters worse, the hospital insisted on making the very ambulatory Abram travel in a wheelchair. This was the "final blow," he stated. "I was perfectly capable of walking, felt no pain or weakness and the wheelchair order was interpreted by me as an insult to my person." Though the civil rights activist had unlikely ever previously imagined cancer patients as an oppressed group, vulnerable to institutions and other power structures, the thought now crossed his mind.[15]

When hospital routine included what Abram saw as sheer incompetence, he grew livid. He had learned from his doctors that a major complication of chemotherapy was infection, which occurred when a patient's white blood cell count was too low. Thus, Abram was stunned to see hospital employees, ranging from doctors to orderlies, entering his room without washing their hands. "I was outraged," he later wrote, "when elementary principles of hygiene and nursing care were violated."[16]

Abram's response to the Mount Sinai bureaucracy mirrored that of his whole career: "I never surrendered to the system." He constantly registered complaints to administrators. Soon, Abram's blood samples were being drawn only once daily to avoid unnecessary needle sticks—and bruises. Abram also found an ally in James Holland, who affixed a sign to his patient's door that read "Do not touch this patient without washing up." The decision to become an activist patient also drew on something else Abram had learned as a lawyer, that "clients, unlearned in the law" sometimes asked questions that forced him "to rethink propositions to my and their benefit."[17]

Abram's active participation extended to his treatment. Just as he had recoiled at Wasserman's paternalism, he saw no reason why he should not learn about his disease and the various therapeutic options. The treatment for AML was in flux as Abram became ill. Specialists had just begun to administer a more intensive "7 + 3" regimen of two chemotherapeutic agents, cytosine arabinoside (Ara-C), given for seven days, and daunorubicin, given for three days. As early data suggested that this regimen was better at prolonging survival, Abram readily agreed to it. Like countless patients before and since, Abram intuitively believed that more would be better when facing such a serious disease. So he was glad when his doctors opted to try to "destroy" this "mortal enemy."[18]

But would the high-dose chemotherapy be good enough? As of 1973, long-term survival for adults with AML was roughly 15 percent for five years, although lower for someone of Abram's more advanced age. The new 7 + 3 treatment, early data suggested, doubled this figure. But these statistics still meant that the vast majority of patients with AML died. And most who died did so nowhere near the five-year mark but very early in their disease.[19]

These gloomy numbers made Abram receptive to treatments that might augment the high-dose chemotherapy. This is where the prominent lawyer's personal connections came into play. In the fall of 1973, a friend of his from Brandeis University, Zmira Goodman, told Abram about a new immunological agent being used in Israel against AML: methanol extract residue (MER). Discovered by immunologist David W. Weiss while working on a vaccine for tuberculosis, MER had supposedly induced remissions in patients with leukemia. Through Goodman, Abram's case became known to Weiss, who was at the Hadassah Medical School in Jerusalem.

When Weiss indicated that Abram was "a perfect case for MER," Abram became eager to begin treatments in conjunction with his chemotherapy. Meanwhile, he was also interested in another immunological intervention: Holland's neuraminidase-treated leukemic cells. But MER was not available in the United States because the Food and Drug Administration had not yet approved it. And Holland was still in the process of setting up a randomized clinical trial of the neuraminidase-treated cells.[20]

Empowered patient as he was, this situation was simply unacceptable to Abram. The notion that he was being deprived of a potentially life-prolonging and possibly even curative treatment for his fatal cancer—again due to bureaucracy—boggled his mind. So Abram did what a politically connected person could. He contacted an old friend, Senator Henry Jackson of Washington State, urging him to use diplomatic channels to obtain MER from Israel.[21]

Abram also confronted his doctors. On March 1, 1974, he wrote a letter to his new hematologist, Janet Cuttner, who had replaced Louis Wasserman, telling her that he did "not want a day to pass for the administration of that immuno-therapy on account of any administrative problems." And, in what bordered on a threat, Abram told Cuttner he was planning to travel to Israel to receive MER if Mount Sinai was "not prepared to administer it."[22]

In pressing his case, Abram then pushed the envelope further. On March 15, 1974, he urged Cuttner and Holland to have a conference call with Weiss, who was willing to treat Abram. Moreover, Abram proposed that he also participate in the discussion. This was surely audacious behavior for a patient circa 1974, something that a person less prominent than Abram could probably never have suggested. But Abram would come to advocate this exact type of physician-patient relationship. As he liked to remind his doctors, "Each physician has many cases, I but one."[23]

After some initial defensiveness, Abram's physicians grew accustomed to—and then comfortable with—his activist approach to patienthood. As far as possible, for example, they scheduled treatments so as not to conflict with Abram's court cases. Part of the physicians' acceptance of Abram's demands stemmed from the fact that they knew he greatly respected them. There were several physicians in Abram's family, including his grandfather,

Morris Cohen, and Abram had grown up admiring doctors. "I do not have to tell you," Abram wrote to Cuttner, "that you have my trust, confidence and gratitude." While Abram surely pushed his doctors, he never refused their advice or shopped for second opinions at other hospitals.[24]

Abram eventually learned that one reason for the delay in his immunotherapy stemmed from its experimental nature. Holland had stated that he would give MER only if and when Abram entered his upcoming controlled trial of the neuraminidase-treated leukemic cells. But Abram could not understand why any of his therapy had to be delayed for the sake of science. As he told Cuttner, "I want my case to be treated as you and Dr. Holland think best without regard to the development of any group statistics."[25]

But here is where Holland, at least initially, put his foot down. In a telling interaction, which Abram documented in *The Day Is Short*, Abram and his eldest daughter, Ruth, pressed Holland to obtain early treatment. Ruth Abram, ably marshaling the increasingly common language of patient autonomy, challenged the doctor: "But it's daddy's body. Why can't he have control over it?" Holland said that Abram could. But when Ruth Abram then informed Holland that it was the doctor's duty to follow his patient's wishes and therefore allow her father to get MER as soon as possible, Holland demurred. "You must bear in mind that I am not your father's physician," he told her. "I am an investigator."[26]

In telling this story, Abram signaled a tension that would become increasingly important, especially with the emergence of AIDS in the 1980s: the blurred line between therapy and experiment. To the degree that sick individuals pursued experimental treatments, they were subjects first, patients second. The experimental protocol, designed to generate scientific knowledge, took precedence. If patients also benefited from the therapy, all the better, but this was a secondary consideration. Well before AIDS activists did so, Abram was arguing that purely scientific concerns should not trump the task of saving lives.

Having initially rebuffed Abram, Holland finally, in the summer of 1974, agreed to treat him and another AML patient, a 20-year-old boy named T. J. Martell, with MER outside a clinical trial. They thus became the first two patients in the United States to receive MER. Abram also concurrently began treatment with the neuraminidase-treated cells, also outside a for-

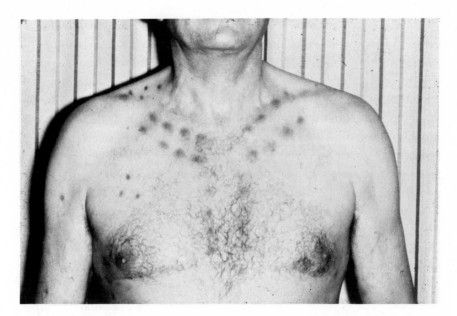

Morris Abram's neck and upper torso after he received his monthly injection of neuraminidase-treated leukemia cells. It is unlikely, in retrospect, that these highly taxing injections were a cause of his recovery. Courtesy of James Holland.

mal trial. Both of these treatments, given roughly once a month, were extremely arduous. The MER, injected into Abram's chest and legs, caused painful ulcers. And the cells were injected into fifty different lymph glands, producing a collar of inflammation around Abram's neck as well as a swollen groin and underarms.[27]

Meanwhile, Abram continued his active involvement in his medical care. In September 1976, when the Mount Sinai doctors began to lower the dosage of his MER, Abram penned a confidential letter to David Weiss. Emphasizing that the missive was not meant to be a complaint about Mount Sinai, he nevertheless wanted Weiss "to be kept up to date on what has happened." Abram told Weiss that he did not want the MER discontinued "without good justification." What, Abram asked, should he do? Weiss offered some opinions in his reply, but urged Abram to discuss the matter with Holland, which he did.[28]

Abram continued to politely query his physicians about the novel combination of chemotherapy and immunotherapy he was receiving. (The doctors stopped the MER later in 1976, believing it might have begun to cause more harm than good. But he was still receiving the neuraminidase-treated cells.) In a September 1977 letter to Cuttner, Abram posed a series of sophisticated questions about whether one or both of the treatments should be discontinued. "Is there any evidence that chemotherapy is suppressing the 'blast' formation?" he asked, referring to the appearance of new leukemic cells. "If chemotherapy does any appreciable harm to my immune defenses, am I really better off with this dual therapy?"[29]

Cuttner's reply to this letter does not exist, but six months later, with Abram still undergoing chemotherapy and the neuraminidase treatment, Cuttner wrote to Holland, Wasserman, and George Bekesi (also now at Mount Sinai) reminding them that their mutual patient had been under treatment for four and a half years without signs of a relapse. "The question now," she wrote, "is should he continue on chemotherapy and the immunotherapy?"[30]

This document was notable for two reasons. First, respecting Abram's earlier desire to be included in the 1974 conference call, Cuttner copied him on the letter. Second, Cuttner was figuratively throwing her hands in the air. Abram was truly an "n of 1" case, having successfully been treated for AML with a truly novel regimen. (Abram's much younger counterpart, T. J. Martell, had long since died.) What to do was far from clear. Yet Abram appreciated his doctors' admission of uncertainty. To him, the truth outweighed false hope or posturing.

Shortly thereafter, when Abram suffered his third bout of hepatitis from contaminated blood products, the doctors stopped the chemotherapy. And when Abram appeared for his neuraminidase shots in January 1979, nearly five years after beginning his treatment for leukemia, he received a surprise. Rather than being greeted only by Holland's technician, Holland himself was there, along with Abram's other doctors. Abram recounted the dialogue in *The Day Is Short:*

> "What's going on?" he asked.
> "These are your last shots," Bekesi stated.
> "Why?" queried Abram.
> "Because you're cured" was the reply.[31]

The unthinkable had thus happened. A man given his death sentence five years earlier had beaten the odds and somehow survived.

Given this outcome, and Abram's prominence, his story was a natural for the press. And so, in the summer of 1977, Morris Abram officially became a famous patient. He agreed to an interview by Pranay Gupte, a *New York Times* staff writer who had met Abram while an undergraduate at Brandeis and had learned about the illness. Gupte's article, "Noted Lawyer Free of Symptoms 4 Years after Getting Leukemia," appeared on the front page of the August 15, 1977, issue of the paper.[32]

The *Times* article forced Gupte and Abram to provide a cohesive narrative of what had been an extremely complicated and rocky illness. Given that Abram had survived a highly fatal leukemia for more than four years, how could this unexpected success be explained? Like Jimmy Piersall and Margaret Bourke-White, Abram crafted an account of his experiences—which he later expanded upon in *The Day Is Short*—that had a coherence and trajectory that had never existed. Although he was surely trying to be as truthful as possible, the outcome of the story necessarily affected how it was told.[33]

Abram attributed his survival, Gupte reported, "to his own determination to live and to the extraordinary treatment formulated by a team of physicians led by Dr. James F. Holland of the Mount Sinai School of Medicine of the City University of New York." In the article, Abram discussed his initial psychological reaction to the diagnosis of AML. "I resolved that, in my case, the disease was not going to be fatal," he told Gupte. "I was not going to give in, and firmly resolved to defeat the disease, even though I had been told by my physician that there was no hope, or very little of it." The piece then went on to describe in great detail the exact nature of Abram's treatment, including his chemotherapy and the two immunological treatments.[34]

As letters written to Abram after the *Times* article demonstrate, this version of events generated a highly positive response among readers, many of whom had leukemia or knew someone with the disease. As with those people who wrote to Bourke-White, many of Abram's correspondents wanted more information about his treatment. For example, a woman from Indiana asked about MER for her leukemic son, who had experienced severe reactions to chemotherapy. A man from Florida inquired as to whether MER might also be effective for his disease, chronic myelogenous leukemia (CML). Another writer, a woman from Ossining, New York, asked about the possibility of trying MER for her brother, whose lymphoma was worsening despite chemotherapy.[35]

The notion that Abram had somehow willed his way to a cure elicited the most correspondence. Cancer patients like herself and Abram, wrote a Chicago woman, survived "because of an attitude and assuming the responsibility to stay alive." A Washington, D.C., man wrote that he "was determined not to give in to the disease." As with Abram, long-term survival—especially when unexpected—could retrospectively foster the idea that personal determination had played a decisive role. "Like you they told also me I didn't have long to live," a New Jersey man wrote, "but I told the doctors who poked me with needles that I was not going to die." "Miracles," said another man, "are often the lasting result of the power of will."[36]

Despite the optimistic messages that Abram's story generated about the importance of the will to live, there were potential downsides to such an assumption. For one thing, doctors who believed that optimism produced better outcomes might oversell certain therapies to their patients. As one hematologist wrote, Abram's story had validated his belief in a positive outlook, "no matter how hopeless the conventional wisdom is." And a New Jersey woman warned against blaming patients, stressing that many courageous people with cancer nevertheless died from the disease.[37]

To what degree, if any, can we attribute Abram's survival to his positive outlook and the immunotherapy? First, we might ask about the degree to which Abram's emphatic insistence on living truly existed at the onset of his illness. In fact, the word *leukemia* had been especially ominous for Abram. He knew four people who had recently died from the disease, three of them within weeks of receiving the diagnosis. His internist Hyman Ashman, according to Abram, had been highly pessimistic, flatly telling his patient that the disease was fatal. In addition, Ashman had stated that chemotherapy would do nothing but make Abram's final days miserable.[38]

It is not surprising, therefore, that when Ashman first told him the diagnosis in June 1973, Abram's response had been "terror, mixed with disbelief." When repeat blood and bone marrow testing showed worsening of the disease in August of that year, Abram was given materials to read about the diagnosis, which confirmed its very high fatality rates. "I foresaw horrible, lonely weeks leading up to an inexorable death," Abram recalled. So the idea that Abram immediately and unequivocally decided that he would beat the AML is an overstatement.[39]

Still, Abram was, by nature, an optimist. His daughter Ruth recalls a childhood vacation in which the Abrams inadvertently rented a shabby, broken-down hut. As the rest of the family panicked, Morris rubbed his hands together and declared, "Isn't this wonderful!" And it was natural to equate the "moral courage" that had characterized Abram's legal career with his "titanic struggle" with cancer. As a reviewer of his book would later state, "The man who beat leukemia learned to fight as a young liberal in Georgia."[40]

In addition, Abram did have a long-standing belief that the psyche affected health. For example, when he received the diagnosis of leukemia, he identified psychological stressors—most notably the breakup with his wife, Jane—as a potential cause of his disease. The corollary to this belief, that positive thinking could benefit one's health, made great sense to Abram.

Thus, while Abram did experience gloom right after his diagnosis, his perspective soon evolved. In a hopeful gesture for a man facing death, he dated and later married an old girlfriend, Carlyn Feldman, another basically optimistic person who had pledged to stay by his side. And gradually, Abram began to formulate—and articulate—the idea that his leukemia was curable. His life was "incomplete," he believed, and thus it was not his time to die. Abram told Steven Teitelbaum, a Washington University pathologist whose brother, Herbert, was married to Ruth Abram, "Steve, I'm going to beat this thing." Teitelbaum was highly skeptical.[41]

But once Abram had convinced himself of this point, positive developments, such as his quick remission, the availability of promising experimental therapies, and, as time went on, his continued survival, could not help but validate the apparent value of his willpower. And once Abram was pronounced "cured," it was only natural to look back and formally credit his fighting spirit as causative. This logic is, of course, a fallacy. Since dead leukemia patients are not alive to describe how they fought their diseases, it seems, in retrospect, that only survivors had enough willpower to live.[42]

Is there any scientific validity to the claim that Abram's will to live helped him survive? Studies that aim to prove a mind-body connection are notoriously hard to perform, in part because it is so difficult to quantify things like willpower or optimism. One randomized controlled trial of women with metastatic breast cancer, published in 1989, found that women who regularly attended support groups, and thus presumably had a superior psychological outlook, survived longer. But subsequent studies have failed to confirm this finding or other similar claims that a positive outlook improves medical outcomes. These studies do not disprove the possible impact of willpower in *individual* cases, such as that of Abram, but they do not prove it either.[43]

What about the value of Abram's immunological treatments? Once again, his assumption that they helped is understandable. Enjoying good health in December 1974, almost a year after he was supposed to be dead, he wrote to David Weiss to thank him for facilitating the MER treatment. "I am apparently in good health," he said, "and I owe so much to you." But this cause-and-effect relationship was purely speculative. Indeed, while immunotherapy is still a focus of leukemia research, no randomized trials have ever shown that either MER or neuraminidase-treated leukemic cells prolong life.[44]

It is most likely that Abram's survival should be credited to the new 7 + 3 chemotherapy regimen that he received. As his oncologists had assumed in 1973, this more intensive treatment did indeed raise five-year survival rates, including cures, into the 35 to 40 percent range. These results have been achieved without the immunotherapy that Abram received. Of course, the chemotherapy does not alone explain Abram's case, as most of the patients treated for the disease still die. Why do some patients who have a given cancer and undergo a particular treatment survive, while others do not? According to growing evidence, specific cases of AML, like those of other cancers, are biologically different even though they carry the same name. Some are simply more treatable than others.[45]

This finding introduces another important element into Abram's story: luck. Whereas he was certainly unlucky to get leukemia, he was fortunate to get a treatable form of the disease. It remains true that certain choices Abram made—such as his hand-washing edict, his careful selection of doctors, and his active role in medical decisions—may have played a positive role in his case. Yet the fact remains that much of Abram's survival was attributable to luck. "It may be a miracle that I have survived leukemia for five years," he acknowledged in 1979. In many instances, he added, the

course of his treatment "seems to have been influenced as much by seren-
dipity as plan."[46]

But luck does not make for good headlines. What patients and their families want to know—and what newspaper editors want to report—is that
something concrete can be done in the face of dreaded illness. Margaret
Bourke-White's brain surgery to alleviate her Parkinson's symptoms was
one such example, but Morris Abram's story packed a much bigger punch.
He was cured. In this sense, definitive proof that the interventions Abram
chose had saved his life was less important than his seeming demonstration that patients who took the initiative could greatly improve their
chances of survival. That the media outlet that published his story was the
New York Times mattered, too. If the country's paper of record suggested
that a strong will to live and the latest experimental therapies could cure
cancer, then didn't it have to be true? And it wasn't just the *Times*. When
the *Boston Globe* ran a feature on *The Day Is Short* after its publication in
1982, the headline read: "How Morris Abram Said No to Death."[47]

Thus, it was Abram's story of perseverance and hope, as much as its scientific accuracy, that provided meaning for the public. The wife of a
leukemia patient made this exact point. She wrote that learning how Abram
attacked his problem "helped [her husband] more than the treatment." "If
Morris Abram can do it," a New York man with cancer announced to his
family, "I can at least try, and so can all of you." The Florida man with CML
wrote that, like Abram, "I cannot and will not accept the opinion that there
is little or nothing that can be done."[48]

That Abram was a prominent figure also mattered, making his story even
more powerful. "I do believe it is important for people like you, Hubert
Humphrey, and others to write of their experiences," wrote the man from
Washington, D.C., "so that people who are told that they have cancer, and
their families and friends, will not immediately consider it a death sentence,
which increasingly does not have to be so." "Thousands afflicted by the
malady," a New York man wrote after seeing the *Times* article, will now
"attempt to duplicate your extraordinary courage." Abram never said no
when Cuttner or Holland asked him to call another leukemia patient to
provide moral support and hope.[49]

In 1978 Abram was contacted by Irving Rimer, vice president of public
information of the American Cancer Society, asking him to describe his

experiences at a national meeting. The meeting, Rimer explained, brought together the top experts in the country to discuss the latest scientific developments in the world of cancer. But Abram would participate in a special part of the program, one that emphasized "the inspirational motif" and the progress that had been made in fighting diseases such as leukemia. As Rimer wrote, "There is a need to build confidence in the tempo of the cancer advances. Obviously, the public wants more. With the kind of disease we are dealing with our role is to point up evidences of progress over and over again. The stories of individual experiences is [sic] a key way to do this." Abram's high profile, which made him an "extraordinary" person, thus encouraged the ACS to publicize his story to very "ordinary" patients. In this manner, Abram's highly individual experience, with its unexpected outcome, became emblematic of what all other AML—and cancer—patients might reasonably expect.[50]

Abram's story played itself out in one other important way when fellow Georgian Jimmy Carter appointed him as chairman of the President's Commission for the Study of Ethical Problems in Medicine and Behavioral Research from 1980 to 1983. One of the main goals of the commission was to emphasize the importance of informed consent, which had been violated during the Tuskegee experiment and in several other research scandals of the 1970s. Having been a cancer patient and having received experimental agents, Abram was ideally situated to help craft a policy that would protect patients and subjects without stifling scientific progress. Foremost in Abram's mind was the responsibility of the physician to provide honest information about the risks and benefits of proposed interventions. "It shall be the duty of the physician," he wrote, "to deliver to the patient in comprehensible form the purpose of medical intervention as well as the known probable adverse consequences."[51]

But realizing that others would not be as outspoken or empowered as he had been, Abram reminded his fellow commission members that "it shall be the further duty of the physician to invite the patient to inquire of possible consequences of the intervention, desirable or adverse, as well as the alternative courses of medical intervention and finally, the consequences of taking no action." That is, physician-patient communication was key, even when the patient was reluctant to instigate it. In this sense, Abram and his commission would underscore, patients themselves had a duty to become informed.[52]

Yet, while the presidential commission ably spelled out the gold standard for consent practices, Abram's personal experiences with informed consent were perhaps more revealing. In a passage written for *The Day Is Short*, excised from the final book, Abram had frankly discussed the limitations of the consent process in his own case: "The documents in which they informed and I granted 'informed consent' to these treatments never explicitly said 'You are about to undergo a life-threatening ordeal in order to attempt a complete remission,' but looking back I see that the plan was to take me to the valley of the shadows." In justifying his choices to a correspondent in 1977, Abram clearly favored doing something, rather than nothing. "It is a risk in experiment," he wrote, "but the other risk is greater." Later, he wrote of his decision to "go for broke" in the search of a cure. "I theoretically had a choice," Abram stated, "but there actually was none."[53]

Abram's own case, therefore, demonstrated how the neutral language of informed consent often had little applicability, especially when physicians and patients were dealing with last-ditch interventions for life-threatening conditions. After all, the same doctors whose omission of gruesome details had helped convince Abram to accept very aggressive treatment had cured him. While a dispassionate discussion of risks and benefits might be acceptable intellectually, it did not suitably address the emotional aspects of the decision-making process.

Abram's advocacy for last-ditch therapies ultimately extended even further. In contrast to his own case, in which he had emphasized the potential of personal therapeutic benefit over the collection of scientific data, Abram increasingly defended a more utilitarian approach to experimentation. At another ACS conference, held in Washington, D.C., in April 1981, Abram argued that human subjects who agree to "high risk intervention," despite little or no chance of success, are "valuable societal resources." It was his personal view, he stated, "that the patient should elect the alternative which will most likely add a final meaning to life, even at great risk."[54]

Interestingly, only one year later, a Seattle dentist named Barney Clark would invoke the same rationale in agreeing to be the first human implanted with a permanent artificial heart. The subsequent outcry over Clark's prolonged suffering would call into question Abram's calculus. Thus, what happened to the patient in the long run inevitably colored how the event was, in retrospect, understood and interpreted.

But before examining Clark's story, there is a third cancer case from the

1970s to be explored: that of Steve McQueen. If Morris Abram was the quintessential insider patient, working within the system to get his way, McQueen increasingly pursued unorthodox options as his cancer worsened. Doing so in the late 1970s was verboten; McQueen was harshly criticized for his actions, both by the medical profession and by the cancer establishment. But from the perspective of 2006, the paths that he and Abram chose were not quite so divergent.

Chapter 7

Unconventional Healing

Steve McQueen's Mexican Journey

Why, asked a reader of a 1980 *Newsweek* article on actor Steve McQueen's cancer, was treatment that "leaves the patient not only intact, but in good health and better educated about keeping his or her body free of disease" derided as "strange"? McQueen was the first major celebrity whose pursuit of unorthodox cancer therapy was avidly followed by the press. His course of action revealed—and in turn promoted—a vibrant underground network of alternative specialists who, depending on your opinion, either snookered vulnerable cancer patients or provided them with viable options.[1]

McQueen had not gone public willingly. He had been outed by the *National Enquirer*, one of the increasingly powerful tabloids that thrived on their ability to pierce the privacy of celebrities. That McQueen's case was first reported by a tabloid raised concerns about its accuracy. Did Steve McQueen really have terminal mesothelioma, a rare cancer of the lung lining? Was he really in Mexico undergoing treatment with vitamins, minerals, laetrile, and coffee enemas?

By explicitly alerting the public to complicated questions about end-stage cancer, McQueen's case built on that of Morris Abram. Might it actually make sense to try untested, unapproved remedies if no other hope existed? Were unorthodox treatments, which generally sought to restore balance and improve patients' immunity, perhaps at times superior to standard toxic interventions, such as radiotherapy or chemotherapy? And what was one to make of the claims of patients who swore that they had been cured of a deadly cancer by alternative therapies?

None of these questions could be divorced from the fact that this particular patient was Steve McQueen, "the coolest guy who ever lived," who had built a Hollywood career on playing disaffected rebels who somehow proved themselves right in the end. Like his film characters, did McQueen know something we didn't?[2]

Steve McQueen was born in Beech Grove, Indiana, a suburb of Indianapolis, on March 24, 1930. He had a troubled childhood. His father, William McQueen, a stunt pilot, left McQueen's mother, Jullian, shortly after their son was born. Jullian McQueen was an alcoholic, and she deposited Steve for long periods with an uncle, Claude Thompson. By his early teenage years, McQueen, now living in Los Angeles, had become a gang leader and committed several crimes. Eventually, he was sent to Boys Republic, a reform school in Chino, California.

After leaving Boys Republic, McQueen left home and tried a series of odd jobs. Then, in 1954, after a stint as a Marine, he moved to New York City to pursue an acting career. McQueen's rugged good looks, with blond hair and blue eyes, helped him land roles in several off-Broadway plays. There he met Neile Adams, a successful actress, whom he married in 1956. Next followed a three-year starring role in a hit television show, *Wanted: Dead or Alive*. During these years, McQueen was also working in Hollywood, where he would become one of America's most famous film stars in the 1960s.

McQueen's film credits were impressive, including *The Magnificent Seven* (1960), *The Great Escape* (1963), *The Sand Pebbles* (1966), *The Thomas Crown Affair* (1968), and *Bullitt* (1968). After several flops, McQueen again had a series of successes in the 1970s with *The Getaway* (1972), *Papillon* (1973), and *The Towering Inferno* (1974). During the filming of *The Getaway*, McQueen had an affair with costar Ali MacGraw, who became his second wife in 1973.

In most of these films, McQueen played a man's man, one who rejects authority for something he believes in. For example, in *The Great Escape*, the McQueen character is Virgil Hilts, a cocky soldier who engineers an escape from a Nazi POW camp. In *The Sand Pebbles*, McQueen played Jake Holman, the moody chief engineer of a U.S. gunboat in China. Holman sacrifices his life to save a group of American missionaries, including a schoolteacher with whom he has fallen in love. Bullitt is Frank Bullitt, a rebellious police detective who, in the course of investigating the death of a Mafia mobster, ultimately confronts his own corrupt boss. In his movies, the *New York Times* wrote, McQueen "personified a nonconformist and underdog, battling to survive in a hostile society."[3]

Bullitt featured what was then the most famous car chase in Hollywood history, and McQueen insisted on doing the stunts himself. When a Ford Mustang was shown careering around San Francisco at 100 miles per hour, it was McQueen at the wheel. His biographers captured this persona. To his friend William Nolan, McQueen was "Hollywood's outlaw hero" who "gave us a vision of life lived at the edge, passionately and without compromise." Writer Penina Spiegel termed him the "bad boy" of Hollywood whose "raw animal magnetism . . . blazed across the screen." Like James Dean, film director Mark Rydell stated, McQueen "took no crap from anybody." Such descriptions indicate the degree to which McQueen's life blurred with his celluloid persona. He was, for example, an inveterate daredevil, racing cars and motorcycles. He took up flying in his later years. "If they were making a movie of my life," McQueen once mused, "they would call it 'The Great Escape.'" As Neile Adams would later reveal, McQueen was also a difficult spouse, prone to moodiness, anger, and infidelity.[4]

Steve McQueen probably had cancer for a long time before he knew it. In the summer of 1978 he developed a persistent cough, which doctors diagnosed as either bronchitis or "walking pneumonia." Eventually, they termed it a fungal infection and prescribed antibiotics. McQueen apparently improved. But when Adams, his ex-wife, visited him in October of that year, she was surprised to see him with a drawn face, leaning on a cane and complaining of body pains. McQueen's symptoms had led him to give up his cigarette habit, which had totaled two to three packs daily.[5]

McQueen's health problems continued into early 1979, when he was directing and starring in *Tom Horn*. Tom Horn is a typical McQueen character: a gunman who fights rustlers in the old West and is hanged, perhaps unjustly, for murder. During filming, according to Spiegel, McQueen was often tired and short of breath. He asked the wife of one of his assistant directors, a nurse, about lung diseases. That summer, McQueen had a lung biopsy, but the results were negative.[6]

McQueen spent the fall of 1979 filming what would be his last movie, *The Hunter*, in which he played an aging bounty hunter. His cough and fatigue persisted, although doctors had made no further diagnosis. By December 1979, when filming was completed, worsening shortness of breath

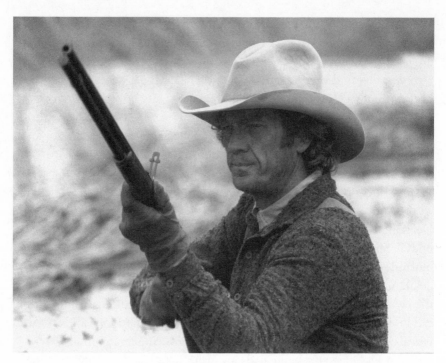

Steve McQueen during the filming of *Tom Horn* in 1979. Horn was a typical McQueen role, a Western gunman heroically fighting rustlers. McQueen would assume a similar role in real life when he began to battle cancer in the months ahead. TOM HORN © Solar Productions, Inc., The First Artists Production Company, Ltd., and Warner Bros. Inc. All Rights Reserved. Courtesy of Warner Brothers Entertainment, Inc.

led a gaunt and bearded McQueen to check himself into Cedars-Sinai Medical Center in Los Angeles. This time, the biopsy was conclusive: mesothelioma, a highly uncommon cancer of the lining of the lungs.

Mesothelioma is strongly related to asbestos exposure. During the early twentieth century, industry began to use asbestos fibers, obtained from mined asbestos rock, to insulate pipes, roofs, and heavy machinery. Its fireproof nature also made it ideal for the lining of oven mitts and protective clothing. But as early as the 1920s, doctors discovered that inhalation of asbestos dust caused scarring of the lungs. Two decades later, epidemiologists identified an association between asbestosis and lung cancer among miners. Finally, in the 1960s, studies showed that asbestos exposure causes mesotheliomas, cancers of the lining of the lungs or abdomen.[7]

How did Steve McQueen develop mesothelioma? After his diagnosis became public, the tabloids had a field day with speculation about where the actor may have encountered asbestos. "Steve McQueen's Love of Racing Cars May Have Triggered His Cancer Crisis," announced the *Star*, a rival of the *Enquirer*. The article posited that the actor had been exposed to asbestos when wearing racing suits. In addition, it noted that he had worked on tanks while in the Marines. McQueen had also apparently served six weeks in the brig, forced to clean the engine room, the pipes of which contained asbestos lining. His smoking, another risk factor for mesothelioma, might have also played a causative role.[8]

Whatever the cause, the medical outlook was gloomy. The physicians caring for McQueen were as forthright as Morris Abram's had been, telling their patient that his cancer was almost certainly fatal. Surgery was not an option, but McQueen's doctors implanted radioactive cobalt into his chest and tried chemotherapeutic drugs, including interferon, a naturally occurring antiviral agent.[9]

But when McQueen returned to see his doctors in late February 1980, the cancer had continued to spread. He was given an even worse prognosis, according to McQueen's friend and fellow pilot, Grady Ragsdale, Jr., who later wrote a book chronicling the actor's last year of life. At that point, the physicians estimated that McQueen would be dead in two months. There was only a 5 percent chance that he would survive into 1981.[10]

It is difficult to know what McQueen actually believed, but to family and friends he seemed to be in denial. After receiving the gloomy news, he announced that he was going to beat the cancer. He even signed a contract to star in an upcoming Hollywood film, *Tai-Pan*, although his condition and prognosis made this a complete impossibility. Some of this rhetoric reflected McQueen's decision to conceal his cancer diagnosis from most of his close acquaintances. Neile Adams and Barbara Minty, a 24-year-old model who became McQueen's third wife in January 1980, knew, but his two children with Neile, Terry, age 21, and Chad, age 19, were deliberately kept in the dark. So were friends and colleagues who had witnessed McQueen's declining health. They were told that he had a fungal infection of the lung.[11]

McQueen had used a pseudonym as a patient at Cedars-Sinai but had been recognized by staff members. Likely through a nurse's aide and her boyfriend, the *National Enquirer* learned that he had terminal cancer. The *Enquirer*, founded in the 1950s, had dispensed with standard fan magazine articles that dutifully praised celebrities. In their place were exposés about Hollywood stars, featuring their affairs, excessive drinking, and volatile tempers. These articles required new types of Hollywood reporters and editors—those willing to aggressively pursue stories, using tips, connections, unnamed sources, and, if necessary, money.[12]

The McQueen story, "Steve McQueen's Heroic Battle against Terminal Cancer," appeared on page 28 of the March 11, 1980, issue of the *National Enquirer*. Although the article listed the diagnosis as lung cancer, as opposed to mesothelioma, many of the other details of McQueen's illness were accurate: the inoperable nature of the cancer, the failed cobalt treatment, and the very poor prognosis. There is no record of how the editors made their decision to go ahead with the piece. But it seems that the tabloid's reporters, Tony Brenna and Donna Rosenthal, having been tipped off about McQueen's illness, had interviewed several hospital employees, including doctors involved in his care. All sources were anonymous, however.[13]

The *Enquirer* story epitomized a new trend in the history of celebrity illness. Whereas Brian Piccolo and Morris Abram had willingly gone public with their cancer diagnoses, McQueen had hoped to keep his a secret. And the actor was no John Foster Dulles, a high-ranking political figure whose illness could potentially interfere with his diplomatic duties and thus was "fair game" for the media. But the *Enquirer*'s editors decided that the apparent diagnosis of terminal cancer in a major Hollywood celebrity was newsworthy enough to outweigh McQueen's right to keep his illness private.

Articles like the one by Brenna and Rosenthal left the more mainstream press in a bind. In order to sell their product, the supermarket tabloids were often willing to print stories based on highly questionable information. Some articles, such as those on UFO sightings, were patently untrue. And the tabloids' willingness to pay sources raised the odds that any information obtained was false. To the degree that newspaper, magazine, and television reporters pursued similar stories, they would be validating the ethos of the tabloid press. This type of decision was especially worrisome when new journalistic lines, such as the outing of ill celebrities, were being crossed.

At the same time, however, non-tabloid publications were understandably wary about being scooped on a "real" story. If Steve McQueen was indeed dying, maybe the public did have a right to know. After all, he was a public figure. And rumors about the actor's seemingly poor health had freely circulated around Hollywood during the filming of *Tom Horn* and *The Hunter*.

So the more mainstream press did pursue the story, albeit gingerly. For example, syndicated gossip columnist Liz Smith quoted McQueen as saying he did not have terminal cancer but rather "terminal fury" at the false claims. *People* magazine, a more reliable and upscale version of the tabloids, also printed a disclaimer by McQueen: "It's ridiculous. I'm fine." Similar untrue stories also appeared in the tabloid press. For example, in April 1980 the *Globe* printed a one-page article quoting McQueen's lawyer and Neile Adams as denying that the actor had cancer.[14]

There was also some degree of backlash against the *Enquirer*. According to Adams, television personality Barbara Walters not only declined to do a story on McQueen's illness but alerted the actor's press representatives that she had been approached. McQueen announced that he planned to sue the tabloid, although he never did. But in retrospect, the fact that the *Enquirer*, as opposed to its more legitimate rivals, had gotten it "right" validated what it had done. True, one could debate the privacy issue, but the tabloid press had proven its ability to expose and fairly accurately describe the illness of a major celebrity. From this point on, all famous patients would have to confront the fact that any of their friends or caretakers were potential sources of information for the press.[15]

As McQueen issued his public and private denials, he was still aggressively pursuing treatment. In June 1980, a doctor in the San Fernando Valley tried one last experimental therapy, most likely intravenous vitamins and minerals, which McQueen received five days per week for seven weeks. To hide his identity, the medication was administered in a camper parked outside the doctor's clinic. Barbara Minty injected the vitamin and mineral mixture. But when McQueen returned to Cedars-Sinai at the end of July 1980 for additional testing, he learned that the cancer had not shrunk.[16]

Meanwhile, unbeknownst to his doctors, McQueen had begun to explore the possibility of unorthodox treatments similar to those recommended to John Foster Dulles. During the 1950s, as orthodox medicine was enjoying great prestige, advocates of alternative methods had largely been dismissed as quacks. But two decades later, with the medical profession under fire and growing public interest in holistic models of health, the time was ripe for new approaches to cancer treatment. California, with its emphasis on the "New Age" lifestyle, became a center for alternative therapy. Its proximity to Mexico, home to a growing number of freestanding cancer clinics that could not be regulated by U.S. agencies, helped to foster such interest. Mexico, according to one writer, was "The Court of Last Hope."[17]

McQueen, living in California, took note, exploring numerous alternative cancer treatments. One jumped out at him: the enzymatic approach preached by William D. Kelley. In 1962 Kelley had been a practicing dentist and orthodontist in Texas when he developed a mysterious disease involving weight loss, body pains, and depression. As he later recounted in his 1969 book *The Answer to Cancer*, his disease went undiagnosed for several months. Finally, a doctor ordered a series of x-rays, which revealed cancer of his liver and pancreas. The outlook was dismal. Kelley was told that he had only months to live and that there was no treatment for his condition. "I freaked out," he later recalled. "All your friends and relatives are ready to put you in a box when they hear the word 'cancer.'" A confirmatory biopsy was considered, according to Kelley, but was not done because the surgeon believed he was too sick.[18]

Even though he had received his dental degree at Baylor University, Kelley had a long history of skepticism toward standard medical practices. One particular interest was cancer. "There were actually very few people," he believed, "who survived the medical establishment's chemicals, surgical procedures, and radiation treatments." Recalling nutrition lectures that he had attended at Baylor, Kelley formulated a theory on why cancer grew and how it could be treated: "Wrong foods caused the malignancy to grow, while proper foods allowed natural body defenses to work and [absorb] the malignancy."[19]

In emphasizing the relationship of metabolic balance to cancer, Kelley's approach was consistent with the work of earlier unorthodox healers, such as Max Gerson, as well as the new emphasis on holistic care. Kelley's ideas also built on another familiar mantra of alternative medicine: cancer was not a monolithic disease, but different from one person to another. Treatment of the disease needed to reflect each individual's distinct metabolic profile.

Kelley went on to devise a highly complicated treatment for his condition. Once he was "cured," he began to recommend his regimen to other cancer sufferers. Central to Kelley's approach was the use of pancreatic enzymes. He believed that cancers arose and grew due to the lack of such enzymes, which normally break down protein. Ingestion of supplemental enzymes, conversely, led to the "digestion" of existing cancers. Added to the enzyme treatment was an individualized diet of minerals, vitamins, and other nutrients carefully selected for patients after they had completed a supposedly 2,500-question survey. Finally, Kelley stressed detoxification, advocating Gerson's daily coffee enemas, to cleanse the liver and gallbladder. He also believed that the enemas, like the dietary treatment, stimulated the body's immune system to fight the cancer.[20]

Like other alternative therapists, Kelley was highly controversial. *The Answer to Cancer*, which he self-published, enabled him to spread the word about his personal recovery and his treatment method. Over the next several years, officials in Texas tried to forbid him from treating cancer patients or distributing his book. In 1971, the American Cancer Society, believing that Kelley was a complete quack, added his regimen to its list of "unproven methods" for treating cancer. Five years later Texas suspended Kelley's dental license, and he moved to Winthrop, Washington, although he retained his affiliation with the International Health Institute of Dallas. Despite his legal troubles, Kelley apparently gave treatment recommendations to thousands of cancer patients in the 1960s and 1970s, perhaps becoming "the nation's leading authority on non-toxic cancer therapy." Interestingly, one of the many physicians who wrote to the American Medical Association requesting more information on Kelley was Harold C. Habein, Jr., the son of the physician who had diagnosed Lou Gehrig's ALS.[21]

It was in Winthrop that Barbara Minty and McQueen, using the alias Don Schoonover, first tracked down Kelley in April 1980. Kelley extensively described his strategy to his visitors, emphasizing that since he was not a doctor, he would only serve as a consultant to whichever doctors were treating McQueen. With at least one other experimental therapy, the intravenous vitamins, still ahead of him, McQueen was only cautiously receptive. But once the vitamin treatment failed, McQueen decided to pursue the Kelley regimen in its entirety, starting with a "body-cleansing diet" of vitamins and organic foods. At the end of July 1980, he and Minty quietly traveled to Rosarita Beach, thirty miles south of the border in Baja California. There McQueen was admitted to the Plaza Santa Maria, a clinic where Mexican and American doctors treated patients using Kelley's regimen. The dentist was listed as a consultant.

McQueen began intensive treatment. In addition to his specially prescribed diet, which consisted of more than fifty daily vitamin and mineral pills, he received massages, shampoos, prayer sessions, psychotherapy, coffee enemas, rectal enzyme implants, and injections of a cell preparation made from the fetuses of sheep and cattle. And although it was not usually part of Kelley's regimen, McQueen was also was treated with laetrile.[22]

Just as Krebiozen had dominated the alternative cancer world in the 1950s, laetrile did so in the late 1970s—with even more fanfare. Also known as amygdalin or, to enhance its legitimacy, vitamin B_{17}, laetrile had actually been used for decades as a cancer treatment. But by the 1970s, the substance, consisting of a mixture of plants and seeds, including apricot pits, had become a cause celebre. The harder the cancer establishment tried to suppress laetrile, the harder its advocates fought. In a decade that saw the emergence of consumerism in medicine, access to laetrile became a way for cancer patients to assert their right to unconventional therapy. By 1978, seventeen states had passed legislation ensuring access to the substance. It was estimated that as many as seventy thousand Americans had chosen laetrile over orthodox cancer treatments. Debates over the substance filled the pages of the *New England Journal of Medicine* and the *New York Times*.[23]

Why did Steve McQueen, a wealthy and prominent actor with access to the best medical treatment in the country, surreptitiously travel to Mexico to pursue therapy from practitioners widely condemned as charlatans and frauds? Perhaps there would be a definitive answer to this question had McQueen left some type of diary or unpublished correspondence. But because all of the information available on this subject—whether from McQueen himself, his friends, or his biographers—was meant for public consumption, it is hard to distinguish the truth from the stories that interested parties sought to create.

Nevertheless, there is some seemingly reliable testimony from the time. Biographer Marshall Terrill said that McQueen was impressed that Kelley treated "the body that has the disease, not the disease that has the body."

Grady Ragsdale reported having heard the following justification directly from McQueen: "The doctors here say I'm a goner. They don't give me any hope. But Dr. Kelley does and he's the *only* one that does. That's why I'm going to Mexico." Such language would have rung true to other famous patients, such as Margaret Bourke-White and Morris Abram, who pursued innovative therapies. But in their cases, the hopeful intervention had existed within the system. McQueen, having been told at Cedars-Sinai that there were no more treatment options, had to look elsewhere.[24]

His response to his physicians is instructive, especially given the changes occurring in the world of death and dying in the 1970s. Patients like Brian Piccolo, who received aggressive and futile treatment until the very end, had not benefited from the teachings of progressive physicians Cicely Saunders and Elisabeth Kübler-Ross, who were urging the public and the medical profession to think of death as a part of life. Assuming that McQueen's doctors did not plan to abandon him, but simply wanted to tell him the truth about his prognosis, their advice that he get his affairs in order seemed straight out of the new teachings on death. But McQueen wanted no part of this. He traveled to Mexico, one doctor there later reported, because his American doctors had "told him just to go home and die." It is unlikely that they used such language, but McQueen remembered it this way. And this was unacceptable to him. "I don't believe that bullshit," he supposedly said. "I believe I can make it."[25]

McQueen's objections had everything to do with who he was and who he thought he was. Whether or not his upbringing and personality first led film directors to cast him as a rebel, it seems clear that his screen roles reinforced McQueen's inclination to assume this persona in real life. Sayings approvingly attributed to the real-life Steve McQueen—"When I believe in something, I fight like hell for it"; "I live for myself and I answer to nobody"; and "Life is a scam"—sound much more like the lines of a movie character than a real person.

So it should come as no surprise that McQueen reacted to a hopeless prognosis by becoming, in effect, one of his film characters, defiant and confident. When asked about his condition, McQueen was relentlessly upbeat, announcing that he would beat the cancer. "I am going to make it, you know," he told Neile Adams. And true to form, McQueen was convincing. Despite knowing his actual prognosis and being highly skeptical of unorthodox therapies, Adams found herself believing her ex-husband.

"So many events that had happened in his life would have broken a lesser man, but not him," she later recalled thinking. "I expected this wouldn't either."[26]

After receiving even more bad news from the doctors in July 1980, and being explicitly told there was no hope, the next page in McQueen's script was thus obvious: the clandestine and courageous trip to Mexico, where Kelley, himself a renegade opposing the establishment, would give McQueen one last chance at beating the odds. That Kelley's regimen was so arduous only added to the challenge. "Steve had made a private bargain," Penina Spiegel reported. "He would bear any torment in exchange for his life."[27]

Although McQueen tried to keep his presence in Mexico under wraps, he was again unsuccessful. By late September 1980, the *National Enquirer* had tracked him down and was preparing another story. Finally, on October 2, 1980, McQueen decided to come clean, issuing a joint statement with his doctors that he indeed had mesothelioma, "a rare, generally incurable form of lung cancer." He apologized for the earlier deception, which had been done "to save my family and friends from personal hurt and to retain my sense of dignity as, for sure, I thought I was going to die." The press release identified Kelley, of the International Health Institute, as one of McQueen's doctors, but the actor's exact location in Mexico was not disclosed.[28]

The other notable aspect of McQueen's announcement was its optimism. During his six weeks in Mexico, it said, his condition had improved. In an interview conducted the day of McQueen's statement, Rodrigo Rodriguez, one of his doctors, stated that his patient had exhibited "shrinkage of the tumor, partial cessation of discomfort, weight gain and significant improvement in appetite since he began the new treatments." Later, Rodriguez and his colleagues would estimate that the tumor masses had shrunk between 60 and 75 percent. The headline of the Associated Press wire story was even more sanguine: "Tough-Guy Actor's Terminal Cancer Reported in Remission."[29]

Once this news got out, there was a snowball effect. Kelley appeared on the *Tomorrow* show with Tom Snyder and gave another hopeful account. Kelley predicted that McQueen would popularize metabolic therapy just as Winston Churchill helped popularize penicillin, which had cured the British prime minister's pneumonia in the 1940s. On October 8, 1980, an audiotaped message made by McQueen was played on Mexican television.

In it, he thanked Mexico and its doctors for enabling him to recover. "Mexico is showing the world a new way of fighting cancer through non-specific metabolic therapies," McQueen stated. "Again, congratulations and thank you for helping to save my life."[30]

Little is known about the circumstances under which McQueen recorded this message. Some listeners said that he sounded very short of breath. Although McQueen may have truly believed what he said, the staff of the hospital surely had an interest in portraying its efforts in a flattering light. So McQueen may have been urged to make what sounded a lot like a commercial for Plaza Santa Maria and the Kelley method.

Indeed, when the Los Angeles Press Club hosted a press conference the day after McQueen's announcement, roughly a dozen of Kelley's "cured" patients, some carrying their medical charts, attended. Rodriguez claimed that 85 to 90 percent of the fifteen hundred patients treated at the clinic over the past eighteen months, many of whom had cancer, were still alive. Kelley, who was also present, stated that he and his colleagues had developed a paradigm that would alter the course of medicine for the next two hundred years. "I'm coming out smelling like a rose and I am proud of the battle scars I have," he added. "It's a hard fight to change the course of medicine."[31]

Naturally, McQueen's family and friends were thrilled. Neile Adams was quoted in the Los Angeles Herald-Examiner as saying that "he really is getting better, but I'm honor-bound not to say anything else." Ralph Thorson, the real-life bounty hunter McQueen had depicted in The Hunter, said that McQueen had confounded the predictions of nay-saying doctors, adding that "miracles do happen." Even Irving Selikoff, the New York physician who helped to establish the causative role played by asbestos in mesothelioma, seemed to countenance the decision to go to Mexico. "I can understand Mr. McQueen's casting about for anything that might benefit him," Selikoff said. A get-well letter from an admiring fan attributed McQueen's apparent improvement to his having "had the courage to live the way he knew was right."[32]

By this point, journalists' traditional misgivings about covering the illness of a famous person had long since disappeared. The notion that McQueen had bucked the system and found some type of miraculous therapy in Mexico made for a great story. People magazine ran an admiring profile of Kelley, referring to him as "McQueen's Holistic Medicine Man."

Still, the media were appropriately skeptical, and plenty of cancer specialists proved willing to pillory Kelley, his treatment, and even his patient. On the *Today* show, a physician charged Kelley with "rank quackery." A spokesperson for the American Cancer Society, which had long maligned Kelley, termed his treatment a hoax. It was estimated that McQueen was paying at least $10,000 monthly for his treatment. Critics also reminded the media and the public that not only was Kelley not a physician but he had been the subject of multiple investigations. Rodriguez, it was claimed, was a radiologist with no particular experience in treating cancer.[33]

As this debate raged, McQueen was going stir crazy in his bungalow at Plaza Santa Maria. Against his doctors' wishes, he and Barbara drove to their ranch in Santa Paula, California, on October 24, 1980. There they were met by their friend Grady Ragsdale. McQueen told Ragsdale that he had not lost faith in Kelley but just needed a break. He was doing better, aside from a persistent mass in his abdomen that was causing severe pain. McQueen had also grown frustrated with the limited diet prescribed by his doctors and had designated October 30 as his "junk food day." He had actually gotten the clinic staff to acquiesce to periodic junk food days for all of the patients.[34]

On Monday, November 3, 1980, McQueen had a visitor: the Reverend Billy Graham, the famed evangelist. Sometime in 1979, before being diagnosed with cancer, McQueen had discovered religion and been "born again." He had begun reading the Bible regularly and attending church with his wife, Barbara. So the opportunity to meet Graham, who had read of the actor's plight in newspapers, was enormously exciting for McQueen. The two men prayed together and read from the Bible. They also discussed McQueen's illness.

Graham was surprised to learn that McQueen had decided to fly that very night to Juarez, Mexico, just across the Texas border. There McQueen would undergo surgery to remove the abdominal mass that was causing so much pain. Graham accompanied his new acquaintance to the airport, even boarding the plane and saying one last prayer with him. After landing in El Paso, Texas, McQueen traveled to the Santa Rosa Clinic and met his surgeon, Cesar Santos Vargas.[35]

A great deal has been written about McQueen's operation, which took place on the morning of November 6, 1980. Surgery is rarely done to remove isolated tumor masses in patients with widespread cancer, especially if they are debilitated. Most accounts suggest that his Mexican doctors favored surgery in part because the abdominal tumor was pressing on other organs and causing McQueen significant discomfort. Kelley also believed that removing the large tumor would help his patient's immune system attack the rest of the cancer. McQueen agreed to go ahead, even though he knew it would be a risky undertaking. He apparently told Billy Graham that he had only a 50 percent chance of surviving the operation. The actor's supposed statement at the time—"I got nothing to lose. Roll 'em"—is surely how one of his screen characters would have consented to the procedure.[36]

McQueen did survive the surgery, but not for long. During the several-hour operation, Vargas removed a small tumor from his patient's neck and the larger one from his abdomen. Grady Ragsdale, who had flown to Juarez and watched the surgery, later wrote that the abdominal mass was roughly the size of a baseball.

According to Ragsdale, the operation went well. Barbara Minty and McQueen's two children were allowed to visit the patient shortly thereafter. Ragsdale said that McQueen joked with his wife, asking her if his stomach had become flat, although it seems likely that he would still have been on a respirator and thus unlikely to talk. During the day, McQueen slept off and on. Vargas told Minty that her husband was doing well and that she and the rest of the family should go to their hotel and sleep. Minty did so, only to be awakened at 4 a.m. to be told that McQueen had suddenly died. The doctors later concluded that he had experienced a fatal heart attack, probably due to the stress of the surgery on his weary body.[37]

The subsequent events were unseemly and represented the worst behavior of the tabloids. Immediately after McQueen's death, reporters converged on the Santa Rosa Clinic to try to interview his doctors and family. That was reasonable, but someone also took a picture of McQueen's corpse as it lay in a local funeral home. The photograph was sold to the press and quickly published throughout the world.[38]

In retrospect, was McQueen's decision to travel to Mexico and embark on the Kelley treatment reasonable or preposterous? Is there a chance that the unorthodox regimen, with its innumerable components, actually caused the cancer to regress? Lacking McQueen's medical chart from Mexico, which may itself have been of dubious accuracy, it is almost impossible to answer these questions accurately. But the existing historical record allows some conclusions, including three that support what McQueen did.

First, McQueen's story underscores how the divisions between orthodox and alternative therapies are never as sharp as advocates of either approach claim. The fact is that the earlier experimental treatments given to McQueen—interferon and intravenous vitamins—were probably as much of a shot in the dark as his Plaza Santa Maria cocktail. But because these interventions (at least the interferon) were administered by supposedly reputable clinicians, this automatically gave them a legitimacy that they may not have deserved. And to McQueen's credit, he did not pursue unorthodox therapy until he truly had exhausted other options. One should be careful about criticizing what desperate people choose to do.

Second, it may be necessary to widen the criteria with which we evaluate unconventional therapies. Among the claims made by Kelley and his colleagues was that the pancreatic enzymes "digested" the cancer and rendered it inactive. According to this theory, the large mass of cancer that McQueen had in his abdomen was thus "dead" tumor. If this was indeed true, surgical removal of the mass might have been justified. This idea of inert tumor masses is unknown in orthodox medicine, but it is at least theoretically conceivable that a radically different type of treatment could produce a new type of anatomical entity.

Third, while McQueen received varying estimates of how long he was likely to survive, he did seem to outlast most predictions. At the end of July 1980, when the Los Angeles cancer specialists threw up their hands, they had apparently estimated his survival in terms of weeks. But McQueen lived for more than three months and, according to some observers, really looked better for a time. And he probably would have lived longer had he not opted for surgery. Considering that McQueen began a modified Kelley diet in April 1980, it might be that he lived for more than six months as a result of unorthodox treatment. The Plaza Santa Maria doctors offered some proof for this theory when they showed Grady Ragsdale the x-rays taken shortly before McQueen died, which supposedly showed much less cancer in the actor's body. In addition, according to biographer William Nolan, cancer blood markers sent to an independent laboratory had shown "unbelievable" improvement.[39]

But, as in the case of Morris Abram, any claim that a particular treatment regimen—orthodox or alternative—extended the life of a given individual must be viewed skeptically. Doctors can provide only a range of prognosis for patients with a specific disease. With or without treatment, some patients will do better than others. Assessing how a therapy has influenced the outcome of a given patient is very difficult. This is why physicians rely on randomized controlled trials, which assess treatments and outcomes among large groups of patients. So it is very difficult to believe that Kelley's regimen prolonged McQueen's life.

Even more dubious was Kelley's assertion, which he made after unexpectedly garnering national attention, that McQueen had been on the road to cure or at least remission. For example, Kelley reported that his patient's tumors had either already disappeared or were disintegrating "like cotton candy." At another point, he announced that had he not undergone surgery, McQueen would have recovered. "A heart attack killed him, not the cancer," Kelley stated. "We had it beaten."[40]

These contentions were belied by two other pieces of evidence: McQueen's own words and what Vargas discovered during the operation. On October 21, 1980, when he was supposedly doing better, McQueen admitted to Brugh Joy, a "spiritual doctor" he had contacted, that his cancer had "grown bigger, not leveled off." This was corroborated by the surgery. The Associated Press quoted Vargas as saying that McQueen "had cancer all the way to his diaphragm, and cancer from the right lung was pushing into the left lung." Vargas added that the cancer had also spread into the patient's neck and intestines. In other words, even the surgeon who removed the large abdominal tumor mass in no way believed that he had addressed the vast amount of cancer still left in McQueen's body. The view from inside the actor's body suggested that the Kelley regimen had not accomplished very much.[41]

The dying McQueen may have assumed the persona of one of his screen characters, but ultimately his life was not a Hollywood movie. He neither recovered from his cancer nor went out in a blaze of glory. He instead had a very difficult last year of life, with periods of joy but mostly pain, depression, and weakness.

In assessing McQueen's experiences after the fact, first wife Neile Adams came down most harshly on his alternative practitioners. In her 1986 book, *My Husband, My Friend*, she concluded that McQueen had simply been the victim of a huge scam. Journalist Ron Rosenbaum agreed. His investigative report on Mexican cancer clinics, conducted around the time that McQueen was being treated, revealed a "murky netherworld of healers, hypnotists, alchemists, etc., seeking a miracle cure." In later years, the McQueen story took on an even odder twist as William Kelley made increasingly outlandish statements, such as the claim that McQueen had been poisoned to death during his surgery to prevent the world from learning how he had been cured by an alternative cancer treatment.[42]

Yet, despite the critical assessments by Adams and Rosenbaum and the lack of evidence that McQueen had been helped, the most enduring legacy of his illness may have been the question of whether unorthodox treatments should remain an option for interested cancer patients. And here the public voted yes. During his illness, McQueen received thousands of supportive telegrams. Letters to news organizations either defended McQueen or sought more information about alternative treatments. One reader wrote to columnist Ann Landers asking why McQueen had to travel all the way to Mexico to find additional experimental treatment after more traditional therapies had failed. And columnist Liz Smith, in discussing William Kelley, reminded her readers of another famous doubter, Galileo, who was at that moment being celebrated in a newly produced Bertolt Brecht play in Washington, D.C.[43]

People with cancer also voted with their feet. "Desperate Cancer Patients Are Flocking to Mexican Hospitals Seeking McQueen's Therapy," read a *Star* headline on November 11, 1980, four days after the actor's death. All of the 152 rooms at Plaza Santa Maria were booked, and "scores" of other people were "clamoring for admittance." Two months later, CBS News reported that thousands of cancer victims, most of them with terminal illness, were "crossing the border into Mexico hoping to stay alive, hoping to escape the death sentences pronounced on them, they feel, by American doctors." "Any chance is better than none," said one such pilgrim, Roy White, of Cincinnati. "A drowning man will try to reach hold of anything." And not all interested cancer patients were traveling outside the country. The same CBS broadcast reported on a recent "Health Freedom" convention in Long Beach, California, where thousands of people had learned about alternative remedies.[44]

Having played a determined, rebellious character in so many movies, it was easy and logical for Steve McQueen to assume the role of a determined, rebellious cancer patient. Yet his choices had great cultural resonance, not because they were fitting ones for an antihero celebrity, but because they were reasonable for many, perhaps even most, dying cancer patients. "Fighting" one's cancer has become the only appropriate response to the disease in American society. Indeed, the metaphor has become so ubiquitous it is almost invisible.

The McQueen case reminds us why such language—and, in some cases, the attendant pursuit of unconventional treatment—remains so popular. "Ordinary" cancer patients may see themselves as Steve McQueens, ready to marshal any possible forces against the dreaded disease. In other words, what assumes value is the fight itself or, more accurately, the perception that one is fighting, or has fought, cancer. This is true whether the treatment leads to a cure, as happened with Morris Abram, or the patient dies, as in Steve McQueen's case. At a private service for McQueen, Leonard De Witt, his pastor, said that his friend "went out like a star." Increasingly, this was becoming a reasonable epitaph for all cancer patients to strive for.[45]

There was one last factor fueling the public's faith in alternative cancer therapy: the apparent survivors. Far beyond the dozen Kelley patients who appeared at the October 9, 1980, press conference, there were hundreds, even thousands, of Americans who claimed to have been cured of a fatal cancer after being written off by oncologists. How could such "data" exist given the American Cancer Society's claims that all alternative cancer treatments were quackery?

This question especially intrigued Nicholas Gonzalez, who, in 1980, was a second-year student at Cornell University Medical School. Working with Robert A. Good, president of the Memorial-Sloan Kettering Cancer Institute, Gonzalez contacted Kelley and got permission to review his medical charts. Between 1981 and 1986, Gonzalez reviewed all of the charts, which numbered over a thousand, interviewed more than four hundred patients and then selected fifty cases for close study. Gonzalez eventually wrote a three-hundred-page manuscript, entitled "One Man Alone," which detailed his findings. Although the monograph was never published, and mainstream cancer specialists who read it objected to some of his data, Gonzalez ultimately concluded that Kelley had treated hundreds of patients with supposedly terminal cancer who lived for five, ten, or more years.[46]

After completing his medical training and an immunology fellowship, Gonzalez hung up a shingle in New York City in 1987. Despite periodic challenges to his credibility by the New York State medical board and other critics, he has continued to treat cancer patients with his own version of Kelley's regimen of enzymes, nutritional supplements, and coffee enemas. Like Kelley, Gonzalez now has a cadre of long-term cancer survivors. But unlike Kelley, he has been able to get the cancer establishment to acknowledge the possibility that he is onto something. In 1999, Gonzalez and colleagues received a $1.4 million grant from the newly established National Center for Complementary and Alternative Medicine, a branch of the National Institutes of Health. Gonzalez's proposed research project, comparing his regimen with standard chemotherapy for advanced pancreatic cancer, is now underway at Columbia University Medical Center in New York.[47]

Members of the public, at least those who believe there is a connection between nutrition and cancer, have praised these developments on various Internet chat sites. Kelley, in turn, has become a folk hero, whom one e-mailer termed "a highly respected alternative cancer healer who had succeeded in 1980 to save actor Steve McQueen from cancer with his metabolic program." As we have seen, such a description is unwarranted. But Kelley's bigger claim, that he could cure some people with "incurable" cancer, is finally getting its day in court.[48]

And even if Gonzalez's regimen shows no benefits, advocates of alternative and complementary medicine have still scored a victory by getting the NIH to establish a center to study such therapies. As people with AIDS and breast cancer would demonstrate in the 1980s and 1990s, a crucial part of disease activism is the ability to obtain research funding from the government. So is the ability to raise private money to establish disease-specific foundations. And the best way to obtain both types of funding is to have a celebrity face associated with a disease. Rita Hayworth's very beautiful face ably fulfilled this task, although she never knew it.

Chapter 8

Medicine's Blind Spots

The Delayed Diagnosis of Rita Hayworth

It was Rita Hayworth's unfortunate problem that the medical profession had largely forgotten about the disease—Alzheimer's—that was causing her to lose her memory. By 1971, when she was in her early fifties, and probably earlier, she was already showing signs of the disease. But it would go undiagnosed for almost a decade, until a physician finally paid more attention to her symptoms than to the labels she already carried. The diagnosis was revealed in 1981.

The reasons for Hayworth's misdiagnosis were complicated, reflecting the difficult nature of distinguishing among diseases, the tendency to blame people for their illnesses, the unsatisfactory care that famous patients may receive, and the well-meaning, but ultimately ill-advised, intentions of her Hollywood friends. Still, the fact remained that doctors had consistently missed the diagnosis. As a result, Hayworth's daughter, Princess Yasmin Aga Khan, like Morris Abram and Steve McQueen before her, concluded that the public deserved to know about the apparent limitations of the medical profession.

Princess Yasmin became a highly prominent activist, helping to propel Alzheimer's disease into America's consciousness and raise tens of millions of dollars for research. Her mother became the public face of Alzheimer's, reminding Americans of both the tragedy of the disease and the need to fight it. In 1982, President Ronald Reagan, with the princess standing behind him, signed legislation proclaiming the first National Alzheimer's Disease Awareness Week (it later became a month). By 1994, when Reagan announced that he had the disease, Americans knew exactly what he was talking about. But in 1981 they had no clue.

Rita Hayworth was born Margarita Carmen Cansino in New York City in 1919, the daughter of a dance instructor and his wife. When she was 9 years old, the family moved to Los Angeles, where she began appearing in dance acts. Hayworth's talent and her father's connections to Hollywood studios landed her a role in *Dante's Inferno*, a 1935 film starring Spencer Tracy. Thus began an extremely successful career as an actress.

By her early twenties, Hayworth had appeared in thirty-two movies, but it was three 1941 films that made her a star: *Strawberry Blonde, Blood and Sand*, and *You'll Never Get Rich*. The last of these, costarring Fred Astaire, enabled Hayworth to display her remarkable dancing ability and landed her on the cover of *Time* magazine. Her most famous movie role, in *Gilda*, followed in 1946. In the film, the sultry Hayworth performed the erotic showstopper "Put the Blame on Mame."

Hayworth's looks also propelled her career. With her long, wavy hair now dyed red, she appeared in one of World War II's most famous pin-ups—in a sleeveless negligee, beckoning American soldiers. A copy of the picture, originally a *Life* magazine cover, was reportedly taped to a peacetime atomic bomb dropped on Bikini Island in 1946. Other successful films followed in the 1950s, including *Pal Joey* and *Separate Tables*. Hayworth appeared on the cover of *Life* four times, more than anyone besides Franklin D. Roosevelt.[1]

Hayworth's personal life was much less happy. She was married and divorced five times. She had children with two of her husbands, the actor and director Orson Welles and the wealthy playboy Prince Aly Khan, son of the Aga Khan, the spiritual leader of the world's Ismaili Muslims. In explaining her difficulties with men, Hayworth liked to say that most men fell in love with Gilda but woke up with Rita. In a 1989 biography, Barbara Leaming attributed Hayworth's erratic lifestyle—which included drinking and emotional lability—to childhood sexual abuse by her father.[2]

Hayworth's medical deterioration can be briefly sketched as follows. Throughout her career, she had been a quick study, able to memorize her lines and dance steps with little difficulty. But by the early 1970s, and probably earlier, Hayworth could no longer do so. Her ability to remember people's names and her daily activities suffered as well. In one especially difficult episode in 1972, she agreed to appear in the Broadway musical

Applause, but had to quit before ever taking the stage. Meanwhile, Hayworth's behavior was becoming increasingly erratic, culminating in a 1976 episode in which she lost control on an airplane. The press widely transmitted pictures of the actress, looking disheveled and disoriented as she left the plane. The cause of her behavior, it was most often stated, was alcoholism.[3]

In 1977, Hayworth's family, notably her second daughter, Yasmin Aga Khan, arranged an admission to Silver Hill, a rehabilitation facility in Connecticut. Hayworth gradually grew worse, although she continued to make public appearances. Finally, in 1981, her lawyer, Leonard H. Monroe, announced that she had Alzheimer's disease, a degenerative disease of the brain. Sacrificing her own emerging career as a singer, Princess Yasmin lovingly took care of her mother until her death on May 14, 1987, at the age of 68. For the last years of her life, Hayworth recognized no one, including her daughter, and was prone to terrors and agitation. She became bedbound and lost considerable weight.[4]

Perhaps the most commonly asked question about Rita Hayworth's Alzheimer's is why it took so long to diagnose. There are several explanations, which I will examine in turn: (1) the limited medical awareness of the disease in the 1970s; (2) the role played by concurrent illness, in this case alcoholism; and (3) the response of Hayworth's friends and colleagues to her condition.

One could argue that it should have been simple to make a diagnosis of a disease that had been described decades earlier. In November 1901, the German physician Alois Alzheimer examined a 51-year-old woman whose husband was concerned by her angry outbursts and memory problems. During the examination, Alzheimer observed severe disorientation, reduced comprehension, paranoia, hallucinations, and very poor short-term memory. When he asked the woman to write her name, she could barely do so, despite repeated attempts. "I have lost myself," she told the doctor.[5]

The woman gradually worsened, becoming bedridden, incontinent, and mute. Alzheimer gradually ruled out a series of possible diagnoses, which included paresis (syphilis of the brain) and dementia praecox (now known as schizophrenia). The patient's disease most closely resembled so-called senile dementia, a condition named by a French psychiatrist in 1838, characterized by worsening short-term memory. But as indicated by the word *senile*, this dementia occurred in the elderly, presumably due to normal aging of the brain. Alzheimer's patient, in contrast, was a relatively young woman.[6]

When the patient died in 1906, Alzheimer received permission to perform an autopsy. What he saw under the microscope was something that had never been described. The brain contained numerous brown plaques, occupying space that should have been filled with normal nerve cells. When Alzheimer applied a specific stain, he saw a second type of invader, what he called "a tangled bundle of fibrils." These tangles, too, seemed to be obliterating the normal nervous tissue.[7]

Alzheimer regularly discussed his findings at scientific meetings and published them in a medical journal. The most enthusiastic response came from Emil Kraepelin, a renowned psychiatrist and Alzheimer's supervisor at the Royal Psychiatric Clinic in Munich. Kraepelin was the world's foremost advocate of the theory that many mental illnesses had an organic basis. This claim put him at odds with the Austrian psychiatrist Sigmund Freud, who was propounding his influential views on the relationship of childhood trauma to future mental disturbances. It was Kraepelin, in his classic text, *Handbook of Psychiatry*, who coined the term *Alzheimer's disease* in honor of his colleague. After all, if the brain findings on autopsy had indeed caused the patient's symptoms, Alzheimer's disease was a prime example of how a damaged brain could result in mental illness.[8]

Although Alzheimer's disease continued to be included in most neurological textbooks of the twentieth century, it was largely forgotten, characterized as a very rare cause of memory loss in young people. Authors distinguished it from the much more common dementia of the elderly, believed to be caused by cerebral atherosclerosis—the accumulation of fatty material in the aging arteries of the brain. This latter condition was popularly known as "hardening of the arteries."

This distinction, however, proved faulty. Benefiting from the new technology of electron microscopy, pathologists in the 1970s who examined brain tissue from deceased elderly patients with dementia saw the same plaques and tangles that Alzheimer had first witnessed. Atherosclerosis was not always present. This finding was potentially revolutionary. It meant that senility among the aged was probably also Alzheimer's disease, not the natural deterioration of an aging brain, and that Alzheimer's was potentially a very common—not an obscure—disease. Robert Katzman, a New York City neurologist, became the strongest advocate of this theory. Like

Alzheimer, he announced his findings at meetings of medical societies and in medical journals.[9]

For a series of reasons, this dramatic news received little attention from the media. In contrast to today, when medical journal editors and public relations departments of medical centers routinely trumpet new research findings, the 1970s were a more modest time. Doctors preferred to debate new issues among themselves and often criticized colleagues who prematurely went to the press. In addition, old concepts die hard in medicine. Physicians taught about senile dementia in medical school were not about to immediately abandon the concept. As a result, Alzheimer's disease remained largely invisible to the public. When Katzman presented some of his research at a 1973 meeting, the only newspaper to cover it was the *National Enquirer*.[10]

Much has been written over the past twenty years about how social and cultural factors can affect the ways in which diseases are labeled over time. Alzheimer's provides an excellent example. In 1906 Alzheimer identified a previously undescribed pathological process in a 51-year-old patient with memory loss. But it remained a rare and obscure disease because doctors, generally psychiatrists, caring for patients with senile dementia did not think they might also be encountering Alzheimer's. When this connection was understood, it gradually became clear to physicians—at least to those attending neurology meetings—that Alzheimer's was probably the most common cause of dementia in all age groups. But the reported incidence of the disease would not increase until doctors, often with the encouragement of patients and families, began suspecting and then making the diagnosis. As we shall see, this new awareness of Alzheimer's disease occurred in large part due to Rita Hayworth.[11]

Of course, the debate over senile dementia had little direct relevance to the actress. Even if physicians had guessed wrong for decades about the cause of senile dementia, the actress was in her early fifties when her obvious symptoms began, the same age as Alois Alzheimer's original patient. So Hayworth was actually a quintessential case of Alzheimer's. But the disease had simply been overlooked.

The second explanation for the confusion in Hayworth's case stemmed from her troubled personal life and reputation as a heavy drinker. While the press found her to be irresistibly charming and loved to feature her in elaborate photographic spreads, it also paid close attention to her marriages and divorces. In such pieces, Hayworth was often portrayed as a victim, either of womanizers, such as Welles and Aly Khan, or of physical abusers, as in the case of her fourth husband, the singer Dick Haymes. But she was not seen as blameless. Her 1949 affair with Prince Aly Khan, which began when he was still married, earned her the enmity of the press, which declared it "a very sordid business." Hayworth's fitness as a mother was also questioned when she took her 4-year-old daughter, Rebecca Welles, on her clandestine European trips to meet the prince, who soon became her third husband.[12]

Hayworth's personal life turned especially seamy in 1954 during the waning days of her marriage to Haymes, a drinker in trouble with the law for unpaid debts. Hayworth, dutifully supporting him, had sent her two children to stay with a babysitter. At one point, sheriff's deputies arrived at the Hotel Madison in New York to arrest Haymes, who refused to cooperate. The press learned of the standoff and reported on it widely. Reporters found the children in White Plains, New York, living in a shabby house with questionable supervision. Eventually, the Westchester County Society for the Prevention of Cruelty to Children filed neglect charges against Hayworth, and the girls were placed in protective care. The media covered the subsequent custody hearings with gusto.[13]

Hayworth's mother had been an alcoholic, and Rita began drinking heavily in 1945 as her marriage to her second husband, Orson Welles, was deteriorating. Her mood swings, including wild rages, also worsened. Hayworth's drinking later increased as she tried to cope with Haymes. And during her fifth and final marriage—to Hollywood producer James Hill, from 1958 to 1961—alcohol "was clearly becoming a serious problem."[14]

Several months after Hayworth and Hill divorced on September 7, 1961, she was offered her first Broadway role, as a former vaudevillian, in *Step on a Crack*. The role had been arranged by the actor Gary Merrill, who was both starring in the play and dating Hayworth. Rehearsals began uneventfully on August 14, 1962, but seven days later the actress was hospitalized at New York's Flower and Fifth Avenue Hospital. There were variable stories as to what had happened. The *New York Times* reported that the actress, suffering from nervous exhaustion, was "too physically and emotionally exhausted" to continue. A physician diagnosed her as "anemic" and told her to quit the play.[15]

While Hayworth may have been anemic, and while the tight rehearsal schedule was surely more arduous than that of a Hollywood movie, why she should have been physically unable to continue is less clear. The term *nervous exhaustion*, like *nervous breakdown*, has long been used as a generic excuse for actors and other performers looking to get out of commitments. Still, the whole episode might have been forgotten as a bad casting idea had not Hayworth's problems persisted.

In 1963 Hayworth traveled to Spain to work on *Circus World*, a film starring John Wayne, which had a rocky production and opened to poor reviews. It was during the making of this film, according to biographer Leaming, that Hayworth first had difficulty remembering her lines. There was drinking as well, and temper tantrums, often for unclear reasons. In one instance, Hayworth screamed obscenities at an American tourist she encountered. Interestingly, however, critics picked out Hayworth as giving the film's best performance.[16]

The next year Hayworth appeared on the Academy Awards, where she misstated the director Tony Richardson's name as Tony Richards more than once. Perhaps this was simply an innocent mistake, but it was surprising enough to generate attention in the press. Hayworth's next film was *The Money Trap*, costarring Glenn Ford and released in 1966. There were again stories of Hayworth's drinking off the set, but this habit may only have enhanced her performance as a worn-out alcoholic waitress. Hayworth, reviewers raved, was "the best of all" and had never looked like "more of an actress."[17]

Hayworth made a series of unmemorable movies over the next several years. She evidently functioned well enough to complete the films, and nothing about her behavior made the newspapers. In early 1971 Hayworth appeared on the *Carol Burnett Show*. She had seen the comedienne do a skit called "Golda," a takeoff on Hayworth's famous Gilda, and got in touch with Burnett.

But 1971 also saw another disaster. Hayworth agreed to be the summer replacement for Lauren Bacall in the Broadway musical *Applause*. But, as with *Step on a Crack* nine years earlier, Hayworth was forced to withdraw. The show's producers and her friends were quick to put a predictable spin on the event: Hollywood actresses need more time to learn Broadway roles. "She is going back to California to work on the part," announced producer Larry Kasha. "Then she will head a national company." Shades of the truth, however, did seep out—specifically, that she simply could not remember her lines. Hayworth vehemently denied this claim when asked. And she also resented any implications that drinking was responsible for her poor performance.[18]

Hayworth continued to receive offers, including one as a gun-slinging mother in *The Wrath of God*, a spoof of action films. She flew to Mexico in late 1971 to begin filming. By this time, there was no denying Hayworth's inability to memorize lines, even on a film set. She made it through the production only because the director, Ralph Nelson, allowed her to memorize line by line, filming each sentence of dialogue separately. "Her memory had just gone," Hayworth's hairdresser, Lynn Del Kail, later reported. "You'd be talking to her about a subject and all of a sudden she was talking about something else." Reviews of the film were mixed, but no critics cited anything abnormal about her performance. Despite Rita Hayworth's severe problems, her film characters continued to function excellently in the dream factory of Hollywood.[19]

The Wrath of God proved to be Hayworth's last completed role, although she did have one additional embarrassment, periods of severe agitation and an inability to learn her lines during the filming of *Tales That Witness Madness* in 1972. She did not finish the movie. The next several years were very difficult. Hayworth was not working—the word was out—and she continued to exhibit erratic behavior. For example, misinterpreting an innocent remark made by Adele Astaire at a dinner party, she threw a drink in the dancer's face. One of the most disturbing events took place when she invited her friends, choreographer Hermes Pan and actress Ann Miller, to dinner. When they arrived, Hayworth came to the door with a butcher knife and screamed at them, "I'm not signing any autographs today!" She chased them away. The next day, Hayworth called Miller on the phone to ask why she had not come.[20]

But the most grisly event occurred in January 1976. A British television show had invited Hayworth to appear and was flying her and her agent, Bud Burton Moss, to London. Hayworth, who never liked to fly, had a tranquilizer and at least one drink. As the flight progressed, she became increasingly agitated, shouting at the other passengers and even slapping a stewardess. Word got out about what was happening, and when the plane arrived at Heathrow Airport, several dozen members of the press were waiting. Moss tried to disperse the reporters, but Hayworth eventually had to leave the plane. Photographers snapped pictures of a disheveled woman in clear distress.[21]

The power of such photographs was enhanced by the fact that Hayworth was such a beautiful woman. Illness often causes visible physical damage, and Hayworth's condition, it seemed, had struck a mighty blow to the actress. Handsome male celebrities who became sick also cared about their appearance, of course—think of Brian Piccolo's embarrassment over his emasculating surgery and Steve McQueen's persistent reclusiveness. Yet, while the media were revealing how a bout of illness particularly altered the looks of celebrities, ordinary patients experienced many of the same transformations. The distraught actress in the pictures was both Rita Hayworth and everyone struggling with addiction or psychiatric illness.

What rules applied to the publication of such photographs? The British tabloids, if anything, were more brutal than their American counterparts. Pictures of a celebrity having a public breakdown were fair game and graphic headlines were the rule: "When a Love Goddess Finally Crumbles" and "The Agony of Rita." But the mainstream press also covered the event and published the photographs, something that once would have been taboo, given Hayworth's evident distress. "Rita Hayworth Ill, Needs Help Deplaning," announced the *Los Angeles Herald-Examiner. Newsweek* featured the Hayworth episode in its "Newsmakers" column, saying that she looked not like a dazzling actress but like the title of her last picture, the "Wrath of God." Moss downplayed the event, citing a combination of fatigue and the tranquilizer as having caused a self-limited problem.[22]

But it was hard to make what had happened disappear. The rumor was that alcohol had caused Hayworth to go crazy. A stewardess from the flight was quoted as saying that "Miss Hayworth had been drinking when she boarded the plane and had several free drinks on the flight. She made a bit of a nuisance of herself." And the tabloids refused to let the story drop. An article in the February 1, 1977, issue of the *National Enquirer*, for example, quoted a friend who said that Hayworth was "the most tragic figure in Hollywood today." Her behavior, the article continued, was characterized by pathetic loneliness, heavy drinking, and bizarre behavior.[23]

Finally, in March 1977, Hayworth was forced to obtain medical attention. An artist named Bill Gilpin had met her on a California golf course and they had begun a relationship. Having worshiped Hayworth's poster as a World War II soldier, Gilpin was thrilled to be dating this beautiful actress, but it was also clear that she needed help. He took Hayworth to a hospital in Newport Beach, California, where she was diagnosed as "gravely disabled as a result of mental disorder or impairment by chronic alcoholism and . . . unwilling to accept, or incapable of accepting, treatment voluntarily."[24]

Based on this report, the Orange County superior court appointed a temporary conservator to manage Hayworth's affairs. Princess Yasmin Aga Khan, then a 27-year-old aspiring singer living in Manhattan, flew to California to see her mother. While she recognized her daughter, Hayworth did not know either the date or the name of the president. In an arrangement made with the court, Princess Yasmin took her mother to the Silver Hill Clinic in Connecticut, a well-known alcohol detoxification facility whose celebrity patients have also included Joan Kennedy and Truman Capote.[25]

Although Hayworth seemed to cut out liquor after her hospitalization, her overall condition never really improved. The actress went back to California, where she continued to live alone but now under more careful watch by friends or attendants. She continued to participate in the Hollywood nightlife and received several honors over the next few years. Typical was a November 1977 event sponsored by the Thalians, a group of celebrities who raised funds for various charities, that honored Hayworth at a dinner in Los Angeles. The salute, attended by dozens of Hollywood stars, was entitled "You Were Never Lovelier," the title of a 1942 Hayworth film. Yet, while Hayworth looked radiant, she was bewildered when she had to go to the dais to accept her statuette. There was a period of awkward silence until the actress Debbie Reynolds, then the president of the Thalians, rushed to the microphone to rescue her. "Our Rita is very shy," Reynolds announced, "and we promised her she wouldn't have to make a speech."[26]

In 1978, friends introduced Yasmin Aga Khan to Ronald Fieve, a psychiatrist at New York's Columbia-Presbyterian Medical Center, who was best known as a pioneer in using lithium to treat manic depression, the illness that afflicted ballplayer Jimmy Piersall. At some point Yasmin began to describe her mother's symptoms and Fieve became interested. In early 1978 he recommended further testing of Hayworth to try to make a definitive diagnosis. Hayworth, who had already seen numerous doctors, was never fond of doing so, in part because they would lecture her about her drinking.[27]

Fieve interviewed Hayworth, tested her ability to understand and memorize, and ordered a series of x-rays. Fieve also referred her to several of his colleagues, who generated some interesting findings. Two neurologists, H. Houston Merritt and Eugenia Gamboa, noted that there was no evidence of nerve damage from alcohol, such as numbness, which one might have expected with a diagnosis of alcoholic dementia. Next, in September 1978, Rita Rudd, a specialist in formal neuropsychiatric testing, saw Hayworth. Rudd found extreme memory impairment, with deterioration of function since an earlier testing in May 1977, despite the patient's supposed abstinence from liquor. These findings led Rudd to suggest a possible diagnosis of Alzheimer's disease, which Fieve communicated to Yasmin Aga Khan in an April 1979 letter.[28]

Over the next two years, Fieve excluded other possible diagnoses. When Yasmin filed a petition in June 1981 to become her mother's conservator, the newspapers announced that Rita Hayworth had Alzheimer's disease. Indeed, Hayworth had a classic case, remarkably similar to the one initially described by the German scientist. It had just taken a remarkably long time to figure this out.

Was alcoholic dementia ever a plausible explanation for Hayworth's symptoms? Perhaps, but this diagnosis was itself controversial. In 1955 a Los Angeles neurologist named Cyril B. Courville had posited that alcohol caused a series of pathological changes in the brain that caused dementia. Subsequent studies, however, had called into question the specific role of alcohol in causing these lesions, even though the patients were heavy drinkers.[29]

Since there was a legitimate argument for the existence of alcoholic dementia, and since Hayworth had been a heavy drinker, giving this diagnosis for her condition made some sense, even after she apparently cut out alcohol in 1977. But if one looks at the types of patients who generally received this label, many of them differed from Hayworth, suffering not only from nerve damage but from cirrhosis of the liver. Moreover, the problems that became worse over time, such as the actress's short-term memory deficits, bursts of angry confusion, and agnosia (inability to recognize familiar people or things), were classic for Alzheimer's disease.

Thus, the doctors who saw Hayworth throughout the 1970s were most guilty of having blinders or, to quote Yasmin Aga Khan, being "trapped in a box." When evaluating the patient, whose history of drinking had been reflexively linked to her worsening memory, they simply corroborated this diagnosis. And the press, whether covering Heathrow Airport or other mishaps, invariably listed alcohol as a predisposing factor. So it was not until Fieve revisited Hayworth's case that another diagnosis would be seriously entertained. The major reason that Yasmin Aga Khan ultimately decided to lend her name to Alzheimer's education was her amazement—and, to some degree, anger—that physicians could have misdiagnosed her mother's disease for so long. "I wish I could have found her the right doctor," Yasmin later stated.[30]

Perhaps due to the so-called VIP syndrome, in which prominent patients supposedly receive worse medical care, Hayworth's physicians had jumped to the wrong conclusions. But so had her friends and colleagues. This is the third reason for Hayworth's delayed diagnosis. Throughout the 1970s, even after the embarrassing episodes at the *Applause* rehearsals and at Heathrow Airport, Hayworth's close acquaintances continually minimized her problems. For example, her agent, Bud Moss, continued to book engagements for her, although these became less ambitious over time. Hayworth's lawyer, Leonard Monroe, helped stave off any legal proceedings that might have named a formal guardian to monitor Hayworth's affairs. And her friends continued to take her out to restaurants and parties, despite the very real possibility that she would create a scene.[31]

In retrospect, one can rightly ask what these people were thinking, parading around such a gravely impaired woman. Yet such an assessment is somewhat unfair. We now know that Hayworth had Alzheimer's, but members of her coterie did not know this. Indeed, given the invisibility of presenile dementia during the years in question, they surely could not have conceived of such a diagnosis. Moreover, Hayworth, not unlike many Hollywood stars, was temperamental by nature and a drinker. As the actress Ruta Lee later recalled, "We had no idea she had Alzheimer's. She didn't know she had Alzheimer's. The people around her didn't know. They were very protective of her and somehow the world and us included thought 'Uh, she's been swilling too much vodka. She's been doing strange things to herself. Living a very hard life.'" Given this ignorance, getting Hayworth to drink less alcohol, and thus potentially control her mood swings, seemed like a viable strategy. That Hayworth's problem might be remediable was probably a comforting notion for those around her.[32]

Moreover, Hayworth's friends were encouraging her to do what she loved to do: act, dance, mingle, and be a star for her public. "We were trying to keep *the image* of Rita as alive as we possibly could," Moss later reflected, "without embarrassing her in public." And when things went well, this decision didn't seem to be so unreasonable. Experts in Alzheimer's disease speak of a so-called zone, a range of behaviors that an afflicted individual can exhibit. Thus, in the early stages of the disease, when clear memory deficits become apparent, there can also be periods of lucidity. It seems logical to take advantage of such windows before further deterioration occurs.[33]

There is also the possibility of what might be termed "seeming lucidity," in which someone with Alzheimer's is able to give the appearance of functioning normally. In the case of Hayworth, given her very public existence, we can find many documented episodes of this phenomenon. If one watches her guest appearance on the *Carol Burnett Show* in 1971, for example, there is no suggestion that Hayworth was already quite impaired, even if one looks for such evidence. In point of fact, she required much more assistance and guidance than other guests, but she carried off comedy skits and a charming duet with Burnett, "Mutual Admiration Society," with remarkable aplomb in front of a live audience. Watching this with the retrospective knowledge of what was occurring is undoubtedly sad, but there is also something wonderful about salvaging a few more brilliant moments from a once-great performer. The same was true for *The Wrath of God*, in which, according to one critic, she was "elegant and beautiful," lending the movie "a note of dignity." If, as Neal Gabler suggests, life has become a movie, why shouldn't Hayworth have been entitled to do in front of the camera what she could no longer do in real life?[34]

Off camera, Hayworth also managed to play her parts well. Many people with early Alzheimer's devise strategies, such as changing the subject, poking fun at their bad memory, or uttering vague platitudes, which can conceal their deficits. Hayworth was adept at such maneuvers. Indeed, newspaper coverage from the time suggested there was nothing amiss. In a March 1977 feature in the *Los Angeles Times*, for example, she was quoted as saying: "I feel better now than I ever have and I'm a better actress than

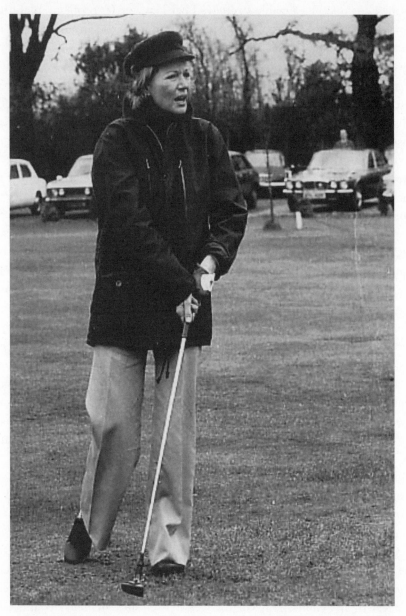

Rita Hayworth golfing shortly after her notorious airplane incident in 1976. Her continued ability to perform certain activities led people to downplay her dramatic memory loss, later diagnosed as Alzheimer's. Courtesy of Caren Roberts-Frenzel and Globe Photos.

ever before." In June 1978, the *Los Angeles Herald-Examiner* reported that Hayworth was "reborn and working again . . . swinging a golf club on the westside of town each day." Later that year she attended the Valentino film festival in Italy, where she was given a lifetime achievement award and had to appear before the press. A reporter later complimented Hayworth for doing "herself and Hollywood proud." As late as 1980, it was reported that the "radiant" actress was back on the show business "party circuit" and planning a comeback.[35]

It is not entirely clear what the writers of such stories were thinking. Some seem to have been duped, just like Hayworth's doctors. Others, however, clearly sensed significant problems. While they never came out and said that Hayworth and her people were pulling a fast one, at times they implied it. For example, Shearlean Duke, who wrote the 1977 *Los Angeles Times* article, noted that in the middle of the interview Hayworth became nervous and anxious, responding with "quick, one- or two-sentence responses." And, Duke reported, Hayworth completely forgot about an earlier discussion they had had about a recent *National Enquirer* article.[36]

Often Hayworth's friends or advisors accompanied her on these interviews, coaching and making excuses for her. At some point, this exercise must have become macabre. Whether it was due to alcohol or some other unexplained problem, the Rita Hayworth they had known was no longer there. She often did not even recognize them or was unable to remember their names. Getting her through an interview or public appearance without a disaster must have become almost a game. And the game, by the 1970s, required outright deception. After Orange County had filed papers to obtain a guardian for Hayworth in 1977, her lawyer, Leonard Monroe, stated that the actress was "perfectly capable of being in charge of her own affairs." Shortly thereafter, Hayworth's friend Gloria Luckenbill told Los Angeles journalist Dorothy Manners that the "nightmare" was over and that Hayworth was herself again. Her friend, Luckenbill added, wanted "to forget everything about this horrid ordeal." As Hayworth's crowd very well knew, this would surely happen, but not for the reasons implied. By this point, continuing to show Hayworth off in public, even if done to give her some joy and ensure her financial security, had become misguided. In the late 1970s, Moss and Yasmin Aga Khan mercifully declined Barbara Walters's request to do a nationally televised interview with the actress.[37]

Once Rita Hayworth's diagnosis of Alzheimer's became public in June

1981, she ceased being a public figure, except in memory. By this point, the word was getting out about the disease. The medical profession, building on the work of Katzman and others, had reached a consensus that Alzheimer's, and not normal aging, was the major cause of senility among the elderly. And voluntary associations devoted to publicizing the disease had formed in several cities. In October 1979, working with Robert Butler, the head of the National Institute on Aging, these groups had merged to form a national organization, the Alzheimer's Disease and Related Disorders Association.[38]

The ADRDA had gotten a major boost in October 1980, when Abigail Van Buren plugged it in one of her "Dear Abby" columns. "Desperate in New York" had written to describe how her 50-year-old husband, who had become increasingly forgetful, had just been diagnosed with Alzheimer's disease. "I feel so helpless," the woman wrote. "How do others cope with this affliction?" The ADRDA received roughly twenty-five thousand inquiries after the column was published, flooding its small Manhattan office.[39]

But Alzheimer's remained a faceless disease. There was no one to do for dementia what Betty Ford did for breast cancer and alcoholism—until the June 1981 announcement about Hayworth. Now the media, having chronicled the actress's public mishaps and her alcoholism, turned their attention to her new diagnosis. Over the next several years, newspapers, magazines, and television shows told and retold her story, often interviewing Yasmin Aga Khan, who was becoming active in Alzheimer's fundraising. "The Tragedy of Rita Hayworth," the *Ladies' Home Journal* told readers in 1983, was "a story that will make you weep." The cover of the June 1, 1987, issue of *People* magazine, which featured a story authored by Yasmin, read: "Princess Yasmin fondly recalls her glamorous mother and her brave fight against Alzheimer's Disease."[40]

One of the facts that Hayworth's family and the media learned about Alzheimer's disease was that it was usually present for at least ten years before diagnosis. That is, well before the disease becomes obvious, early anatomical changes in the brain cause problems with memory and behavior. The question thus arose, For just how long had Rita Hayworth had Alzheimer's disease?

There was, of course, no way to know. The tests that might have revealed the diagnosis five, ten, or fifteen years before had not been done. But this did not prevent people from making estimates about the duration of Hayworth's Alzheimer's. What were these speculations and why did they prove to be so compelling?

It was certainly reasonable to assume that Hayworth's behavior at the time of the *Applause* debacle in the early 1970s was due to Alzheimer's disease. Her inability to remember lines and her mood swings, interspersed with periods of clarity, are characteristic of the early stages of the disease. What, then, of Hayworth's sometimes heavy alcohol use during these years? To her credit, Yasmin Aga Khan has not ignored this reality, admitting that her mother did have a lifelong drinking problem. Suggesting that Hayworth had probably turned to liquor to deny "the painful realities of her sickness," Yasmin believed that the memory and behavior problems likely stemmed from a mixture of alcoholism and Alzheimer's disease.[41]

But at the same time, the members of the media were creating another narrative, one that selectively used history to create a mythical version of Hayworth's illness. All of the actress's long-standing problems, they suggested, had been attributable to Alzheimer's. "Movie Star's Irrational Behavior Was Caused by a Disease All Along" announced one headline. Hayworth had originally been diagnosed as an alcoholic, reported *Variety*, but "it was only some time later that the true nature of her ailment was discovered." "Finally came a diagnosis," film critic Stefan Kanfer wrote in the appropriately titled *Memories* magazine. "Hayworth wasn't an alcoholic; she had Alzheimer's disease." Hayworth's former agent, Bud Moss, agreed: "Whenever she would go into her lapses or what people used to think were drunken stupors, it was Alzheimer's setting in."[42]

In conjunction with this reading of Hayworth's story, the date when she supposedly developed Alzheimer's disease kept getting pushed back further and further. For example, in describing Hayworth's problems during the rehearsals for *Step on a Crack* in 1962, biographer Barbara Leaming wrote that the actress already "had fallen victim to a dementing disease that sooner or later inevitably interferes with job performance." Quoted in the *Ladies' Home Journal* article, Yasmin pushed the date back a few more years, suggesting that her mother may have had the disease for twenty-five years, beginning when Yasmin was a child and Hayworth was about 40 years old. "I can go back and all of it connects now," she stated, recalling her mother

throwing out perfectly good food and putting clothes in the wrong clos-
ets. While symptoms of Alzheimer's exist for many years before diagnosis,
twenty-five years is on the long side.[43]

In attempting to understand what made this version of Rita Hayworth's
illness so appealing, we need to understand the story in its historical context. As of the early 1980s, Katzman and other neurologists were actively
trying to change how the medical profession and, by extension, society
understood dementia. As noted earlier, Alzheimer's disease, as it affected
younger persons, had fallen off the radar screen. In the case of old people,
it was believed not to be relevant. The doctors who sought to put Alzheimer's front and center, the media that began to cover this story, and family members seeking definitive diagnoses had little interest in ambiguity.
Indeed, one of the first decisions made by the fledgling ADRDA was to
focus primarily on Alzheimer's—as opposed to all causes of dementia—so
as not to muddy the waters.

Thus, the more straightforward version of Hayworth's saga, which
downplayed her longtime alcoholism and emotional lability, made it an ideal
tutorial for publicizing this old—but now new—disease. If the actress's earliest symptoms had truly represented undiagnosed Alzheimer's, the same
possibility applied for other people experiencing incipient memory loss.
Such a suspicion might be the impetus for an early doctor's visit and possible interventions.

This reading of events had another great virtue. Even though alcoholism
was technically a "disease," it could not help but raise issues of Hayworth's
culpability in the whole scenario. Alzheimer's, in contrast, exonerated her.
"But it's upsetting that we all thought that she was drinking and we attributed all of her behavior to her being an alcoholic," Hayworth's nephew
Richard Cansino later recalled. "I feel guilty I perceived it that way." Even
Princess Yasmin, who has consistently been open about her mother's drinking problems, stated that "I want to communicate that my mother is a victim of this horrible disease and not some sort of wretched alcoholic."[44]

The dominant narrative that emerged about Rita Hayworth's case also
jibed seamlessly with the mindset of the Alzheimer's activists. Many of the
founders of the first groups had become energized due to their anger and
frustration over the delayed diagnosis of a loved one. For example, Robert
Wollin—the father of Lonnie Wollin, who founded the New York group
in 1972—had seen doctors all over the city, who had diagnosed only "hard-

ening of the arteries." Chicago businessman Jerome Stone, who became the first president of the ADRDA in 1979, had to travel to the Massachusetts General Hospital to get a definitive diagnosis for his wife, Evelyn. He was also stunned to find out just how little information existed about presenile dementia in neurology textbooks.[45]

When the announcement was made in 1981 that Rita Hayworth had Alzheimer's disease, Rhonie Berlinger, a member of the New York chapter of the ARDRA, had an idea. Why not approach Princess Yasmin and urge her to become active in the association? When Berlinger, Wollin, and Alzheimer's education specialist Miriam Aronson went to visit the princess, Wollin recalls, "she was as scared a caretaker as I have seen." The visitors wound up spending most of their time telling her about adult diapers, hospital beds, and other equipment that could ease her burden. They also provided Princess Yasmin with emotional support. In turn, Yasmin told her visitors that she was only too glad to join them in their mission. "I didn't hesitate at all," she stated. "It was a natural flow."[46]

There were only a couple of caveats, Yasmin told them. First, in contrast to her mother, she was quite shy and did not like public speaking. And second, she was not interested in doing fundraising. But the princess soon changed her mind on both scores. In the early 1980s she approached Jerome Stone with the idea of doing an annual fundraising gala in honor of Rita Hayworth. Now held twice a year, in Chicago and New York, these events have been extremely successful, raising more than $40 million to date for research into Alzheimer's. And Princess Yasmin, who subsequently became the president of Alzheimer's Disease International, is now a highly visible activist.[47]

Central to this dramatic success was the fact that Rita Hayworth was a beloved celebrity and her daughter a wealthy, socially connected heiress. (Yasmin's father, Aly Khan, died in an automobile accident in 1960 and left her a substantial sum of money.) The connection between celebrity and disease activism had existed for decades. For example, Mary Lasker, wife of the prominent advertising executive Albert Lasker, had energized both the National Institutes of Health and the American Cancer Society in the decades after World War II. And as we have seen, certain celebrities, such as Brian Piccolo, had given their names to foundations attacking specific diseases.

But the relationship between Yasmin Aga Khan and the ADRDA, which became the Alzheimer's Association in 1988, took this process to new heights. Princess Yasmin, by dint of her Hollywood connections, could attract very generous donors to the Alzheimer's cause. And because of who she and her mother were, the media took note. So did Congress, where Yasmin testified and met personally with legislators, helping to increase federal funding for Alzheimer's research from $146 million in 1990 to $679 million in 2004. This money has helped to produce a series of scientific breakthroughs, including improved diagnostic tools, the identification of genetic markers for the disease, and the development of several drugs that may slow the progression of the disease.[48]

Just as in the case of Lou Gehrig, Lonnie Wollin notes, the name Rita Hayworth "personalized the disease and gave us name recognition." Jerome Stone agrees. Rita Hayworth, he says, gave the Alzheimer's Association "cachet." When another Alzheimer's caregiver, "Desperate in Long Island," wrote to "Dear Abby" in June 1983, indicating her feelings of helplessness in caring for her father, Van Buren not only provided information about the Alzheimer's Association but also wrote: "Do you remember Rita Hayworth, the beautiful actress who married Prince Aly Khan? She is a victim of Alzheimer's." Activists for other diseases, notably AIDS and breast cancer, have subsequently emulated the Alzheimer's model, recruiting celebrities and building bonds in Hollywood.[49]

Beyond the biannual Rita Hayworth galas, images of the actress have become a familiar part of Alzheimer's awareness. In 2001, for example, the Alzheimer's Association aired a public service announcement across the country that showed an old clip of Hayworth dancing with Fred Astaire. The message: "Alzheimer's afflicts even the world's prettiest and most famous faces." Yasmin Aga Khan has participated in many educational ventures, such as narrating a film, *Losing It All: The Reality of Alzheimer's Disease*. Although Ronald Reagan may now be the best-known victim of the disease, Hayworth has remained indelibly associated with Alzheimer's for over twenty years.

And so has her daughter, Yasmin Aga Khan. Perhaps in no other disease is the role of caregiver so important, and so potentially neglected. Princess Yasmin's decision to sacrifice her own career to tend to her increasingly demented mother, and her continued activism long after her mother's death, have made her even more of a celebrity in the Alzheimer's community than Rita Hayworth. "Rita may have been a star known by the world," Patricia A. Sprague, whose mother had Alzheimer's, wrote in response to Yasmin's 1987 *People* article. "But in my opinion the real stars are the care givers who daily witness the ravages of the disease." As with the other cases in this book, it was often the ordinariness of famous patients—and their loved ones—that made their stories so compelling for nonfamous Americans confronting the same medical and emotional issues.[50]

And, as the cult of celebrity in America increasingly came to include the lives of nonfamous individuals, ordinary people who became sick might find themselves on the front page of newspapers across the country. This was the case with Barney Clark, a Seattle dentist who became the world's first recipient of a permanent artificial heart in 1982. Clark would spend his last 112 days with this heart in his chest, tethered to a nearly 400-pound machine that enabled it to function. During this time, his family members struggled mightily with a series of problems. How aggressive should they be in prolonging his life? Who should make the decisions, the doctors or the family? And was it ever acceptable to "pull the plug," to turn off the machines that were keeping Clark alive? In publicizing these questions, which applied to countless dying patients, the Barney Clark case provided Americans with an unexpected crash course in medical technology and human experimentation.

Chapter 9

Hero or Victim?

Barney Clark and the Technological Imperative

Most applications to institutional review boards to obtain permission for medical research do not quote Theodore Roosevelt. But one exception was the request submitted by William C. DeVries, who eventually became the first surgeon to implant a permanent artificial heart. "Far better it is to dare mighty things, to win glorious triumphs, even though checkered by failure," Roosevelt had said, "than to take rank with those who neither enjoy nor suffer much, because they live in the great twilight that knows neither victory nor defeat."[1]

The quotation was removed from the revised version of the application, but the sentiment was not. DeVries and his colleagues saw the artificial heart not merely as a treatment for congestive heart failure but as a revolutionary approach to stave off death. However, the University of Utah Medical Center was not San Juan Hill. The doctors there well knew that the old days, in which paternalistic and sometimes arrogant physicians simply told patients what to do, were gone. The revamped system was one that valued patient autonomy, in which the sick person was entitled to make his or her own medical decisions. Extensive, detailed consent forms, drafted with the help of the new medical center employees, bioethicists, sought to ensure that modern research subjects, unlike those in the past, were fully informed about their options.

The form that Barney B. Clark signed before receiving an artificial heart was eleven pages long. Clark, well-educated and medically sophisticated, had devoted a tremendous amount of time to learning about the new technology. At first glance, therefore, his willingness to receive the heart represented a triumph of patient autonomy and thus the new bioethics.

But when Clark died four months later, after an incredibly rocky medical course, almost nobody agreed with this assessment—at least on the record. Commentators, including bioethicists, were highly critical of the University of Utah. Meanwhile, members of the Clark family, caught up in an unexpected maelstrom of publicity, tried to make sense out of questions they never thought they would have to confront. The one person who might have provided some answers to these questions—Barney Clark—had very little to say before he died. And even when he spoke, it was hard to know what he was really feeling.

Clark was born to Mormon parents in Provo, Utah, on January 21, 1921. He graduated from high school in 1939, eventually joining the military during World War II. In 1944 Clark married Una Loy Mason, with whom he would have three children, Gary, Stephen, and Karen.

After World War II, Clark enrolled at and graduated from Brigham Young University. He then matriculated at the University of Washington Dental School in Seattle. He worked as a dentist in the Seattle area for twenty-five years, until poor health forced him to retire in 1978. The tall and strapping Clark had developed congestive heart failure, meaning that his heart muscle did not pump effectively. This led him to become short of breath when playing golf, his favorite pastime. Clark's breathing problem was exacerbated by some degree of emphysema, a form of lung disease.

By 1980, Clark's heart condition had worsened. His Seattle cardiologist, Terence Block, referred him to Jeffrey Anderson, a cardiologist at the University of Utah Medical Center. The Clarks still had family ties in Utah and had remained members of the Church of Latter-day Saints (LDS). Anderson entered Clark into an investigational study of a new drug, amrinone, but without much effect. Clark was too old for a heart transplant, but in October 1982, Anderson told him that his colleagues were researching the implantation of artificial hearts for patients with severe heart failure. The Clarks had heard about this procedure on television. They agreed to meet with the surgeon in charge of the project, William DeVries, and toured a facility containing dozens of animals that had successfully received artificial hearts. Among these was a sheep, named Ted E. Baer, who had survived for more than five months. Clark also learned about a calf, named

Lord Tennyson, who had survived 268 days. He returned to Seattle without having decided about trying the new device.

At the end of November 1982, Clark's heart situation drastically deteriorated, leaving him too short of breath to walk. At that point, he chose to go to Salt Lake City to receive an artificial heart. After meeting with hospital staff and signing a specially designed consent form twice within twenty-four hours, Clark went to the operating room on the night of December 1, 1982. There, doctors removed his natural heart and replaced it with an aluminum and polyurethane Jarvik-7 heart, the latest version of a device under development for years. The heart was connected via plastic tubes to a 375-pound air compressor that Clark would have to "wear" for the rest of his life.[2]

The surgery took nine hours, longer than expected due to difficulties getting the heart to work and the fragility of the tissue in Clark's chest. Postoperatively, as discussed extensively below, Clark suffered a series of setbacks. But he also had periods when he seemed to be recovering. On March 2, 1983, he appeared on national television being interviewed by his surgeon, DeVries. But on March 21, Clark's condition took a major turn for the worse, including a blood infection and kidney failure. He died on March 23, 1983, 112 days after the initial operation. The artificial heart was functioning well, but the rest of Clark's organs had stopped working.[3]

The media coverage of the Clark case demonstrates the remarkable degree to which illnesses of famous patients had gone public over the previous decades. When Lou Gehrig was discharged from the Mayo Clinic in 1939, the hospital had issued a brief press release. By the time of John Foster Dulles's cancer twenty years later, Walter Reed Hospital was holding daily news conferences and providing details of his treatment and prognosis. In Clark's case, the University of Utah made a conscious decision to emphasize open disclosure; the publicity that resulted can only be described as enormous. Journalists from around the world attended well-orchestrated press conferences twice daily.[4]

This is not to say that Clark had no privacy. Reporters were not allowed onto the wards of the hospital or to see him directly (although a few tried to get access surreptitiously or hired hospital staff to do so). His family members were largely protected from reporters, except when they willingly appeared at press conferences or gave interviews.

The reason for the intense excitement, of course, was the novelty of the procedure. In 1969 and 1981, Texas heart surgeon Denton A. Cooley had implanted his version of the artificial heart into patients as a bridge to transplantation. In Clark's case, however, the device was meant to be permanent. Not surprisingly, some of the media coverage addressed philosophical aspects of the operation, including speculation that replacement of the natural heart, long seen as the emotional center of a person's being, might somehow change the patient's personality.[5]

But most newspaper articles and television stories focused on Clark's medical progress and the enormous burden that had been placed on him and his family. As with the Karen Ann Quinlan case of the mid-1970s, which had sparked a nationwide debate on the right to die, Clark's situation was "an educational case study for the American public" on a series of crucial issues, such as the benefits and risks of medical technology and the use of informed consent as a prerequisite to medical experimentation. As Clark's condition worsened, the issue raised by the Quinlan case—when is it time to say "enough"?—recurred, but in quite a different fashion.[6]

Early on in Clark's saga, the media relied on the press conferences for information. The two main sources were Chase Peterson, vice president for the University of Utah Health Sciences campus, and John Dwan, director of public affairs for the medical center. Thus, on December 2, 1982, the press dutifully reported that Clark had become the first recipient of a permanent artificial heart. By December 4, newspapers were quoting Peterson as saying that Clark's color had gone from an underoxygenated blue before surgery to a healthy pink. Clark, the *Washington Post* reported, was "In the Pink." The patient's vital signs, including his blood pressure and temperature, were normal.[7]

Of course, it was hard for both the hospital staff and journalists not to be excited about what had occurred. A man with an artificial appliance circulating his blood was very much alive, even requesting a drink of water. "Surgeons Stand in Awe as Implant Defies Death," headlined the *Portland Oregonian*. Even the usually staid editorial page of the *Wall Street Journal* announced that the "miraculous" had been achieved. Analogizing Clark's operation to the American space program, which had freed mankind from the constraints of gravity, the editorialist wrote: "That same window on freedom is the thrill of the artificial heart."[8]

But the Utah spokespeople tried assiduously to contain their optimism, warning that complications could still develop. And they soon did. On

December 4, DeVries and his colleagues repaired air leaks in Clark's lungs. The press reported this complication, as well as a severe bout of brain seizures Clark suffered on December 7. The seizure episode, however, also demonstrated the limits of allowable candor. In the weeks following the seizures, Clark's mental status remained clouded. The possible connection of the two events was not discussed publicly, nor was the belief of some of the physicians that they had inadvertently caused the seizures by turning up the output of the artificial heart. Clark required two other operations. On December 14 he underwent replacement of a broken left ventricle, and on January 18, 1983, he had surgery to stop severe nose bleeding.[9]

In the coming weeks, the press would report on Clark's many ups and downs. Yet, while reporters continued to rely on Peterson and Dwan, they increasingly sought other sources, such as the Clark family or other physicians across the country. A few doctors, most notably Denton Cooley, objected to what had occurred, stating that the device had not been ready for elective implantation. Journalists also penned the typical human interest stories that accompany major events—features on the valiant yet grandfatherly Clark; the tall, "frontier" surgeon DeVries; the handsome physician-bioengineer Robert K. Jarvik, who had designed the Jarvik-7 heart; and Willem J. Kolff, the senior member of the Utah team who had championed the artificial heart for decades. Una Loy Clark, petite, tough, and unfailingly pleasant, was also a favorite of reporters. The public responded avidly to the story, sending many thousands of letters of encouragement to the Clarks. "God bless and keep you," wrote President Ronald Reagan and Nancy Reagan. "Our hearts and prayers are with you and your family. You have given us all a great lesson in courage and faith."[10]

Clark's saga inspired a variety of other news stories. For example, William J. Broad of the *New York Times* reported that the operation had been a financial windfall for the University of Utah and Kolff Medical, the company that developed the Jarvik-7 heart. And Broad's colleague, physician-journalist Lawrence K. Altman, educated readers about congestive heart failure and other medical topics. DeVries was especially pleased about this type of coverage. "I think medicine has gotten a lot out of [the artificial heart]," he later stated, "because suddenly people are aware of what the heart is, what it does, how it works, where it is and things like that from listening to the news.[11]

Journalists also asked how Clark had agreed to become the first recipient of the Jarvik-7. Their articles described how Clark had met DeVries, learned about the artificial heart, and, when his condition worsened, contacted the surgeon to begin the process. In addition, reporters detailed what had happened when Clark arrived at the University of Utah Medical Center on November 29, 1982. He had met with several members of the artificial heart team, including DeVries, two cardiologists, a psychiatrist, a social worker, and a nurse, who screened him for fitness to proceed. They were all impressed. As social worker Margaret (Peggy) Miller told the *New York Times*, "He had a strong will to live, had an intelligent, thorough understanding of his disease and what his option was, was a flexible person and had a loving, supportive family." Chase Peterson agreed, noting that Clark was bright, articulate, and knowledgeable.[12]

The press also reported that the consent form signed by Clark had been blunt in its language, with a "doom-laden" last sentence indicating that there were no guarantees. Just before signing for the second time, reporters wrote, Clark had made a joke, noting that "there sure would be a lot of long faces around here if I backed out now." Finally, reporters wrote that the doctors had decided to do the operation earlier than expected, on the night of December 1 rather than the morning of December 2, since Clark's condition had apparently worsened.[13]

Given the early optimism following the operation, the press had not raised the topic of Clark's likely mode of death. But Willem Kolff did. Kolff had wended his way to Utah as part of a remarkable career in developing medical technology. During World War II, as the Nazis occupied his native Holland, he had built the world's first artificial kidney dialysis machine with his own hands. Kolff later joined the staff of the Cleveland Clinic, where he began his work on an artificial heart. In 1967 he moved to the University of Utah as head of the Artificial Organs Division.

In contrast to other members of the artificial heart team, who carefully stuck to a prearranged script when speaking with the press, the straight-shooting Kolff said what was on his mind. On December 4 he remarked that Barney Clark would be given a key to turn off the artificial heart if he so chose. "If the man suffers and feels it isn't worth it any more," Kolff said, "he has a key that he can apply."[14]

Kolff's comments caused a major stir, not only because he had raised the uncomfortable issue of the experiment's failure but because the notion of a patient using a key to end his own life seemed macabre. Indeed, some members of the press began to refer to Clark's "suicide key." Peterson quickly moved to defuse the situation, stating that there was little chance the key would be used, by either Clark or a staff member, to terminate Clark's life.[15]

But by raising the issue of how Clark would actually die, the key controversy prepared the public for his inevitable death while attached to the machine. Thus, when Clark began to deteriorate seriously at the end of March 1983, there was frank discussion of how his unexplained fever and kidney failure were life-threatening. And when the rest of his organs failed on March 23, the press reported that DeVries had indeed turned the key shutting off the artificial heart, which was still functioning well.[16]

Ultimately, the University of Utah's openness about its "tragic and triumphant research-patient celebrity" allowed for a remarkable degree of scrutiny of what had happened. Given that the artificial heart raised profound issues about human experimentation, bold new medical technology, and the doctor-patient relationship, Clark's saga became a sort of test case for the new bioethics. After all, when Clark went under the knife in late 1982, the President's Commission for the Study of Ethical Problems in Medicine and Behavioral Research, chaired by Morris Abram, had just issued its report on medical decision-making. Not surprisingly, therefore, bioethicists and other critics closely scrutinized the Clark experiment.[17]

Perhaps the topic that generated the most interest was informed consent. Ensuring that subjects gave true informed consent before entering research studies had been one of the commission's foremost concerns. So how well had the system worked? In volunteering to be the first recipient of a permanent artificial heart, had Clark really known what he was getting into? Or was he another victim of a scientific establishment that hoodwinked subjects into participating in inappropriate experiments?

The overwhelming evidence is that Clark was, as university spokespeople had claimed, fully informed. Some worrisome things had occurred, such as the way in which he had become familiar with the artificial heart. By taking Clark to the animal barn to view the large number of animals living satisfactorily with the same device, DeVries and his veterinary colleagues may have too strongly implied that a human would necessarily do as well. And DeVries had provided another, not so gentle, push, telling Clark in October 1982 that if he, DeVries, were in the same position, he would go ahead with the implant. "I said I wouldn't hesitate," DeVries later told Earl and Miriam Selby, who were writing a book on the Clark case. "And if I didn't feel that way about it I wouldn't have ever offered it to patients."[18]

Still, DeVries had cautioned Clark that his own willingness to enter such an experiment did not imply that he thought it would be successful. "Barney," he recalled telling Clark, "I can't tell you that you are going to live any longer with this device. In fact, you may live shorter." The consent form that Clark signed twice had clearly stated this as well. It read, in part:

> No representations have been made to me with respect to whether the procedure will be successful, nor the length of time which the artificial heart device will function, nor the level at which it will function. I recognize that if the artificial heart fails, death or serious injury is the near certain result. I nevertheless accept the risk of substantial and serious harm, including death, in the hope that beneficial effects of the implantation of the artificial heart device can be demonstrated. No guarantees have been made to me concerning the result of the operation or procedure.

The consent form also spelled out a large number of possible complications, including emboli (blood clots), infection, hemorrhage, pneumothorax (air in the chest cavity), and "other risks which are not foreseeable at this time and may arise."[19]

Hospital staff had read the entire eleven-page document along with Clark to make sure he understood what he was signing. To the degree that Clark, who was quite ill, was able to pay attention during this process, he surely knew that there were not only no guarantees but an extremely high likelihood of problems. What made the argument that Clark was fully informed even more compelling, however, were his statements and behavior before he actually consented. Clark and his family, including his son Stephen, an ear, nose, and throat physician, were medically savvy people. Clark had signed consent forms for other research projects, including one for the amrinone study. And he had actively sought second opinions about his heart failure.[20]

Moreover, in discussions with his physicians, family, and friends about the artificial heart, Clark consistently stated that he knew he was entering wholly uncharted waters. Clark's Seattle cardiologist, Terence Block, had told his patient that instead of being the first to try the new device, it made more sense to be the one-hundredth. But Clark had decided to go ahead for two reasons. First, he had been told that his heart failure would soon proceed to a point where there were no other options except certain death. Second, he indicated his sincere interest in making a contribution to science before he died, echoing the utilitarian philosophy that Morris Abram espoused in his later writings. Clark was grateful to the medical profession, which he believed had extended his life, and he repeatedly stated that he wanted to give something back. After his first meeting with DeVries, Una Loy Clark said, her husband had stated that it would give him "a great deal of satisfaction if he could receive the heart and make a contribution to Medical Science." When Clark decided to go ahead in November 1982, he said: "I would like my life [and] even perhaps my death to count for something."[21]

Clark thus said and did all the right things to demonstrate that he consented to the artificial heart with full knowledge and without coercion. But some critics raised a larger philosophical question. Was it truly possible to give informed consent to an experimental procedure when the other option was certain death? As the bioethicist Albert R. Jonsen cogently argued at a conference on the Clark case held in Alta, Utah, in October 1983, the misleading notion that the artificial heart was somehow a therapy for Clark had masked the boldly utilitarian goal of the procedure—which had been to acquire scientific knowledge. Even William DeVries, when asked, admitted that "disease is coercive."[22]

The frank Willem Kolff had a particularly interesting take on the matter. Noting how the consent form had gone into excruciating detail about likely complications, he remarked that he was amazed that anyone at all would sign up. Kolff's European colleagues had told him that their patients would have "run out of the hospitals in fear" after reading even one-third of Clark's consent form. In other words, it was almost as if signing such a document was itself evidence of a lack of judgment.[23]

The notion that it was irrational for Clark to have agreed to receive an artificial heart led to scrutiny of the process by which the experiment was allowed to proceed. Approval by the University of Utah Institutional Review Board (IRB) for Research with Human Subjects was necessary. The federal government, in addition to forming Abram's commission, had responded to the medical research scandals of the 1970s by mandating that all institutions conducting human experimentation establish internal review panels to approve research projects. By the time of the Clark case, there were between five hundred and a thousand such boards. Members generally consisted of some combination of research physicians, nurses, chaplains, lawyers, and lay representatives.[24]

Because the artificial heart was a new medical device, approval by the federal Food and Drug Administration's Bureau of Medical Devices was also necessary. In September 1981 the FDA gave the University of Utah permission to implant the heart in seven patients who had undergone heart surgery and could not successfully come off the heart pump—in other words, patients who would have otherwise died within minutes. But when no such patients became available, the FDA, in May 1982, expanded the pool to include patients like Clark with "end stage chronic congestive heart failure secondary to idiopathic (cause unknown) cardiomyopathy." The local IRB at the University of Utah also approved both sets of patients.[25]

As with all IRBs, the deliberations at the University of Utah were kept private, but worrisome details about the process gradually became known. One scholar who wrote extensively on this issue was University of Pennsylvania sociologist Renee C. Fox, who conducted research on the Clark case with her longtime colleague Judith P. Swazey. Fox and Swazey had been studying clinical trials for decades when they arrived in Salt Lake City shortly after Clark's death. They performed copious research, reviewing the media coverage of the case, conducting interviews with the major participants, and examining unpublished documents. Fox and Swazey conducted their study as "objectively" as possible, but ultimately rendered several opinions about what had occurred.[26]

Those approving the experiment, they concluded, had inadequately scrutinized DeVries's earlier research. For example, there had been objections by certain national heart specialists, who had urged the FDA not to approve the artificial heart but rather approve a left ventricular assist device that was inserted directly into a failing heart. Some of this concern stemmed from published articles documenting a large series of complications witnessed in animals with artificial hearts that were likely to also occur in human subjects. At some of the early Utah IRB meetings, those in attendance, even Robert Jarvik, had expressed reservations as to whether the Jarvik-7 was ready to go.[27]

The Utah IRB, Fox wrote, had established an artificial heart subcommittee to work with DeVries to revise his application into a suitable form, including removing the Theodore Roosevelt quotation. In so overstepping its role, she believed, the IRB had not been able to function as an effective guardian of the review process. This situation had resulted, interviewees told Fox, because DeVries lacked the experience and expertise to design and conduct clinical research. Fox and Swazey even later analogized De-Vries, whose ambitious visions for the artificial heart never came to fruition, to Willy Loman, the tragic protagonist of Arthur Miller's play *Death of a Salesman*.[28]

After the Clark case, the Utah IRB declined to approve a second implan-tation, which raised questions about other improprieties that it may have discovered. One issue being discussed was the procedure by which Clark had been given medical clearance to receive an artificial heart. During the 112 days he survived after surgery, he had persistent lung problems, which the doctors attributed to emphysema, likely caused by his twenty-five-year history of smoking cigarettes. Clark had carried this diagnosis for several years, and breathing tests performed in both May and November 1979 had shown "severe obstructive airway disease." One of the stated disqualifica-tions for an artificial heart in the Utah protocol was severe lung disease.[29]

Although it was true that Clark had never needed medication for the condition, it does seem that the magnitude of the lung problem got lost in the excitement of the consent process. The suggestion that he might not have been an appropriate medical candidate just added to the sense that Clark's doctors had received insufficient oversight.

Another issue that Fox and others found problematic was the behavior of Ross Woolley, an engineer and University of Utah faculty member who was vice chairman of the IRB. Most IRBs perform little or no surveillance of the research projects they have approved, rather relying on the integrity of the investigators to do what they said they would. Although some crit-ics believe that IRBs should be more hands-on, few would countenance what Woolley, at the invitation of DeVries, did. He saw Barney Clark every day, read his chart, made rounds with the artificial heart team, and became a confidante of Una Loy Clark.[30]

How did Woolley assume such a role? At the Alta conference, Renee Fox pointed to the culture of Mormon Utah as an explanation. Woolley, she stated, was a Mormon elder, a highly respected senior member of the LDS church. He thus was able to assume a "priestly" function as the "moral watchman" in the case. Fox noted that Woolley's role was especially worrisome because, as a member of the IRB that approved the implant, he had a logical interest in seeing the experiment "succeed." DeVries and Chase Peterson later agreed that Woolley's efforts had been inappropriate.[31]

Fox noted two other salient characteristics of Mormonism that had influenced the Clark case. First, the faith's strong sense of kinship, which saw the family as the "basic unit of society," led to a remarkable degree of personal interaction between Barney Clark and hospital staff members, many of whom were LDS church members. Woolley and his colleagues bonded especially deeply with Una Loy Clark, who was enormously respected for her dedication, strength, and compassion. Fox described how the doctors frequently brought their families, including children, to visit the Clarks during the hospitalization. One physician's children, she added, had become so close to the Clarks that they considered them to be an additional set of grandparents. Fox's concern about this situation was implied: such an interaction, while commendable in its warmth, represented a conflict of interest for the physicians, who needed to retain a healthy objectivity about the medical condition of their patient.[32]

Second, Fox noted how the history of Mormonism was infused with a sense of "manifest destiny," in both a secular and spiritual sense. Fleeing religious persecution, the charismatic Mormon leader Brigham Young had established a frontier outpost in 1847 in what would become Utah. Mormonism, Fox wrote, placed a high emphasis on "personal and collective achievement, accomplishment, mastery, and progress through vigorous human effort, animated by rationality, knowledge and intelligence." Science and research were thus a way to honor the glory of God. Nearly all of the major players in the Clark case, it seemed, represented this ethos: DeVries, who was raised a Mormon and was married to a devout Mormon; Clark, whom Chase Peterson, also a member of the LDS church, termed "a pioneer to match these Western lands"; and even Kolff, who, although not a Mormon, was analogized to Brigham Young for having brought the artificial heart program to Utah.[33]

In sum, according to Fox, Mormonism had helped shape the artificial heart team's values, vocabulary, leadership, and organization, as well as its relationships to the Clark family, the IRB, the press, and the public. That is, the cultural setting of the experiment had led to unrealistic expectations about what could be achieved. Putting an artificial heart in Barney Clark,

Fox and Swazey ultimately concluded, had been "fundamentally unethical" and "profoundly disquieting," characterized by "dangerous excesses" and "misconduct."[34]

The last concern raised by critics addressed not the decision to proceed with the experiment but the events after Clark received the artificial heart. Didn't 112 difficult days in a hospital, marked by multiple complications as well as frequent confusion and persistent shortness of breath, "prove" that the implant had been a terrible mistake?

Several representatives from the world of bioethics weighed in on this issue. For example, Arthur I. Caplan of the Hastings Center, a New York ethics think tank, argued that implantation of the heart in a human had been premature. Something about the case, wrote University of Alabama ethicist Gregory E. Pence, "seemed fishy." Boston University lawyer and bioethicist George J. Annas agreed, terming the experiment a "halfway success." True, Clark had survived for a time, but with "severe confusion, mental incompetence, or coma." Because Clark had not been adequately prepared for this possibility, Annas believed, the consent process was not truly informed.[35]

Others who emphasized what they saw as Clark's suffering included a Seattle cardiologist, Thomas A. Preston, and University of California historian Barton J. Bernstein. Preston wrote that rather than experiencing a peaceful death from heart failure, Clark had instead undergone a series of painful medical procedures that increased his discomfort. Bernstein argued there was no evidence that the massive federal investment in artificial hearts would ever truly improve the quality of life of patients like Clark.[36]

Among the most virulent critics of the artificial heart was the editorial page of the *New York Times*. On December 16, 1982, right after the emergency surgery to repair Clark's heart valve, a *Times* editorial asked: "But can all that pain and exertion be worthwhile?" The purpose of medicine, the writer continued, was to improve the quality of life, "not to make Methuselahs of us all." The *Times* would later continue its criticism when DeVries performed three additional implantations of the Jarvik heart between November 1984 and April 1985 at the Humana Hospital in Louisville. Calling the artificial heart a "Dracula" project that sucked tens of millions of dollars out of the National Heart, Lung, and Blood Institute, the *Times* editorial writer said that it provided "dismal quality of life at vast expense."[37]

Additional ammunition for the argument that Clark had suffered too greatly came from two other sources. First was the two-and-a-half-minute video interview that was aired on March 2, 1983, at which point Clark had been living with the artificial heart for 91 days. He was seated, wearing pajamas and a dressing gown. DeVries asked Clark ten questions, all of which he answered in short sentences. Speaking seemed to make him more short of breath. When DeVries sympathetically asked whether his experience had been a "hard" one, Clark said yes. But Clark also reaffirmed his earlier decision to participate, even adding a plug for future volunteers. "It's worth it," he stated, "if the alternative is they either die or have it done."[38]

Like any other piece of film, what the interview demonstrated could be interpreted in many different ways. Some commentators marveled that a man who had lived for three months with an aluminum and plastic heart was interactive and communicative. But some critics savaged what they had seen, even describing Clark as "zombie-like." Clark's performance was not a "ringing endorsement," wrote Joe Morgenstern of the *Los Angeles Herald-Examiner.* "Clark seemed to be in so much pain," Morgenstern added, "that he sounded like a gallant press agent when he [said]: 'All in all, it has been a pleasure to be able to help people.'"[39]

DeVries and the University of Utah countered these negative assessments by stating that they had mistakenly interviewed Clark at the end of the day, when he was exceptionally tired. In addition, Clark's seeming lack of attention to DeVries stemmed from the fact that it was the officious Ross Woolley, off camera, who had actually been asking the questions. Nevertheless, the zombie accusation was hard to shake off.

Then, in September 1984, eighteen months after Clark's death, two University of Utah psychiatrists, Claudia K. Berenson and Bernard I. Grosser, published a controversial review of the case in a medical journal, the *Archives of General Psychiatry.* Berenson was the psychiatrist who had assessed Clark preoperatively; she also saw him occasionally during his hospitalization. Grosser was the chair of the psychiatry department. Among other findings, Berenson and Grosser reported that Clark had experienced organic brain syndrome—that is, mental confusion—during most of the 112 days. And the article reported that, during his worst moments, Clark was quite depressed, announcing that he wanted to die or be killed.[40]

Although aspects of this story had been reported before, this version received wide press coverage. Berenson explained that suicidal wishes were not uncommon among acutely ill patients and that Clark had convincingly denied suicidality on his more lucid days, but the psychiatrists' report nevertheless fostered the image of medical researchers torturing a dying man in order to keep their scientific experiment going. As such, it seemed to corroborate the gloomier assessments of Clark's experiences as reported by Fox and Swazey and the other critics.[41]

Should this version thus be considered the definitive story—that Barney Clark, while knowing what he was getting into, nevertheless submitted to an ill-advised and ultimately harmful experiment? Perhaps, but such an appraisal ignores the unique aspects of Clark's saga. For one thing, it may be inappropriate to use standard outcome measures when assessing a procedure such as the insertion of an artificial heart. While surgeons may usually define success as discharging their patients, with healed incisions, after thirty days, such criteria may not apply to an operation that was, by definition, such a long shot.[42]

If critics potentially disregarded the extraordinary nature of the Clark case, they also ignored what made Clark's 112 days very ordinary. To be sure, the artificial heart was a landmark medical technology. But in the 1980s, as now, certain patients willingly submitted to risky experimental or therapeutic interventions that other patients would decline. And the assessment of such efforts depends not only on the ultimate medical outcome but on the day-to-day ups and downs as experienced by patients and their families.

In Clark's case, there were several periods of time during which he seemed to be getting better. These were dutifully and enthusiastically reported by the press. For example, on December 18, 1982, four days after undergoing repair of his damaged left ventricle, Clark sat in a chair, looking out of a window with a view of the Wasatch Mountains. Doctors reported that it was his "best day in two months." Clark then spent a "joyous" Christmas with his family and members of the hospital staff. He was speaking more and able to take a few steps around his room.[43]

As of mid-February 1983, after his nose-bleeding problems had largely resolved, Clark was standing and walking even more; he was transferred to a private room outside the intensive care unit. By early March, shortly after the videotaped interview, he was doing even better. Una Loy reported that their thirty-ninth anniversary, March 7, 1983, "was one of Barney's best days." "Barney is great," psychiatrist Claudia Berenson told *Time* maga-

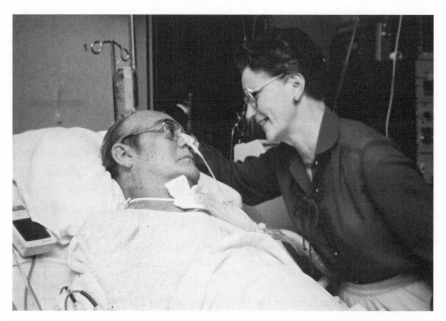

Una Loy Clark at her husband's bedside. The quality of Barney Clark's existence after he received an artificial heart was the subject of heated debate. Photograph from the Barney Clark papers, Special Collections Department, J. Willard Marriott Library, University of Utah.

zine for its March 14 issue. "He is a totally different person." The *Time* article showed Clark undergoing physical therapy and speculated about his leaving the hospital, albeit hooked up to the cumbersome air compressor. Although these assessments, in retrospect, exaggerated what Clark was actually accomplishing, they at least raised the chance that he might get out of the woods. Given that immediate death had been a distinct possibility after implantation of the artificial heart, it was hardly surprising that the media and the public would celebrate the fact that Clark was walking, talking, and reasonably interactive. This remained true, moreover, despite the growing realization of many insiders that he was unlikely to ever truly recover.[44]

Indeed, Clark's postoperative period resembled that of many other patients who undergo extensive surgery with the hope of combating a serious medical condition. Changes in mental status, sometimes permanent, may occur with heart operations, like Clark's, that use a heart-lung bypass machine. Of those patients who survive major surgery, most require extensive physical therapy for weeks or months, often due to setbacks, such as those experienced by Clark. And of those who leave the hospital, many remain semi-invalids for the rest of their lives. As Una Loy commented, her husband was not a zombie but an ill man.[45]

Such cases also often result in disagreements among family members. This was the case with the Clarks. As Barney Clark experienced his roller-coaster ride of complications followed by recovery, it was his son Stephen who first contemplated holding off on further emergency surgery. As a physician, Stephen knew that patients who experienced such difficult post-operative courses generally did poorly. Shortly after his father died, Stephen Clark gave an exclusive interview to the *AMA News*, a weekly newspaper published by the American Medical Association. Clark said that the whole experience had left "an ambivalent taste" in his mouth. "The operation," he stated, "was clearly not worth it for Dad in terms of any useful prolongation of his life, in terms of any added quality of life."[46]

Stephen Clark's comments, coming amidst a torrent of eulogies for his father, rubbed some people the wrong way. But his statements were honest. Una Loy Clark had herself struggled with what to do each time her husband deteriorated. She was well aware that he was suffering, as she revealed in a series of letters to her friends. "Barney continues to be plagued with complications," she wrote in January 1983, "each one seeming to be brought on by the complication preceding it." Una Loy was also very candid in a series of interviews she gave to the Selbys. For example, she admitted that she had felt very discouraged at the time of the surgery for the nose bleeding. "I think I was beginning to feel like Barney had had enough," she said.[47]

But ultimately, weighing advice from DeVries, the other physicians, social worker Peggy Miller, and her family, Una Loy Clark did what she thought her husband would have wanted, which was to keep the experiment going. This meant agreeing to aggressive therapy, including the three operations. Another factor that helped Una Loy was her religion. Before Barney had agreed to the implant, she and he had contemplated the meaning of the artificial heart in the context of Mormon teachings. After Clark had become ill, he had returned to his religious roots, praying more regularly and "sealing" himself to Una Loy within the LDS church for eternity. The Clarks concluded that the artificial heart embodied two of God's most precious gifts to man: life and the desire to gain knowledge. When Beth Ann Cole, a nurse on the University of Utah IRB, discussed Clark with a woman's group, mostly composed of Mormons, they strongly supported the implant, telling her that science should be given the opportunity to advance life. Thus, within the context of her individual life—which is, after all, how people make medical decisions—it made sense for Una Loy to continue trying to prolong her husband's life as long as possible.[48]

At least until March 21, 1983. On that day, with her husband going into kidney failure, Una Loy strongly considered withholding hemodialysis, detoxification of the blood with a machine. By this point, Clark was sicker than ever before and had almost no chance of recovery. Most of the doctors, as well as Stephen Clark, argued against dialysis. Una Loy never had to make the decision because her husband deteriorated so quickly, dying on March 23.

It is possible, therefore, to view Barney Clark's decision to undergo an experimental medical procedure and his 112-day attempt to return to an acceptable quality of life as not especially remarkable. Members of the public agreed. For example, Dorothy Gilliam told *Washington Post* readers about her father's premature death from a heart attack at the age of 51. "What if an artificial heart had been available when we stood helplessly by and watched someone we cared about slip past the physician's skill?" she mused. Technological progress must come in stages, Howard S. Miller explained in the *New York Times*. "The first stage may be undignified and painful, but until we have mastered the basics and the mechanics, we cannot move on to the complex and esthetic." Responding to one of his own newspaper's negative editorials on the artificial heart, the *Times* columnist William Safire remarked that "I'm glad that editorialist is not my doctor." The purpose of medicine was not only to improve the quality of life, he wrote, but to save lives. "If, in the process of averting death, a patient chooses to become a human guinea pig or to marry a bulky machine, the patient has the right to demand that the medical profession let him make that choice."[49]

Even Joe Morgenstern, the journalist who had chided Clark's video interview as unconvincing, had to admit that the prospect of any life at all was alluring. "I'd take it," he wrote, "for just one or two of the right days, when you're so precariously and amazingly alive that you truly comprehend the difference between being and not being." At the Alta conference, science writer Joann Ellison Rodgers reported that ten of eleven seriously ill heart patients interviewed at the time of Clark's surgery said they would have tried the implant.[50]

Letters sent to Una Loy Clark after her husband's death made many of the same points. One school-aged child sent a paper he had written, which stated that "the artificial heart is part of the gift of life that God has given us." "I lost a brother to heart disease and suffer from a serious heart problem myself," wrote another correspondent. "Dr. Clark has given us all hope."[51]

It was this hopeful message that Una Loy Clark came to embrace as a spokesperson for the American Heart Association. For four years after her husband died, she traveled the country, speaking on her experiences and the topic of heart disease. She often focused on cigarettes, which cause not only heart problems but also the lung disease that she believed had ultimately caused Barney Clark's death. Her late husband, she told audiences in her forthright fashion, should not have smoked for twenty-five years.[52]

When Una Loy Clark spoke of the artificial heart, she never denied what an ordeal the 112 days had been. But, she repeatedly said, she would do it all over again. So would her late husband, who, as Una Loy reminded audiences, had said so on tape two weeks before he died. Over the years, she remained friendly with and strongly supportive of Willem Kolff and Donald Olsen, the veterinarian in charge of the animal experiments at the University of Utah. At a Barney Clark Memorial Race held in June 1983, Una Loy stated that "in my estimation, the artificial heart is a huge success." At her heart association appearances, she told audiences that "my heart is really with the artificial heart."[53]

The story of the artificial heart after Barney Clark is complicated. Two of the three patients who received Jarvik-7 implants from DeVries at Humana survived for more than a year, but experienced very turbulent medical courses. In 1990 the FDA withdrew its approval for the permanent artificial heart program, stating that the risks outweighed the benefits. By this point, the left ventricular assist device was showing considerable promise and thus deemed much more worthy of funding.[54]

But the artificial heart lived on in two guises. First, Donald Olsen and his Utah colleagues continued to improve their technology, eventually devising the artificial CardioWest heart, which has been successfully used as a bridge to heart transplantation in more than 280 cases. Second, in 1988 the National Heart, Lung, and Blood Institute began to support a new generation of artificial hearts—ones that would be fully implantable in a patient's chest, thereby eliminating the tubes and air compressor of the earlier Jarvik model. One such heart is the AbioCor, developed by Abiomed. Between July 2001 and May 2004, surgeons implanted an AbioCor into fourteen patients. The longest period of survival was seventeen months.[55]

One of these patients was James Quinn, a 51-year-old retired baker who received an AbioCor on November 5, 2001, at Hahnemann University Hospital in Philadelphia. He survived nine months but experienced many complications, including a stroke, water in the lungs, and "excruciating pain." In contrast to Barney Clark, Quinn reported shortly before his death that accepting the artificial heart had been a mistake. "If I had to do it over again, I wouldn't do it," he stated. "No ma'am. I would take my chances on life."[56]

To some degree, Quinn's words were vindication for Renee Fox and Judith Swazey. In 1992 they had announced that they were "leaving the field" of research into human experimentation. One reason they gave was that despite their years of warnings, there was still disturbing overuse of lifesaving technologies, "a rescue-oriented and often zealous determination to maintain life at any cost, and a relentless, hubris-ridden refusal to accept limits." There were limits, they might have added, to the model of patient autonomy that supposedly protected research subjects like Barney Clark.[57]

But it still depended on whom you asked. William DeVries had little patience for his opponents. "The artificial heart was an easy target for critics, especially for the 'ethicists,' whoever and whatever they are," he stated in 1989. Then he played his trump card, commenting from the perspective of a doctor, not a detached academic: "Very few surgeons can turn their backs on a dying patient." For her part, Karen Clark Shaffer was glad that DeVries had not done so. When, on the twentieth anniversary of her father's receipt of an artificial heart, a reporter asked her about the critics who had so vilified the experiment, she became tearful. "I'd like to say," she stated, "that if perhaps it were their father, or their husband, or their wife, they might have a different opinion." Given how particular circumstances can dramatically influence the ways in which individuals respond to illnesses and later recall them, she may have been right.[58]

Like Barney Clark, Libby Zion became famous only because she got sick. Unlike Clark, however, Americans only learned the story of Zion after she had died. Libby's father, Sidney, subsequently embarked on a crusade to fix the problem that he believed had caused her mysterious death: the use of overtired, poorly supervised young doctors to provide patient care. Zion succeeded, leading to the overthrow of yet another of the formerly insular practices of the American medical profession.

Chapter 10

"You Murdered My Daughter"

Libby Zion and the Reform of Medical Education

"Some doctors," wrote a law clerk working on *Zion v. New York Hospital,* "will tell you that *Zion* is a clear case demonstrating the detrimental effect of a lack of supervision [of doctors-in-training], but showing nothing about the harm caused by sleep deprivation. Other doctors will argue precisely the opposite." As well as any other, Libby Zion's case demonstrates how different individuals can craft competing versions of the same historical events.[1]

After 18-year-old Libby Zion died a mysterious death at New York Hospital in 1984, at least five stories emerged that sought to provide a coherent account of what had happened—and why. The five stories, which at times overlapped, were as follows. (1) Libby Zion died because of medical malpractice, for which the doctors and hospital were culpable. (2) Libby Zion was killed by a broken medical system that left overworked and unsupervised young doctors in charge of her care. (3) Libby Zion died an unpreventable death from an unidentified cause. (4) Libby Zion died as a result of illicit cocaine use, which she concealed from doctors. And (5) Libby Zion "died twice," first at the hospital, then as the victim of a vicious smear campaign.

All of these versions had their limitations. Indeed, it is possible to construct a sixth and probably more accurate narrative, one that emphasizes the random nature of disease and how doctors "play the odds" when treating patients. But those involved in the Zion case were less in search of precisely truthful stories than impassioned ones.

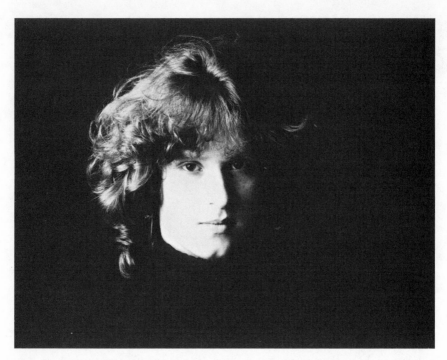

Libby Zion, in a photograph taken shortly before her death. Courtesy of Sidney Zion.

Despite the competing accounts of Libby Zion's death, some facts seem irrefutable. Zion was a student at Bennington College when she became ill in early March 1984, shortly after a tooth extraction. Her symptoms included a low-grade fever and an earache, for which a private doctor prescribed erythromycin, an antibiotic. At home, Zion got worse instead of better and began acting strangely, with agitation and jerking motions of her body. This led her parents, Elsa and Sidney Zion, to take her to the emergency room of New York Hospital on the night of March 4, 1984. Sidney Zion was a well-known investigative journalist and former lawyer.

The emergency room resident physician could not determine a clear source for Zion's temperature, which was 103 degrees, but found an elevated white blood cell count of 18,000, possibly indicative of bacterial infection. He also learned that Zion was taking an antidepressant known as Nardil, which had been prescribed by a psychiatrist. Aside from marijuana, she denied any use of other illicit drugs, including cocaine. The emergency room physician contacted Raymond Sherman, whom Sidney Zion had called before the family left for the hospital. Sherman, an attending physician on the staff of New York Hospital, had treated both Libby Zion and other family members in the past. The decision was made to admit Zion to the hospital, given her unexplained fever and strange behavior.[2]

When Libby Zion arrived on the hospital floor, a nurse noted that she was lucid at times but had periods of confusion. Two resident physicians, both of whom had been working for roughly eighteen hours—Luise Weinstein, an intern (first-year resident), and her supervisor, Gregg Stone, a second-year resident—evaluated Zion. Weinstein, who had graduated from medical school the previous spring, was covering about forty patients. Neither doctor knew exactly what was going on with Zion, but they were not especially alarmed. Stone's admission note raised several possible diagnoses, but highest on his list was "a viral syndrome with hysterical symptoms." Stone touched base with Sherman. The plan was to give Zion intravenous fluids and Tylenol for her fever while awaiting the results of other tests. The doctors ordered that the patient's vital signs—temperature, pulse, and blood pressure—be taken every four hours, no more frequently than routine.[3]

Having been reassured that their daughter was all right, Sidney and Elsa Zion went home around 3 a.m. on March 5. Although what happened next remains contested, some events seem clear. At 3:30 a.m., Libby Zion was given a shot of Demerol, an opiate medication, to help control her shaking movements. Around 4:15 a.m., fifteen minutes after Weinstein had left the floor to see other patients, Zion grew more agitated, swearing and trying to climb out of bed. One of the nurses, Jerylyn Grismer, called Weinstein and recommended that Zion be restrained. Weinstein, evidently believing that the behavior was more of what she had already seen, gave an oral order to do so. The senior nurse, Myrna Balde, evidently also paged Weinstein to apprise her of the situation. Following hospital protocol, the nurses first applied a Posey restraint that tied Zion's torso to the bed. When the Posey did not control Zion, the nurses next tied down her wrists and ankles. Still believing that the patient was in danger of hurting herself, Grismer called Weinstein again and asked her to come and evaluate Zion. Weinstein declined, indicating that she was with another sick patient and had seen Zion recently. Instead, Weinstein prescribed an injection of Haldol, a tranquilizer, which the nurses administered around 4:30 a.m.[4]

Finally, according to the nurses, Zion fell asleep. At 6 a.m., Balde later said, she awakened Zion and got her to take two Tylenol tablets, although this interaction was not recorded in the chart. One-half hour later, during the routine morning temperature checks, a nurse's aide found Zion's temperature to be extremely high, somewhere between 106 and 108 degrees. The nurses immediately called Weinstein, who ordered cold compresses and a cooling blanket. But ten minutes later, Zion was in cardiac arrest, presumably because her extremely high temperature had caused an irregular heart rhythm. Despite almost an hour of resuscitative efforts, Zion died.[5]

Whereas it is relatively easy to acknowledge flagrant medical mistakes, such as the administration of the wrong drug or dosage, errors of judgment are the least identifiable with the "truth." Thus, they will always inspire multiple and competing stories. This is exactly what happened in the Libby Zion case. The first such story, mainly "authored" by Sidney Zion, emerged in the hours and days after his daughter died. Even though this was the first story temporally, it should not be thought of as the correct, or definitive, account that later got amended. Rather, there was never a definitive story. All of the accounts were spun from the start, both consciously and unconsciously.[6]

The first story began when Sidney Zion received a phone call from Raymond Sherman at 7:45 a.m. on March 5, 1983. Sherman said to Zion, "It's very bad, very bad." He told Zion to come to the hospital immediately. Shortly thereafter, Luise Weinstein, the intern, called the Zion home. Elsa Zion answered the phone. Weinstein, without telling her that Libby had died, said, "I want you to know we did everything we could for Libby. We couldn't get the fever down. We gave her medication. We gave her ice baths." When Elsa Zion asked if this meant that her daughter was dead, Weinstein answered, "Yes."[7]

Like any parents told that their seemingly healthy 18-year-old daughter had died, the Zions responded with a combination of disbelief and sheer anguish. But because one of the parents was Sidney Zion, another emotion surfaced: outrage. According to Natalie Robins, author of *The Girl Who Died Twice*, Sidney Zion immediately announced to his son, Adam: "They did it. They killed your sister."[8]

Sidney Zion was no ordinary individual. He approached his jobs—as a federal prosecutor, reporter, and finally a columnist—more as crusades than as mere employment. Among the subjects he covered as a journalist were the civil rights movement, the Israeli-Arab conflict, and the Vietnam War, all of which raised passionate feelings of right and wrong. Robins attributed Zion's passion to his upbringing. His mother had taught him that "he didn't have to take no for an answer"; he, in turn, taught his children to "never let anybody dominate your life." Zion embraced "the role of disarming the mighty," Robins reported.[9]

But it would be wrong to assume that Zion was itching to take on his daughter's doctors as some type of vendetta against the medical profession. Zion was actually very worshipful of doctors, stemming from his great admiration for his childhood physician. But Zion had reacted angrily both to the news of his daughter's death and to the way in which he had learned about it. That neither Sherman nor Weinstein had come out and actually said that Libby was dead smelled like the beginnings of a cover-up.[10]

One obvious option for the Zions was to file a malpractice lawsuit against New York Hospital and its physicians. Since the early nineteenth century, civil lawsuits had been the primary mechanism for disgruntled patients and family members to obtain recompense—both financial and emotional—for perceived errors that occurred during medical care. Indeed, the frequency of malpractice lawsuits had begun to increase dramatically in the 1970s. In general, in order to win a case, plaintiffs needed to demonstrate that hospitals or physicians had deviated from the standard of care, thereby leading to a bad outcome.[11]

Not surprisingly, therefore, one of the first people Sidney Zion called after his daughter's death was Theodore H. Friedman, an old friend and a prominent malpractice lawyer. At first glance, Friedman thought there was a very strong case, which he sought to confirm by soliciting opinions from several physicians. Those who reviewed the available information were utterly appalled at Zion's care.

For example, Steven Roose, a psychiatrist at Columbia University, wrote that Weinstein's decision not to reevaluate a patient with a high fever and worsening agitation was "inexcusable and negligent." Boston emergency room physician Harvey J. Makadon agreed. The failure of Weinstein to more closely monitor her patient represented "a serious lapse in clinical judgment and a gross departure from standard medical practice." New Jersey physician Jonathan M. Alexander was even more harsh. Sherman, he believed, had been negligent for not coming to the hospital to see his patient. And Weinstein had "violated the most basic principle of human caring and professional conduct by essentially abandoning her patient to the fate of a totally preventable death." Later negative assessments of the case would raise two other issues: that the doctors had cavalierly dismissed Libby Zion as a "crock" and had neglected to send her to the intensive care unit for closer monitoring.[12]

It was these preliminary inquiries that led to the construction of the second story of Libby Zion's death: Zion was not the victim of medical malpractice but was "murdered" by an archaic and dangerous system of patient care. As Sidney Zion learned more about what had happened on the night of March 4, 1984, he grew increasingly amazed. What stunned him was that Raymond Sherman, his daughter's doctor and the senior physician on the case, had not been consulted when Libby worsened and did not see her before she died. Rather, it was Luise Weinstein, an intern nine months out of medical school, who was in charge of her care and had single-handedly made the decisions that either caused or did not prevent the death. Moreover, Weinstein was in the middle of a thirty-six-hour shift of duty and was busy with other patients as Libby deteriorated. Gregg Stone, who had gone to sleep in a nearby building but was still on call, was not roused from his bed. Finally, Sidney Zion learned, it might have been the combination of Nardil and Demerol, known to be toxic, that led to Libby's death.[13]

At this point, the Zion family's story of what happened to their daughter evolved well beyond malpractice. Rather, they concluded, the system by which New York Hospital cared for its patients, at least at night, was gravely flawed. It was routine, apparently, for senior physicians not to come to the hospital at night to see newly admitted patients. House officers (interns and residents) not only had to cover dozens of sick patients at night, but they often did so in thirty-six-hour shifts with little or no sleep.

From a modern vantage point, after more than twenty years of discussion of these topics, such revelations are hardly startling. But in 1984, to most people outside the medical profession, they were. No doubt other aggrieved families had learned this information when researching their loved ones' deaths. It was Sidney Zion, however, who chose to make the issue of overworked, unsupervised residents central to his lawsuit. And he was especially well-equipped, through his political connections, to engineer a crusade to reform how young doctors were trained.

Within the medical profession, the problems with the training system were an open secret. House officers had worked very long hours and covered for attending physicians since the early twentieth century. Those physicians who discussed medical errors, occurring due to fatigue or other causes, generally urged concealment for fear of legal reprisals. But a few researchers, concerned with both patient safety and the well-being of resident physicians themselves, had gently begun to question the status quo. For example, a 1971 paper reported that sleep loss among interns impaired their psychological states and their job performance. "I am so tired," one intern told the researchers, "I forget what the name is on the chart I am writing in."[14]

An occasional popular work featured exhausted young doctors wreaking havoc. The doctor in training, wrote "Doctor X" in the 1965 book *Intern*, "will inadvertently kill the patient who might otherwise have lived, through stupidity, or blundering, or blind inexperience." But no major whistleblowers had emerged from within the medical profession. One researcher working on the issue of house-staff training during these years was Terry Mizrahi, a social worker whose 1986 book, *Getting Rid of Patients*, was a scathing indictment of the system. Mizrahi convincingly argued that residency so brutalized house officers that they routinely used epithets to describe their patients and hoped that patients would die to ease their workloads. In such a universe, a demanding, time-consuming patient like Libby Zion, seemingly overreacting to a mild illness, would have been considered merely a pain in the neck. Mizrahi's book, however, was not published until two years after Zion died, and her research was not widely known outside sociological circles.[15]

Sidney Zion believed he had inadvertently unearthed a "Mafia code of silence" common to groups resisting change or defending themselves against charges. As he increasingly argued, it took nothing more than common sense to realize that something was seriously awry in the world of medicine. "You don't need kindergarten," he wrote, "to know that a resident working a 36-hour shift is in no condition to make any kind of judgment call—forget about life-and-death."[16]

And thus the second story emerged, one not only of misdiagnosis but also of misconduct. Given how teaching hospitals cared for patients, it was less surprising that Libby Zion had died than that anyone lived at all. This new narrative had an added advantage. To the degree that Sidney Zion could get the message out and effect change, his daughter would not have died in vain. "This is a cause, not a case," announced Theodore Friedman, "and I am unabashed about expressing my hope and desire that there be as much press coverage as possible."[17]

To achieve this latter goal, Zion ably used his connections. As an upper-middle-class Jewish New Yorker who had worked for the government and several newspapers, Zion had friends in high places. One connection was New York City Council president Andrew Stein, who had once hired Libby Zion to be an intern. Upon hearing Sidney Zion's jeremiad, Stein convened three public forums on safety and errors in city hospitals. Zion also mobilized several well-known journalists, such as the *New York Times*'s Tom Wicker and the *San Francisco Examiner*'s Warren Hinckle, to write impassioned columns about the need to reform patient care. Zion used his own column in the *New York Daily News* to perpetually remind the public why his daughter's death should not be forgotten.[18]

Zion's publicity efforts reached their pinnacle in 1987, when the top-rated CBS news magazine, *60 Minutes*, broadcast a segment on overworked interns. Correspondent Mike Wallace spent thirty-six hours on call with an intern, who obligingly forgot one of Wallace's questions during his twenty-fifth hour. When interviewees informed Wallace that interns saw patients as their enemies, he told Americans that this was "astonishing." And it was.[19]

But Zion was not content merely with outing a faulty system. His new story was full of venom. Because the attending physician had not seen Libby Zion and the intern had ignored her worsening agitation, tied her down, and caused a fatal drug interaction, New York Hospital, he believed, had killed his daughter. "It is my definition of murder," he said. "They gave her a drug that was destined to kill her," Zion stated, "then ignored her except to tie her down like a dog." What had happened, he concluded, was not a "human mistake," which was forgivable, but an "inhuman mistake."[20]

In promoting his theory of murder, Zion used one additional connection. He and his friends conducted a successful letter-writing campaign that convinced Manhattan district attorney Robert Morgenthau to convene a grand jury to consider criminal charges against Libby Zion's doctors. To Zion, the physicians were as culpable as other public servants, such as police, who could be charged with homicide if they inadvertently killed someone.

Morgenthau agreed to forge ahead. On May 5, 1986, a grand jury was convened to consider charges against the doctors, which would have been unique in the history of American jurisprudence. Although the grand jury ultimately declined to indict the physicians, it did something unexpected. After six months of hearings, on December 31, 1986, it issued a report strongly criticizing "the supervision of interns and junior residents at a hospital in New York County."[21]

This development underscored an important historical point. Even though there had previously been little public discussion of how hospitals trained doctors, the "basic soil for change was present." As the cases of Morris Abram and Steve McQueen demonstrated, consumerism had come to medicine. And just as patients, alerted by the media, had begun to challenge how doctors made medical decisions and ran clinical experiments, so, too, did they now take interest in the medical care rendered by the young doctors who staffed teaching hospitals.[22]

From a political standpoint, the grand jury report came at an opportune time. The governor of New York was a Democratic reformer, Mario M. Cuomo, whose state health commissioner was David Axelrod, a progressive physician willing to confront the medical profession. In response to the grand jury, Axelrod convened an Ad Hoc Advisory Committee on Emergency Services that would recommend a series of dramatic reforms in the training and supervision of doctors in New York. The committee was known informally as the Bell Commission, named for its director, primary care physician Bertrand M. Bell. The affable but outspoken Bell, a longtime critic of the residency system, was an ideal person to ensure that Sidney Zion's reform efforts would not fade away. The grand jury had been convened, Bell opined, because the middle class had finally realized that the care it received in New York's finest hospitals was no better, and perhaps even worse, than that provided at the city's public facilities.[23]

That the ground was fertile for reform was shown by the responses of house officers and medical students to Libby Zion's death and its aftermath. As they told Sidney Zion in a series of letters, he had provided the first outlet for doctors-in-training to voice their concerns about a dehumanizing system. "I protested," one resident wrote, "that it was inhuman and dangerous for the Department to assign us to cover up to 200 patients single-handedly on our on-call nights." A medical student described house officers as "often miserable, hostile people who abused their relationships with medical students, who talked disparagingly about their patients and were bitter about their specialty choice." A mother of a medical resident declared the system "indefensible," with work requirements not seen in sweatshops or prisons. Saddest of all was a letter from the parents of an intern who had killed himself, they believed, due to "his extremely long hours on an understaffed team without available supervisors."[24]

Of course, just because house officers—or their parents—equated long work hours and inadequate supervision with bad outcomes did not mean such claims were true. After Libby Zion died, New York Hospital's doctors reviewed what had happened and came up with their own account, which became the third story of her death. Two words entirely absent from this version were *error* and *mistake*; circa 1984, this type of language was rarely invoked on the wards and almost never with family members. Rather, the physicians characterized Libby Zion's death as a bad outcome, one that might—but hopefully would not—result in a lawsuit. When Sherman and Weinstein initially spoke to the family, they were apologetic but did not indicate that anything had gone wrong.

The crafting of this story began on the morning of March 5, 1984, when the chief medical resident, Joseph Ruggiero, reviewed Zion's unexpected death. He found nothing unusual except that she was taking Nardil, a medication known to have many interactions with other drugs. When Ruggiero checked the *Physicians' Desk Reference* (*PDR*), he learned that Demerol was contraindicated in someone taking Nardil, because the combination of the drugs could lead to malignant hyperthermia, an extremely high, and potentially fatal, body temperature. But the book indicated that this risk had been reported only for doses of Demerol of 50 milligrams or higher. Zion had received 25 milligrams for her shaking. Thus, concluded both the chief resident and the physician-in-chief of the hospital, R. Gordon Douglas, Jr., Zion had not died from a drug reaction. In this manner, one potential medical error was explained away.[25]

Nor did the Department of Medicine, on whose service Zion had been treated, hold a formal morbidity and mortality (M&M) conference on her case. M&M conferences allowed doctors to review cases that had either interesting findings or unfortunate outcomes. The Zion case, with its mysterious death, seemed to be an ideal teaching case. But the possibility of a lawsuit and Sidney Zion's notoriety probably discouraged a semi-public airing of what had happened. Whether or not VIP patients like the Shah of Iran, whose case was mismanaged at New York Hospital in 1979, truly received worse care, the hospital paid especially close attention to how it retrospectively evaluated bad outcomes among its prominent clientele. In the Zion case, feedback was limited to a brief, informal discussion at a regularly scheduled M&M conference.[26]

Over the next months, other aspects of the hospital's story came together. For example, Luise Weinstein denied having been told that Libby Zion had become more agitated after the Demerol. The medical staff defended the use of restraints and Haldol as appropriate management of a patient at risk of hurting herself. And Raymond Sherman continued to believe that nothing wrong had occurred. There was even a growing consensus that Zion had been improving until the time that her temperature dramatically increased. Others in the medical community, such as James Todd of the American Medical Association, agreed. Zion's death, Todd wrote, was "an isolated case."[27]

Nevertheless, three years later, New York Hospital seemed to take some responsibility for what had occurred. In March 1987, after investigating the case, the New York State Department of Health fined the hospital $13,000 for its "woeful" care of Libby Zion. The report cited several errors in her treatment as well as inadequate supervision of Weinstein. In addition, the state required the hospital to file monthly reports on unexpected deaths and submit to periodic inspections. By consenting to this arrangement, the hospital was, in a sense, admitting its guilt, but it had also insisted on a clause indicating that this agreement could not be used in any hearings related to the Zion case. Nor, as Sidney Zion frequently pointed out, had anyone at New York Hospital ever formally apologized to him and his family. The hospital's initial narrative of the Libby Zion case, therefore, was crafted to accept limited blame and, as best as possible, put the matter to rest.[28]

But with a lawsuit on the horizon and the highly critical grand jury report being made public at the end of 1986, the Libby Zion case was not going away. Thus, New York Hospital began to craft the fourth story of Zion's death, one that was more offensive than defensive in nature. And the topic it emphasized was cocaine.

The issue of cocaine had briefly been raised in 1984 when a nasal swab and a blood sample analyzed at Zion's autopsy proved positive for trace amounts of the drug. Subsequent tests had called these findings into question and the subject was dropped. But a January 14, 1987, press release by

New York Hospital, issued in response to the critical grand jury report, brought cocaine front and center. The statement linked Zion's death to those of two athletes, Len Bias and Don Rogers, who had recently died from clear-cut cocaine intoxication. "Certainly," wrote the hospital, "the recent death of two prominent athletes demonstrates the unpredictable effects of cocaine ingestion and points to cocaine, found on autopsy, as the cause in whole or in part of the sudden cardiac collapse of [Libby Zion]."[29]

According to this theory, the cocaine had proved toxic when combined with Nardil and a series of other drugs, including the opiate Percodan, that Zion was taking but had concealed from the doctors despite repeated questioning. It was not known when on March 4, 1984, Zion had used the cocaine, but during *Zion v. New York Hospital*, the malpractice trial that finally took place in 1994–95, defense witnesses would speculate that it was shortly before she came to the hospital. In addition to explaining Zion's sudden deterioration and death, the cocaine theory also provided a basis for her agitation and uncooperativeness. Finally, since she had told neither Weinstein nor Stone about her cocaine use, this story had another virtue for New York Hospital: it placed some (or even all) of the culpability for Zion's death at her own feet.[30]

Since these claims were such a dramatic departure from previous statements made by New York Hospital, they evidently caught some people off guard. One was surgeon and future hospital president David B. Skinner, who termed the cocaine accusation "a real leap." Still, the cocaine story stuck and would become a centerpiece of dispute during the trial. When Gregg Stone finally went public with his story on NBC's *Dateline* in 1997, he stated that Zion had died from a reaction to cocaine.[31]

Accompanying the new emphasis on cocaine was a backpedaling from earlier statements in which the hospital seemed to accept some blame. For example, during testimony at disciplinary hearings for Weinstein, Stone, and Sherman held by the New York State Board for Professional Medical Conduct between 1987 and 1989, New York Hospital's Gordon Douglas stated that the use of both Demerol and restraints had been appropriate and that Zion had not required transfer to the intensive care unit. He added that Weinstein was an outstanding intern. Douglas also defended Sherman's behavior, saying that he "acted appropriately and according to the policies and standards of the state's university hospitals."[32]

Part of the reason that New York Hospital began such a furious defense was the virulence of Sidney Zion's opprobrium. Even though the grand jury had declined to indict the physicians on criminal charges, the taint remained. And Zion's ubiquitous media appearances, in which he regularly charged the hospital with murder, infuriated both its doctors and its lawyers. Francis P. Bensel, an outside attorney hired by New York Hospital, charged Zion with "reckless and malicious attacks on the physicians who took care of his daughter." Zion's grief was understandable, Bensel continued, but his "uninformed invective" was not. Sherman stated that Zion was on a "vindictive witch hunt."[33]

Sidney Zion's response to New York Hospital's "cocaine defense" constituted the fifth and final story of the Libby Zion case. In addition to its original sins of providing terrible care and covering up errors, he now charged the hospital with slandering his dead daughter as a "junkie." The press release had been "so vile in its very being that the most hardnosed newspapermen in this city told me they had never seen such slime." The defendants, stated Theodore Friedman, "have elected to malign the late Libby Zion by 'spreading the word' that she was a cocaine addict and died of that." Friedman analogized this strategy to that used by one of the lawyers in the case of Robert Chambers, who had killed Jennifer Levin in Central Park in 1986. New York Hospital's goal, Friedman wrote, was "to do to Libby Zion what Jack Litman did in the Chambers case, which was to make Jennifer Levin the defendant for her past social life and history." Columnist Warren Hinckle, Zion's friend, compared the press release to the Protocols of the Elders of Zion, the infamous fabricated document used to slander the Jewish people.[34]

In all five of these narratives, the various protagonists, from the very start, emphasized or deemphasized certain facts to suit their own needs. So does this mean there is no real "truth" in the Zion case? Are there ways to extract the facts from how they have been spun? One way would be to revisit the "objective" evidence dispassionately. A possible source of this information would be Libby Zion's hospital chart. But medical charts follow formulas, contain coded language, and omit relevant facts.[35]

Another possible locus for determining the facts would have been the malpractice trial that began in November 1994. But as well as any other example, the Zion case demonstrates why the courtroom setting hinders — rather than fosters — the discovery of the truth.

By the time of the trial, the original stories had become increasingly slanted, with any earlier nuance being replaced with bold assurances that supported either the plaintiffs or the defense. The star expert witness for the plaintiffs was Harold Osborn, who said Zion's death was the worst case of malpractice he had seen in twenty-five years. Even though Osborn was a physician, he was an outsider: a pony-tailed emergency room doctor from Lincoln Hospital in the Bronx with a history of political activism. In contrast, the defense's star expert was Harvard-trained internist Robert M. Glickman, the chief of medicine at Boston's Beth Israel Hospital. The media circus that accompanied the trial, which was covered daily by the Court TV network, only exacerbated the antagonism between the two sides. The issue of cocaine further obfuscated things by deflecting attention from how Zion's case had been managed, regardless of whether she had used cocaine. Not surprisingly, perhaps, the jury ultimately threw up its hands, apportioning equal responsibility for the death to New York Hospital and Libby Zion herself.[36]

Other attempts to provide an "objective" assessment of Libby Zion's death have also failed. For example, as media scholar Joan McGettigan argued in a 1999 article, two documentaries made about the Zion case— by Court TV and NBC's *Dateline*—provided dramatically different accounts of what occurred. "The very existence of these two documentaries," McGettigan concluded, "emphasizes the subjective nature of all interpretation and serves as a kind of admission that there may never be a 'truth' in the Zion case, only multiple meanings."[37]

But by implying that all stories are necessarily equal, this argument may go too far. There is a reality to what happened on the night of March 4, 1984, which can provide some definitive conclusions and even closure to a highly contentious matter. The best way to approach this last "story" of the Libby Zion case is to focus on the randomness of disease and the probabilistic strategies that doctors used at the time to treat deteriorating patients.

When Libby Zion came to the emergency room, she was assessed just like any other young person with an obscure fever and other symptoms, receiving a physical examination, blood and urine tests, and a chest x-ray. When these did not reveal anything specific, the decision was made to admit Zion to the hospital for observation and await additional test results. The possible diagnoses at her admission reflected this mindset. Luise Weinstein suspected there was some type of infection but was not sure what kind. As noted above, Gregg Stone's leading diagnosis was "viral syndrome with hysterical symptoms."

At the trial, plaintiff expert Osborn fiercely criticized Stone for having implied with this phrase that Zion was only mildly ill and, given her psychiatric history, was overreacting. According to Osborn, Stone's words were code language for "a ditsy redhead" who did not require admission and would simply get better. The implication was that Stone and Weinstein did not take Zion's deterioration seriously and thus medicated her and tied her down to the bed. These actions, in turn, led to her death.

While there is surely some truth to this explanation, it ignores the wider population of patients who had likely received similar diagnoses and care. If one could obtain the previous hundred charts of young patients admitted to New York Hospital with similar symptoms, it is likely that they would show that all of them survived. That is, Stone's initial diagnosis, even with its negative implications, may have been reasonable. It is also reasonable to argue that Weinstein was not obligated to make a personal appearance at Libby Zion's bedside every time something changed in her condition. A hospital could not function if this were the expectation for busy interns.[38]

But the Zion case revealed a series of troubling triage strategies routinely employed by doctors called to see patients with potentially worsening medical conditions. For example, it was considered acceptable for physicians to give phone orders for sedating drugs and restraints without actually examining patients. It was considered acceptable to let a supervising resident sleep while an intern was being overwhelmed. Similarly, it was considered acceptable for doctors to write a generic order for routine vital signs when a more worrisome situation actually warranted more frequent checks.

And, most amazingly, it was considered acceptable for house officers to care for patients without necessarily accessing all of the available medical information that might be helpful. This phenomenon became apparent at the trial during a series of remarkable exchanges between defense expert witness Robert Glickman and plaintiffs' lawyer Thomas A. Moore, who had taken over the case from Theodore Friedman. On January 10, 1995, Moore got Glickman to admit that the 1984 *PDR* clearly stated that Demerol should not be given with Nardil. Going in for the kill, the fiery Moore, whose Irish brogue had been termed "the opposite of a fireside chat or a walk in the country," asked Glickman: "And do you still say, knowing that there was this contraindication in the Physicians Desk Reference, do you still hold to the opinion that these physicians did not depart [from standard practice] by prescribing it?"[39]

Glickman, to his credit, told the truth. "Well, I do," he stated. "The reason I hold to that opinion is that we often look up information we feel unsure of and don't know, and I think it's difficult to look everything up in terms of every medication we prescribe, and we would have to have an indication to look up something specific about a medication. So not knowing that such an interaction existed, I don't believe not looking it up was a failure of medical practice."[40]

A week later, Moore returned to this subject. "Is it your testimony," he asked Glickman, "that if somebody didn't know about whether Demerol interacts or doesn't interact with Nardil they wouldn't have the obligation to look it up?" When Glickman did not answer the question directly, Moore became incredulous. "Doctor," he asked, "if you can't answer the question yes or no, you can't answer one of the basic issues in this case, true?"[41]

Moore then asked specifically about Gregg Stone, who, along with Weinstein, had decided to order the Demerol. "Doctor, I ask you again," Moore said to Glickman. "If he did not know of the interaction, wouldn't he have the obligation to look one or both of those drugs up, yes or no?" Glickman was again candid. "I can't answer that yes or no," he stated.[42]

Then Moore went on to discuss Luise Weinstein, reminding Glickman that the intern had actually looked up Nardil in the *PDR* but had not noticed that giving the two drugs together was contraindicated. "And you still hold this case up as an example of good practice?" Moore asked. "I do," Glickman replied.[43]

In other words, Glickman was admitting that it was acceptable behavior, at one of America's finest teaching hospitals, for doctors-in-training to not do their best. The corollary to this admission might have been that New York Hospital, by tolerating a standard in which overworked, undersupervised residents routinely provided less than top-notch care, had caused Libby Zion's death. But the jury did not ultimately interpret the case in this manner.[44]

The larger point is that the care of all patients, including Libby Zion, is based on percentages and hunches, backed up, when possible, by the medical literature. The initial assessment of Zion's condition relied on similar cases that the doctors had seen or learned about. But the main question, which was never explicitly asked either before or during the trial was, When did Zion's case become *atypical* enough to warrant more aggressive intervention? In defending her decision not to see her patient despite the nurses' requests that she do so, Weinstein noted that she had just seen Zion. That is, she already knew the situation. She was still thinking within the initial construct that she, Stone, and Sherman had devised.

In retrospect, of course, the Zion case was anything but typical. We should then ask, At what point, if any, should Weinstein have realized this, gone to see the patient, called Stone and/or Sherman, or sent Zion to the intensive care unit? The answer to this question should have nothing to do with the fact that Zion was a "difficult" patient, that she may have used cocaine, that Weinstein was busy with other sick patients, or that Sidney Zion was seen as a royal pain. The fact is that the doctors at New York Hospital, when urged by the nurses to reassess Libby Zion, guessed wrong—way wrong—and as a result did not do the things that might potentially have saved a seriously deteriorating patient. That Zion's dramatically high fever, which probably caused her heart to stop, may have been due to a drug-drug interaction that the doctors should have known about further implicates the hospital.[45]

The same scenario, of course, might have played out at other understaffed teaching hospitals in New York City or elsewhere in the 1980s. Residents at another New York hospital later recalled hearing the Libby Zion story and thinking to themselves, "There but for the grace of God go I." But this knowledge should not hide the reality that Luise Weinstein, herself a victim of a system that overworked interns and strongly urged them to act macho even when overwhelmed, missed a series of red flags that might have saved her patient's life. "In most instances, interns get away with this kind of corner-cutting," Timothy B. McCall, a Boston physician, wrote about the Libby Zion case. "[Weinstein] did something all interns do, but in this instance was burned badly." The jury's ultimate decision had less to do with this type of analysis of what happened than with the ability of the defense team to shift the focus of the case to possible causes of Zion's death and her purported responsibility for it. The main point had become obscured: Libby Zion should not have died, at least without having received more aggressive treatment.[46]

What is the legacy of the Libby Zion case? A 1989 article in the *Jour-*

nal of the American Medical Association stated that her death "has changed residency training forever." The Zion case is also routinely cited as having sparked a new movement to eliminate medical errors. To what degree are these conclusions correct? How effective are well-publicized individual cases in driving public health policy?[47]

With regard to graduate medical education, the connection of the Zion case to subsequent reform is clear. The case led to the grand jury report, which in turn led to the Bell Commission regulations. The commission recommended that house officers at New York State hospitals work no more than eighty hours weekly, work no more than twenty-four hours on a single shift, and receive on-site attending-level supervision at all times. Lack of supervision, according to Bertrand Bell, was the major flaw in the existing system. New York State adopted the commission's recommendation, although many residency programs violated them for years. In 2003, teeth were put into these reforms when the Accreditation Council for Graduate Medical Education mandated them for training programs nationwide.[48]

But when one looks at what happened during Libby Zion's hospitalization and the subsequent educational changes, the connections are less straightforward. For example, the most vivid image that spurred reform was that of the exhausted intern, perpetually on the verge of falling asleep. Yet, even though Luise Weinstein and Gregg Stone had been working for eighteen hours, it is far from clear that fatigue played a role in the decisions they made. Rather, as suggested above, they just guessed wrong. On *Dateline* in 1997, Stone stated that neither he nor Weinstein felt overworked. Weinstein testified during the trial that it was not fatigue that led her to overlook the contraindication of Nardil and Demerol when she looked it up. She just had missed it.[49]

Nor does it seem that a lack of supervision, at least in the emergency room, affected the Zion case. By drawing a battery of tests on a young woman with a mysterious fever and then deciding to admit her for observation, the resident did what any attending would have done. (It is true that a more senior doctor on the floor might have averted the tragedy.) Rather, it was the fact that the Zion case publicized the very real issues of resident fatigue and inadequate supervision—as opposed to exemplifying them— that propelled reform forward. Changes were needed and Libby Zion's death became the vehicle. Whether or not Raymond Sherman's presence that night would have saved Zion's life, at some point "you just have to get your ass out of bed and come in," as one physician testified at the disciplinary hearings. Or, as one sleep expert has argued, just because it may be possible that extreme sleep deprivation does not impair performance, this doesn't mean it is acceptable.[50]

That the Zion case became the one that finally produced the needed changes had all to do with Sidney Zion. To be sure, even though he was trying to bring constructive reform from his child's tragic death, Zion had more than his share of detractors. His blunt and pugnacious manner at times spawned enormous enmity. One woman, who admired what he had achieved, nevertheless called him "an irritating, egotistical son of a bitch." Another woman termed Zion a "grand stander . . . bellowing about his 'murdered baby.'"[51]

Perhaps the most provocative statements came from writer Anne Roiphe in the *New York Observer.* Roiphe admired Zion's inclination to turn his daughter's death into something constructive and wished him comfort and peace. But she argued that Zion's diatribes against the medical profession masked the "inside-the-story story . . . about what the father didn't want to know or refused to believe." This story was one of a child of well-to-do New York parents who was "caught in the downslide of hope," living a life full of angst, antidepressants, and illicit drug use. The real problem, Roiphe was suggesting, was not that Libby Zion died at the hands of incompetent doctors but that she—and her parents—had created a scenario where such an outcome was possible.[52]

Not surprisingly, Roiphe took a beating from readers in their letters to the editor. These correspondents were among a large number of individuals who passionately embraced Zion and his crusade. When he addressed a group of Canadian medical residents, Zion reported, they cheered him "as if I were the man who had found the cure for AIDS." Sure, Zion was "aggressive, narcissistic, self-indulgent, pushy, persistent and paranoid," wrote psychiatrist Willard Gaylin in the *Nation*, "but that is precisely the stuff successful reformers are made of. I'm not sure I'd want Carry Nation, Florence Nightingale, Ralph Nader or, for that matter, Jesus, as a roommate." Zion, Gaylin added, was "entitled to his rage, unexamined."[53]

Not surprisingly, many people who called or corresponded with Zion had similar horror stories to tell. For example, a Boston man told of his sister's death in an emergency room, "where basically a healthy person suffering an acute and treatable medical problem was left to die." A California nurse wrote that one of her patients had almost jumped out of a window because a doctor had been too lazy to write an order for restraints.[54]

Some of the letters described events that had occurred at New York Hospital—in these instances, involving not VIP patients but ordinary ones. A woman wrote that "no one was aware that mother was dying and I had to shout and insist that the resident call the attending physician." "My husband's death," claimed another woman, "was precipitated by the refusal of the resident to see him for several hours following the onset of severe respiratory distress, and this resident's refusal to give him medication which was used successfully by the previous resident to overcome a similar episode in November." "Please keep up the fight with New York Hospital on York Avenue," urged a Florida man whose wife had died there in 1973. "They killed [your daughter] like my wife," he said. "No service."[55]

Health policy reform, in this instance, had thus been contingent on several factors: a serious system-wide medical problem, a "famous patient" who met a tragic end, a well-connected and highly visible spokesperson unwilling to let the press drop the issue, and a large reservoir of horror stories from an angry public. It ultimately mattered little that Libby Zion's death—or those deaths described in the letters to her father—did not necessarily prove the charges. Nor did one need a randomized controlled trial definitively showing that fatigued residents resulted in higher morbidity and mortality. The existence of apparent victims of such house officers was enough.[56]

Identification of supposed villains also propelled reform efforts. Even though Sidney Zion and his correspondents all wished to reform the system of house-staff training, that there were identifiable people to blame, such as Weinstein, Stone, and Sherman, made the horror stories infinitely more compelling and inexcusable. Many letters to Zion were positively seething with anger at doctors and hospitals. One man described his doctors' unsuccessful treatment of a knee problem, which, he claimed, they then tried to blame on him. "FUCK 'EM FUCK 'EM FUCK 'EM," he wrote to Zion. "Do not give up your fight. Nail these bastards to the wall." "There is a conspiracy of silence among doctors," wrote a woman from Queens. "They lie to dead patients' families. They change the patients' charts to erase any damaging data that a litigant may find. They are disgusting." A California woman told of the death of her son after a liver transplant. "They are murderers and actually should be brought up on criminal charges," she wrote to Zion. And, in language he surely understood, she added: "The fire in me will never die until I do, and join my son, the love of my life."[57]

One person who appreciated the connection of blame to reform was Sidney Zion. "Nobody ever got anywhere by beating heads against 'the system,'" he wrote in 1999. "No names, no accountability." Although he supported the initiatives to combat medical mistakes that began in the early 1990s, he reminded his *New York Daily News* readers that the term *medical error* was a "euphemism for malpractice."[58]

It should come as no surprise, perhaps, that a proposed Hollywood movie on the Zion case planned to play up the issues of blame and innocence, painting what happened in black and white terms. The plan was to do a "full-on story" from Sidney Zion's point of view, showing how he tried to get information about medical practices but was "stonewalled at every turn." Along the way, the grieving Zion would meet "the botched abortions, the orthopedic nightmares, the carpal tunnel syndrome victims, etc., normal everyday things [the] audience relates to which will scare the shit out of them." While the film would portray some individual sympathetic doctors, the American Medical Association would be "like the Great Wall of China." Although the film was never made, its plot shared the characteristics of other cinematic versions of actual stories, which favor swashbuckling heroes and readily identifiable scoundrels. The working title, "First Do No Harm," was intentionally ironic.[59]

It was the unique nature of Sidney Zion's campaign that channeled the passion and anger of individual blame in the service of fixing a severely broken system—the training of house officers. "It is no exaggeration," stated Stanford University professor of medicine Eugene D. Robin, "to say that Sidney Zion has changed medical history in the United States."[60]

So did Elizabeth Glaser and Arthur Ashe. Glaser, the wife of actor Paul Michael Glaser, and Ashe, the tennis star and civil rights activist, both learned in the 1980s that they had AIDS. Although Glaser and Ashe initially kept their condition secret from the public, they were both eventually outed by the media. That both made incredible contributions to AIDS activism before their death is indisputable. But this fact begs the question. Did the public have the right to know they were seriously ill in the first place? Had the growing coverage of celebrity illnesses finally gone too far?

Chapter 11

Patient Activism Goes Hollywood

How America Fought AIDS

For most of their lives, Elizabeth Meyer Glaser and Arthur Robert Ashe, Jr., had little in common. Glaser was raised in a white, middle-class family in the Boston suburbs, became a schoolteacher and museum curator in California, and married an actor, Paul Michael Glaser. Ashe was born into a working-class African American family in Richmond, Virginia, and went on to become a star tennis player who helped to dismantle long-existing racial barriers.

But in the 1980s and early 1990s, their lives intersected. Both Glaser and Ashe developed acquired immune deficiency syndrome through a blood transfusion. Both, after being outed by the media, became eloquent advocates for increasing attention to AIDS and funding for research. And both would be criticized. Why had Glaser and Ashe, as public figures, kept their diagnoses secret? And what was the connection of their atypical stories to those of the many poor, disadvantaged people who contracted AIDS?

More than any disease before or since, AIDS changed the rules of the game. Faced with a fatal disease killing previously healthy people and an indifferent federal government, AIDS activists, many of whom were gay, attacked the medical and social status quo with ferocity. Glaser and Ashe became important players in a turbulent drama.

Elizabeth Meyer graduated from college in 1969 and earned a master's degree in early childhood education from Boston University. After a failed first marriage, she moved to Los Angeles, where she found a teaching job at a private school. Then, on June 9, 1975, at the age of 27, she had a Hollywood moment. While driving, she made eye contact with another driver, Paul Michael Glaser, an actor soon to debut in a new television show, *Starsky and Hutch*. Glaser had also played Perchik in the movie version of *Fiddler on the Roof*. They both stopped their cars, talked, and made a dinner date. By September 1975 they were living together.[1]

Starsky and Hutch, a series about two detectives, proved to be an enormous hit and Paul Glaser became an international star. After the show ended, he continued to act and also began to direct. Elizabeth eventually took a job as exhibits director of the Los Angeles Children's Museum. Paul Glaser and Elizabeth Meyer were married on August 24, 1980, and on August 4, 1981, their first child, Ariel, was born.

The pregnancy, however, had not gone smoothly. At the six-month mark, Elizabeth Glaser started bleeding and was diagnosed with placenta previa, a condition in which the placenta grows across the cervix. The bleeding stopped but resumed in early August. At this point, doctors at Cedars-Sinai Hospital, where Steve McQueen had been treated the previous year, performed an emergency cesarean section, successfully delivering Ariel. All seemed to go well until Elizabeth started bleeding again— dangerously quickly. The doctors were able to stop the bleeding but not before Glaser received transfusions of seven pints of blood.[2]

During the summer of 1981, the press was full of accounts of what seemed to be a new disease, one that rapidly killed otherwise healthy people by damaging their immune systems. The disease was initially labeled gay-related immune deficiency (GRID), because so many of its victims were homosexual men, but in July 1982, officials at the Centers for Disease Control in Atlanta renamed it acquired immune deficiency syndrome, or AIDS. A major reason behind the name change was that the condition was also being discovered in another population: hemophiliacs who had received transfusions of blood or blood products. In her 1991 autobiography, *In the Absence of Angels*, Glaser wrote that she queried her obstetrician about the possibility that she had been exposed to AIDS during her transfusions. Relax, he told her, "Your nightmare is over."[3]

This seemed to be the case. On October 25, 1984, Glaser gave birth to a son, Jake. There was no abnormal bleeding or other complications. But in September 1985, when she was 4 years old, Ariel, known as Ari, got sick. Her first symptoms were diarrhea and abdominal pain. At first doctors assumed she had an intestinal virus, but when the condition persisted, they admitted Ariel to the hospital. They discovered that her hematocrit, or blood count, was extremely low but were unable to make a definitive diagnosis. Several months of inconclusive testing followed.[4]

But Ariel's doctor, Richard Fine, had quietly been suspecting AIDS and had done some indirect tests suggesting the diagnosis. He next persuaded the Glasers to have Ariel tested for antibodies to the human T-cell leukemia III virus, which scientists had by then concluded caused AIDS. (The name was later changed to human immunodeficiency virus, known as HIV.) In late May 1986, Fine called with terrible news: Ariel had tested positive. "I remember walking into the bathroom and screaming as loud as I could," Elizabeth Glaser later wrote. "It was the most traumatic day any human being can imagine." But the news only got worse. Further testing revealed that Elizabeth and Jake were also infected with the virus. They were HIV positive, although they did not, as did Ariel, have AIDS. Only Paul had been spared.[5]

In trying to find an explanation for this catastrophe, all arrows pointed in one direction: the blood transfusions Elizabeth had received at the time of Ariel's birth in 1981. Because Cedars-Sinai was located in West Hollywood, which had a large gay population, blood donated at that time (before it was being tested for HIV) had a higher-than-average likelihood of being infected. Elizabeth, the doctors surmised, had become infected by the transfusions, Ariel through breast-feeding, and Jake while in utero. The Glasers immediately had to confront a series of difficult questions. Whom should they tell? Could Ariel continue nursery school? Did they need to start treatment? And, most horrifyingly, were Elizabeth, Ariel, and Jake, three members of a previously storybook American family, going to die?[6]

Elizabeth Glaser was no activist when she learned she was HIV positive, but when Arthur Ashe was given the same diagnosis, he surely was. By dint of being born in segregated Richmond, Virginia, in 1943 and being an excellent teenage tennis player, Ashe learned early how race erected barriers. At times he was forbidden from joining his high-school teammates on certain public courts or in private clubs. But it was Ashe's performance as a professional tennis player that focused national attention on his race. In 1968 he became the first African American man to win one of the four major tournaments, capturing the U.S. Open title. Then, in 1975, Ashe won Wimbledon, perhaps tennis's most prestigious tournament.[7]

Ashe made a powerful point about racial equality on the tennis court, but he also became an increasingly vocal critic of segregation in the United States. "I had been brought up to think that I myself was obliged to be a leader, and especially to help my fellow blacks," Ashe would write in his 1993 autobiography, *Days of Grace*. But he received his share of criticism, both from whites who resented his use of tennis as a pulpit to promote civil rights and from Black Panthers who believed he was insufficiently strident. Radicals in South Africa called him an "Uncle Tom" because he participated in tennis tournaments in a country whose apartheid laws completely dehumanized blacks. Ashe argued that his presence demonstrated to South Africans how successful a free black man could be. Ashe's racial politics—a pragmatic approach favoring steady pressure and moral suasion—exemplified his reformist ethos. He liked to quote a line from a John Dryden poem: "Beware the fury of a patient man."[8]

Given Ashe's powerful connection to the issue of race, it makes sense that he met his future wife at a fundraiser for the United Negro College Fund, another organization in which he was involved. Jeanne Moutoussamy was a graphic artist at NBC and a professional photographer. They were married on February 20, 1977, only four months after they met.

The couple shared a strong family history of heart disease. Jeanne's father, John, had suffered a major heart attack in 1974. Four years later, Jeanne's aunt underwent a cardiac bypass operation. High blood pressure had contributed to the death of Ashe's mother, Mattie, when Arthur was only 6 years old. And in July 1979, Ashe's father, Arthur R. Ashe, Sr., experienced a severe bout of chest pain, believed to be angina.[9]

The big blow, however, came later that month when Ashe himself, only 36 years old, suffered a heart attack. The verdict from doctors at New York Hospital was serious: Ashe's professional tennis career was over. In December 1979, Ashe underwent surgery to bypass four clogged arteries. But he continued to experience angina and, in June 1983, had a second bypass operation at New York Hospital. It was almost certainly during this surgery that he received the blood transfusion that caused his HIV infection and AIDS.[10]

Although Ashe did retire from professional tennis, he remained actively involved in the sport as captain of the United States' Davis Cup team from 1980 to 1985. During these years, Ashe began an ambitious research project, a history of African Americans in sports. He spent five years researching and writing the acclaimed three-volume book that resulted, *A Hard*

Road to Glory: The History of the African-American Athlete. It was published in 1988.

Ashe also embarked on a series of philanthropic projects. These included the Ashe-Bollettieri Cities program, begun with his friend Nick Bollettieri, which used tennis as a wedge to teach children from poor neighborhoods about crime and drug abuse. Ashe's Safe Passage Foundation sought to help poor young people, especially blacks, get into college and succeed there. Ashe also served on the board of directors of the Aetna Life and Casualty Company, where he took a special interest in its African American clients. In 1985 Ashe became co-chair (with singer Harry Belafonte) of Artists and Athletes Against Apartheid and was arrested in an anti-apartheid demonstration in Washington, D.C. He was, *Sports Illustrated* later wrote, the "eternal example."[11]

But in late August 1988, shortly before the publication of *A Hard Road to Glory*, Ashe encountered another medical problem: an inability to move his right hand. His general physician, William Russell, ordered a CAT scan of the head, which showed an irregular mass in the left side of Ashe's brain. Two weeks later, after neurosurgery and a series of blood tests, the verdict was in. Arthur Ashe not only was HIV positive but had full-blown AIDS; the lesion in his brain was toxoplasmosis, an infection common in immunocompromised patients.[12]

Ashe's response, according to his wife, was merely to say "Aha." As the always pragmatic Ashe later wrote, there was no point in getting hysterical. There was nothing he could possibly do about his maladies "except to treat them according to the most expert medical science available to me." Fortunately, the toxoplasmosis could be cured by antibiotics. But the options for treating AIDS in 1988 were much less satisfactory.[13]

Like Elizabeth Glaser, Arthur Ashe also had to decide whom he was going to tell. Although he was retired from tennis, Ashe remained a well-known and highly respected figure. The press and the public would surely be interested. The same was true of Glaser, since she was the wife of a Hollywood actor.

Ultimately, both decided on the same strategy. To protect themselves, and most importantly their children, from the unfortunate stigma of an AIDS diagnosis, they told only a small group of friends and acquaintances. Some of these people were the parents of their children's friends. On December 21, 1986, twenty months before Ashe's AIDS diagnosis, Camera

Ashe had been born. Happily, both Camera and Jeanne, like Paul Glaser, were HIV negative. By and large, the confidantes of both the Glasers and Ashes kept quiet.

Going public at this time would have been unusual and remarkable. As of the mid-1980s, AIDS represented a double burden for a public figure. It meant not only sacrificing one's privacy but also admitting that one had a disease overwhelmingly associated with homosexuality, promiscuity, and illicit drug use. The best-known celebrity to have AIDS was Rock Hudson, who had tried to conceal the diagnosis and his homosexuality until his death in July 1985. Although both Glaser and Ashe would eventually work tirelessly to eliminate the stigma of HIV infection, the decision to do so would emerge gradually.[14]

For the Glasers, the short-term issue was not the public perception of AIDS but Ariel's health. In the nineteenth and early twentieth centuries, the death of children, from infections such as diphtheria or tuberculosis, was not uncommon. As late as the 1950s, parents of children with acute lymphocytic leukemia took their children home to die rather than enter them in protocols of new experimental chemotherapeutic agents. But as baby boomers became parents, and as consumerism and patients' rights entered medicine, any remaining passivity about trying to save children's lives disappeared.[15]

Even though it was written after the fact, and thus potentially simplified a more complex story, *In the Absence of Angels* provides a vivid and believable account of Glaser's "transition from Hollywood housewife to AIDS warrior." As Glaser recalled, it was at the time of Ariel's sixth birthday in August 1987 that she first took an active role in her daughter's medical care. Ariel was having terrible stomach pains and had much less energy. According to her blood tests, Ariel's AIDS was no worse, but now, what the doctors thought suddenly meant less to Glaser. "As a mother," she wrote, "I knew instinctively that I was losing her."[16]

She called Ariel's doctor, Richard Stiehm, a pediatric immunologist at the University of California, Los Angeles. "We must have AZT now," she said. "She's starting to fail." AZT is azidothymidine, the one available drug that seemed to slow the progression of AIDS and perhaps prolong survival. It was AZT that had produced one of the earliest and most intense political controversies among AIDS activists.[17]

From the beginning of the AIDS crisis, the actions of one group affected by the disease—the gay community—were dramatically different from any previous responses to disease outbreaks in the United States. The fact that the disease struck so many gay men led to the formation of activist organizations that sought to energize the response of the medical profession, government, and the public to AIDS. New York and San Francisco, with large populations of gay men, many of whom were affluent and politically savvy, became the centers of activity. Two of the most prominent groups were Gay Men's Health Crisis, founded in 1982, and its more radical and angry counterpart, ACT-UP, founded in 1987. Whichever AIDS organization one belonged to, business as usual was unacceptable.[18]

As of the mid-1980s, standard drug approval occurred through a conservative process at the U.S. Food and Drug Administration. The FDA insisted on testing new medications for safety (phase I trials) and efficacy (phase II trials) before trying them in randomized controlled studies (phase III trials). This process often took years.

Thus, when the FDA began evaluating AZT in the mid-1980s, it seemed that even if the drug ultimately proved safe and effective, it would not become widely available to AIDS patients for a long time. To the burgeoning ranks of AIDS activists, who were watching lovers, friends, and relatives die daily, such a delay was thoroughly unacceptable. Eventually, AIDS activists would force the FDA to speed up its overall drug-evaluation process.[19]

But the use of AZT in children raised a different issue. In response to her demand, Stiehm told Glaser that AZT was not ready for use in a pediatric population. "Elizabeth," he explained, "we don't even know the dose to give her [Ariel]. We can't just experiment. This is a toxic drug. It could kill her." Shortly thereafter, however, results from the first formal trial of AZT in children became available, showing the drug was safe and effective. Ariel began taking the pill.[20]

But Ariel continued to worsen. She developed pancreatitis, an inflammation of the organ that produces digestive enzymes, and was unable to eat. The doctors had to feed her intravenously. Then, in March 1988, she developed a severe pneumonia. Meanwhile, a scan of her brain showed atrophy: it was being eaten away by the virus. At one point, Richard Stiehm feared the worst and told the Glasers that their daughter was likely to die within forty-eight hours.[21]

Stiehm was wrong. Even though Ariel remained unable to walk or talk, she recovered from the pneumonia and went home from the hospital. But the episode was a reality check for Elizabeth Glaser. "It was not until the doctors told us that there was absolutely no hope," she wrote, "that I confronted the possibility of Ari's death for the first time." As unbearable as the thought of Ariel's death was the notion that it would somehow be due to Elizabeth Glaser's passivity. As a mother, Glaser believed, she was failing her child. This moment was her epiphany. As she announced to her friend Lucy Wick, "If Ari dies, then Jake is going to die. I can't keep sitting here in Santa Monica making a cozy little life for my family if we are all going to die! No one cares if we all die from AIDS. Something is very wrong."

Having taken the first step from parent to activist, Glaser now took a giant leap. "You have to get me to Reagan," she told Lucy Wick. Lucy was married to Douglas Wick, whose family had long been close friends of President Ronald Reagan and Nancy Reagan. So while the notion of the parent of a sick child demanding to see the president was ordinarily laughable, in Glaser's case it was a possibility.[22]

And Ronald Reagan wasn't Glaser's only potential connection. After Ariel returned home from the hospital, Elizabeth and Paul Glaser made a list of other people they might contact. Their UCLA doctors were very prominent; perhaps they could arrange for Elizabeth to meet with Admiral James Watkins, head of Reagan's Commission on AIDS, or C. Everett Koop, the surgeon general. The Glasers also listed prominent politicians who might be sympathetic, such as Senator Edward M. Kennedy and Representative Henry Waxman. High on the Glasers' list were celebrities. Because of where they lived and who Paul Glaser was, very famous people in Hollywood were just one or two phone calls away. For example, Elizabeth had taught Cher's daughter in elementary school. Lucy Wick knew film director Steven Spielberg.[23]

Just what Glaser was doing was now becoming clearer. At one level, she was simply trying to save the lives of her family. "I wanted to save my children," she later wrote, "and only bold strokes could accomplish that." But like any other effort to attract attention and, ultimately, funding, she needed to come up with a definable cause that was at once both sympathetic and compelling. And that cause became increasingly apparent: children with AIDS. No one within the broader AIDS movement, it seemed, had identified children as a separate interest group. "No one was fighting for the children," wrote Glaser. "No one. I felt a mantle of responsibility descend over my shoulders. It was a frightening and unforgettable moment."[24]

Within a few weeks, Glaser had already achieved one of her goals. Her physician, Michael Gottlieb, arranged for her to meet Koop during a trip he was making to Los Angeles in April 1988. Glaser's description of her preparation for the meeting is instructive. Yes, she would soon become "the most effective AIDS lobbyist in the country," but that day she was worried about what she should wear and what Koop would think of her. And she was about to break the careful code of silence that she and Paul Glaser had imposed on their lives, telling a stranger her secret.[25]

Glaser's meeting with Koop, who had himself experienced the death of a child, went well. And, inadvertently, she made a strategic move, mentioning to Koop that her friendship with Lucy Wick might give her direct access to President Reagan. Telling people that she had connections to the president, prominent politicians, or famous celebrities, Glaser was learning, made people view her as a "player." As time went on, Glaser became less and less reticent about using her friends to promote her cause. Within a few weeks, she traveled to Washington, D.C., to meet with Admiral Watkins and several influential members of Congress. Here Glaser learned another key lesson. Simply telling her story, and describing the seriousness of Ariel's condition, could get hardened Capitol Hill veterans to take notice and even cry.[26]

Not just anyone could have accomplished this. Glaser was becoming an extremely effective lobbyist. Once in the door, she was like a terrier latching onto someone's pant leg, passionate and single-minded in her insistence that pediatric AIDS was as much of an emergency as any other issue Congress was facing. Glaser was, one reporter wrote, an effective combination of "brittle" and "intense." Largely as a result of her lobbying, lawmakers would increase the 1989 NIH budget for pediatric AIDS from $3.3 to $8.8 million.[27]

Another event during Glaser's first visit to Washington further radicalized her. One of her meetings was with Philip A. Pizzo, chief of pediatrics at the National Cancer Institute and one of the few prominent researchers working on AIDS in children. Glaser was meeting with Pizzo both to learn about possible new AIDS drugs for Jake and to enlist him in her nascent effort to increase the amount of research funding allotted to pediatric AIDS. But Pizzo seemed more focused on Ariel's condition. He told

Glaser that he was completing a trial of intravenous AZT, which had produced positive results in a series of severely ill children with AIDS. Ariel had been taking the drug in pill form.

Glaser was "so surprised, it was hard to even breathe." Even though she and Paul had been discussing forgoing further aggressive measures for Ariel, what Pizzo was suggesting seemed well worth trying. And how, she asked herself, had Ariel's doctor not raised intravenous AZT as an option? When Glaser returned home, she "stormed in" to Stiehm's office and angrily demanded an explanation. Stiehm told her that because the drug was unavailable outside Pizzo's randomized trial, he had not mentioned it to her.[28]

Glaser's response, as recounted in her autobiography, could not better symbolize the new fervent patient-activist of the 1980s. "I do not fucking believe this!" she screamed. "You are telling me that there is something that may help her and the drug company won't let us use it?" Only months before, Glaser had thought of herself as a mother caring for a sick child. But now, by unabashedly pulling strings among the government officials she had just met in Washington, Glaser managed to obtain the intravenous AZT from a very reluctant Burroughs Wellcome, the pharmaceutical company that manufactured the drug. Ariel Glaser thus became the first child to get the drug outside a clinical trial.[29]

This story is at once both infuriating and inspiring. That it was Hollywood and Washington connections that got Ariel the drug seems inherently unjust. Yet the fact that Glaser had beaten the system made her a populist hero, the type that Henry Fonda or Jimmy Stewart played in the movies. As Glaser herself asked, "What can be more American than one person who tries to make a difference?" Glaser would have been the first to express discomfort at what had occurred and to emphasize how all children with AIDS deserved the same. But, after all, you had to start somewhere. And this was her precious, dying daughter.[30]

What happened next was also pure Hollywood. In June 1988, three weeks after the intravenous AZT was started, Elizabeth Glaser walked into her daughter's room. "Good morning, Mom," said Ariel, who had not uttered a word since before her hospitalization for pneumonia. "I love you." When Paul Glaser appeared, Ariel simply said, "Hi, Dad." Both parents cried.

Ariel Glaser continued to improve dramatically while taking the drug—walking, swimming, and even going to an amusement park. Intellectually, the Glasers knew this respite would only be brief. But it was hard to deny the Lazarus-like miracle. "The focus was always on what we could do," Elizabeth later recalled, "and now, anything seemed possible." Even more important was the apparent explanation behind Ariel's incredible turnaround. "None of us had given up," her mom wrote.[31]

With Ariel better, Glaser turned her attention to a meeting with the Reagans. When she approached Douglas Wick, he told her that he had never before asked the Reagans for anything and had rebuffed similar efforts from other friends. But it was Elizabeth Glaser's great gift to get people to do things they hadn't done before. Wick asked the Reagans, and they agreed to meet with Wick and Glaser on June 25, 1988. The meeting lasted more than an hour and the Reagans cried when they heard Ariel's story. Glaser told the president about her agenda and urged him to become a "leader in the struggle against AIDS."[32]

To Glaser's great chagrin, Reagan never followed through. He left office half a year later having utterly dropped the ball with respect to the AIDS epidemic. But Glaser pushed ahead anyway, beginning a private foundation to raise money for pediatric AIDS research with two of her best friends, Susan DeLaurentis and Susie Zeegen. There was a long tradition of parents starting foundations to publicize and fundraise for their children's diseases, such as cystic fibrosis and muscular dystrophy. For the most part, however, these organizations had been polite, dominated by expert physicians.

In the era of AIDS, however, there was no place for such niceties or deference. Ariel, having gradually lost the benefits of the AZT, died on August 12, 1988. Glaser's mission now crystallized: it was to save her son's life. "I had just lost a child," she wrote. "The last thing I was going to do was lose another." Time, therefore, was of the essence. The Pediatric AIDS Foundation, which promoted basic biomedical research, became a reality in 1989. That same year, the PAF hosted the first of its innovative think tanks, which gathered international AIDS researchers in the same room to share their results and to work together toward new insights.[33]

In a highly symbolic move, Glaser got liberal Ohio Senator Howard M. Metzenbaum and conservative Utah Senator Orrin G. Hatch to cosponsor "A Night to Unite," a PAF fundraiser held in Washington, D.C., on June 21, 1989, which netted more than $1 million. To get attendees to fork over $15,000 or more for a table, Glaser had unabashedly invited celebrities, ranging from Muhammad Ali to Alan Alda, who served as master of ceremonies, to her old friend Cher, who performed several songs.[34]

Glaser herself had to lie low at the event. Despite all of the miles she had logged in behalf of pediatric AIDS, Glaser had still not gone public. Those who knew her story, from the Reagans on down, had kept her confidences. Glaser told those who asked why she was at "A Night to Unite" that she was there in support of her friends, DeLaurentis and Zeegen, who were the public heads of the PAF.

The secret did not last much longer. People using fictitious identities soon began to place calls to the Glaser's home, the PAF, and Richard Stiehm's office, aggressively asking questions about Ariel and Elizabeth. Then, on August 11, 1989, someone from the *National Enquirer* called, admitting that the tabloid was planning to run a "very sad" story about the Glaser family. Knowing that the game was up, the Glasers decided to go public on their own terms rather than speaking with the *Enquirer.* Through a friend, they contacted Janet Huck, a reporter at the *Los Angeles Times.* Huck's article, "Breaking a Silence," which appeared in the August 25, 1989, issue of the paper, told the whole story, including Elizabeth Glaser's transfusions, Ariel's death, and the founding of the PAF.[35]

The Glasers were furious at having been outed, especially because of the harassment that had occurred. "How could any human being be doing this?" Elizabeth Glaser raged. "It was unethical, immoral, a total outrage."[36]

But she also knew better than anyone that her powerful personal story could now be harnessed to energize the pediatric AIDS cause. And it was. On February 4, 1990, CBS's *60 Minutes* aired a segment on the Glasers and the PAF, showing Elizabeth in action, relentlessly lobbying in Washington, D.C. A sympathetic portrayal on *60 Minutes*, which this most surely was, immediately legitimized her cause. Then, on March 13, 1990, the Glasers testified in front of the Budget Committee of the House of Representatives, demanding more money to research a disease that they estimated was affecting more than twenty thousand children in the United States. The media avidly covered the story, which had all the ingredients that would engage the public: a dead child; a doomed mother; an uninfected father, who was a Hollywood star; and a disease that raised issues of

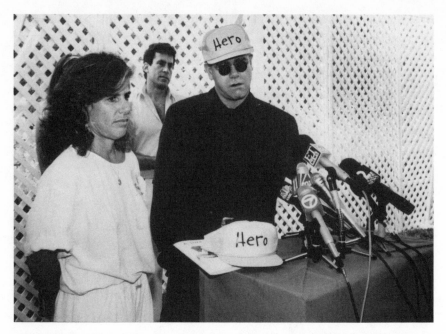

Elizabeth Glaser, with Elton John, at a Pediatric AIDS Foundation fundraiser. Courtesy of Michael Jacobs and the Elizabeth Glaser Pediatric AIDS Foundation.

stigma and blame. And there was also Jake. "If the federal government moves at the pace it is accustomed to," Glaser bluntly told the committee, "my son will probably not live."[37]

In its first five years, the PAF raised $30 million. Once again, the role played by the rich and famous was central. Among the celebrities who attended the PAF's annual fundraising picnics, which received extensive media coverage, were Whoopi Goldberg, Billy Crystal, Robin Williams, Billy Dee Williams, Florence Griffith Joyner, and Ronald and Nancy Reagan. The PAF, now the Elizabeth Glaser Pediatric AIDS Foundation, has continued to expand its purview, including delivering HIV drugs to developing countries.[38]

Glaser's remarkable achievements exemplified the new paradigm for disease advocacy that had emerged in the United States thanks to people like herself, Joy Piccolo, Betty Ford, Yasmin Aga Khan, and Ryan White, the HIV-positive Indiana teenager who became an AIDS activist in the late 1980s. If you wanted attention paid to a particular disease, you needed to scream loudly and where someone would hear you. And if you could equate inaction with death, so much the better. Attention meant money, and money meant hope. Mobilizing the press was utterly essential. As Edward Bernays and the other founders of public relations knew, there is no such thing as bad publicity.

The pinnacle of Glaser's crusade came when she spoke at the Democratic National Convention on July 14, 1992. Although public figures with AIDS, including Earvin "Magic" Johnson and Arthur Ashe, were becoming more commonplace, the presence of someone with the fatal disease addressing the entire country was still a news event. Glaser used the opportunity to hammer home one theme: the Reagan and Bush administrations had neglected AIDS and had thus let down their country. "We *must* have ACTION," she implored, "a President *and* a Congress who can work together so we can get out of this gridlock and move ahead."[39]

But it was because Glaser was an HIV-positive mother whose daughter had died of AIDS that her words were so compelling. The most frequently reproduced paragraph of her speech includes the following:

> My daughter lived seven years, and in her last year, when she couldn't walk or talk, her wisdom shone through. She taught me to love when all I wanted to do was hate. She taught me to help others, when all I wanted to do was help myself. She taught me to be brave, when all I felt was fear.[40]

These words added little to the health policy implications of Glaser's speech. But because they were so moving, they propelled her cause forward. How could you not support this courageous mother whose beautiful daughter had died? Glaser ended her speech differently than did most speakers at the convention, with a deep, conspicuous bow. My cause, pediatric AIDS, is not going away, her body language said, even if I do not survive. Indeed, Glaser died of AIDS on December 3, 1994.[41]

Glaser also used her speech to note the irony that she, a heterosexual woman, was serving as the public face of AIDS. She was a "strange spokesperson" for the disease, she noted, which by 1992 had become increasingly prominent among injection drug users and poor and minority populations. But to Glaser, how she or others had become infected with HIV was infinitely less relevant than what the government was going to do about it.

Arthur Ashe could not have agreed more. As an African American who had grown up in a family of modest means, he knew as well as anyone how dangerous it was to cast HIV-positive individuals either as "innocent" victims or as deserving of what had happened. Moreover, when he learned of his infection in 1988, Ashe knew that AIDS was increasingly becoming an issue for the black community.

Nevertheless, the man who had been a lifelong activist for problems affecting African Americans did not initially choose to become an AIDS crusader, even behind the scenes, as did Glaser. For one thing, by 1988, Ashe could benefit from a series of advances that scientists and activists had already achieved. After his toxoplasmosis was cured, he began to take AZT and then, in 1992, added the second effective HIV drug, didanosine (ddI). Also, Ashe's plate was full with numerous other charitable enterprises. But mostly Ashe did not act because of his family. The unfortunate reality was that the diagnosis of AIDS still carried a tremendous stigma as of the late 1980s, and Ashe did not want to add to the burden that his illness already placed on the lives of Jeanne and Camera. He knew he would have to go public some day, but wanted to do so on his own terms.[42]

Like most AIDS patients, Ashe, always slender, was losing weight and appeared gaunt. When somebody asked about his frailty, he was able to cite his serious heart disease as a cause. Rumors about a more grave diagnosis abounded, but remained rumors.

Thus, what happened on April 7, 1992, came like a jolt. A childhood friend of Ashe and a tennis writer at *USA Today*, Doug Smith, had asked if he could visit. After some small talk, Smith cut to the chase. With obvious discomfort, he told Ashe that his newspaper had gotten a tip that Ashe was HIV positive. Smith's editor had asked him to find out. "Is it true?" Smith asked.[43]

According to *Days of Grace*, Ashe acted with his usual equanimity. "I try hard to keep calm and subdued at all times," he wrote. "But the anger was building in me that this newspaper, *any* newspaper or any part of the media, could think that it had a right to tell the world that I had AIDS." Still, in the weeks after the episode, Ashe and Jeanne would actually provide emotional support to Smith, who felt very guilty over what had occurred.[44]

Rather than answering Smith, Ashe called his boss, *USA Today* sports editor Gene Policinski. Policinski did not back down, asking Ashe, "Are you HIV-positive, or do you have AIDS?" Rather than lying, Ashe said: "Could be."[45]

The confrontation between Ashe and *USA Today*, which would soon be front-page news, was perhaps the most prominent public debate about an issue that has arisen throughout this book: does the public have the right to know when celebrities become seriously ill? As of 1992, the answer was yes in the case of elected officials, but was less clear for professional athletes, such as Magic Johnson. If such people wished to remain active in sports, then disclosure seemed appropriate. One might also argue that someone like Elizabeth Glaser, by dint of her behind-the-scenes role as an AIDS fundraiser, had also sacrificed her right to privacy. But as Ashe told Policinski, he was simply a retired tennis player, a private citizen minding his own business.

Policinski, of course, disagreed, telling Ashe that his tennis career and political activism made him a public figure: "And any time a public figure is ill, it's news. If he has a heart attack, as you did in 1979, it's news. We have no special zone of treatment for AIDS. It's a disease, like heart disease. It is news."[46]

With their backs to the wall, Arthur Ashe and Jeanne Moutoussamy-Ashe decided, as had Elizabeth and Paul Glaser, that it was better to go public on their own terms—specifically, to hold a press conference at which Ashe would announce that he had AIDS. Meanwhile, he called numerous family members and friends to give them advance warning. Finally, he asked his friend, sportswriter Frank Deford, to help him draft a statement.

Ashe awoke the next morning, April 8, to one piece of good news. *USA Today* had not published the story. When Ashe, accompanied by his wife, doctors, New York City mayor David Dinkins, and friends, stepped to the podium at Home Box Office headquarters at 3:30 p.m., the room was packed with sports and medical reporters. Ashe began with a joke, saying that he had been asked to manage the New York Yankees. But he then recounted his medical history from his heart bypass operations to learning in 1988 that he had AIDS. Ashe then explained his original decision to keep quiet and why he could no longer do so. To sports fans watching, Ashe's dignified public admission of a fatal illness had to bring back memories of Lou Gehrig's words fifty-three years earlier. But a symbolic, vague statement about a "bad break" was no longer sufficient. Forty-five minutes of questions from reporters followed Ashe's remarks.[47]

And there was another major difference between Ashe and Gehrig. The media had become a visible player in the story of Ashe's illness. Journalists across the country and the globe asked themselves, Had their colleagues at *USA Today* made the right decision? What would they have done in the same situation?

The ethics of journalism, as much as Ashe's illness, dominated the news for several days. Television programs that discussed the outing included *Nightline, 20/20*, the *Today* show, *Geraldo* (with Geraldo Rivera), and *First Person* (with Maria Shriver). Most programs featured commentators on both sides of the issue. Newspapers and magazines also ran extensive coverage on the ethical debate.

Not surprisingly, *USA Today* defended its decision, underscoring the duties of the fourth estate. "When the press has kept secrets . . . that conspiracy of silence has not served the public," editor Peter Prichard wrote. "Journalists serve the public by reporting news, not hiding it." Another argument was that the enormous public interest in the Ashe story had retrospectively validated the decision. "Unfortunately, it is a story that's bigger than the individual," stated Paul McMasters, executive director of Vanderbilt University's Freedom Forum First Amendment Center. "The reaction to this whole thing is the best proof possible." In other words, the ends justified the means.[48]

Other critics pushed the issue further, arguing that Ashe deserved to be outed because he was not doing enough to promote AIDS awareness. Bryant Gumbel, a longtime acquaintance of the Ashe family, raised this uncomfortable issue when he interviewed Ashe on NBC's *Today* show the morning after the press conference. Gumbel quoted one AIDS activist as stating that Ashe could have saved lives had he announced his diagnosis in 1988. Ashe addressed the issue in typical fashion, without anger or defensiveness. "I will responsibly get involved the way I see fit," he told Gumbel.[49]

The majority of commentators, at least publicly, took Ashe's side. A typical comment came from essayist Lance Morrow in *Time* magazine, who chided his peers for treating Ashe's story as "juicy gossip" and "red meat." "There was no public need to know, or right to know," Morrow intoned. "The fact that Arthur Ashe was a great and renowned athlete who established milestones for blacks is no reason to treat his personal struggle as a peep show," opined syndicated columnist Mona Charen. The *Washington Post's* Jonathan Yardley agreed. "No public issues were at stake," he stated. "No journalistic rights were threatened." "This story makes me queasy,"

New York Times columnist Anna Quindlen wrote. "Perhaps it is the disparity between the value of the information and the magnitude of the pain inflicted."[50]

Indeed, the image of Ashe, a seemingly decent human being with so much bad luck, now being subjected to unwanted public scrutiny made some people change their minds about the outing. *Philadelphia Inquirer* editor Acel Moore, for example, said that he initially believed that the story should be published. In retrospect, however, "the personal human side . . . outweighed the news value." NBC anchorman Garrick Utley apologized for his profession: "Journalists are not perfect. Sometimes we make mistakes. And this was one of them."[51]

What did the public think? It was hard to tell. Those who registered formal opinions mostly objected to what had happened. *USA Today* received roughly seven hundred calls, 95 percent of which were critical. Similarly, Ashe received hundreds of letters in the weeks and months after his announcement, which overwhelmingly chastised the media. Typical was the letter from a New York man: "I was very saddened to see you and Jeanne have to stand up in front of a firing squad and have them invade and reveal your private life." "I felt my blood pressure hit the ceiling," wrote a woman. "Anger at the paper and all reporters who feed upon other people's tragedies." Those who agreed with *USA Today*, of course, would have been much less likely to write to Ashe.[52]

Beyond the issue of outing, the letters to Ashe revealed continuities with those sent to earlier ill celebrities. First, as had been the case with John Foster Dulles, Ashe received considerable correspondence urging him to embrace God to help him get well. Many of these letters came from African Americans. "What I am getting at," a pastor from Queens told Ashe, "is that God has made provision for your healing, even of the aids [*sic*] virus." Other correspondents told familiar, usually uplifting "n of 1" stories about their own illnesses or those of loved ones. "My older brother, Mark, contracted HIV in 1983," wrote a man from South Carolina, "and is still going strong."[53]

But different themes emerged as well. The spectacle of Ashe being forced to reveal his diagnosis in front of the entire world genuinely moved people. Letter after letter, many from individuals who had never previously written to a celebrity, commented on Ashe's grace and dignity. Ashe, a Long Island man opined, was someone "who has authenticity, true character, integrity, and the most rare of all traits: elegance." "Listening to you answer those most difficult questions with honesty, integrity and intelligence," a New Jersey man wrote, "reaffirmed my belief in the resiliency and power of the human spirit to manage adversity." "I suppose you will never know how many people you have helped by appearing on TV," wrote an HIV-positive man, "but here is one."[54]

The fact that Ashe was going public about a stigmatized disease did not go unnoticed. Many people announced that they would view Ashe no differently now, an attitude that he surely wished would be applied to everyone with AIDS. A woman from Locust Valley, New York, sent a note "to let you know you are still, to me, the same person you have always been." "Yes, there will be people who fear your Aides [sic]," wrote a woman from Alabama, "but I won't be one." While Ashe had not intended to educate the public about AIDS—yet—he was already doing so impressively. "When a family like yours is hit with this disease, the public has to change its perception of the whole situation," wrote Ashe's friend George W. Haywood. "It becomes harder for people to hold on to old prejudices against people with AIDS."[55]

Ashe's race also mattered. Whites who wrote to him often stated their race, presumably to demonstrate how Ashe's tragedy transcended racial boundaries. "As a white Richmond woman," wrote someone from Ashe's hometown, "I have always been so proud of Arthur." A Jewish woman in California proposed starting an Ashe fan club for grandmothers. "You have made a greater difference already than most people can ever hope to make," wrote a "white, female, country club tennis player."[56]

African American correspondents identified with Ashe's plight even more intensely. A "young, black American" woman from Florida told Ashe that he had long been one of her idols, and a woman from Illinois wrote that "we are proud of our black men." A group of African American students from Brooklyn's Bishop Loughlin Memorial High School sent letters as part of a class assignment. "This is sad that another brother has fallen to a deadly disease," one wrote. "You are a strong blackman [sic]," wrote her classmate, "and I have no doubt you will continue to be strong."[57]

But AIDS had also splintered the black community. Some commentators questioned the standard account that HIV had emerged in Africa, an explanation, it seemed, that indirectly blamed the epidemic on African Americans. Another set of blacks being singled out unfairly as potential vectors of AIDS, critics charged, were Haitians. More radical writers, noting the growth of AIDS in poor and black communities as the 1980s progressed, claimed that the disease had been created by scientists as a means of genocide. Fueling such allegations were very real historical episodes, most notably the Tuskegee experiment, in which African Americans had been victimized by the largely white medical establishment.[58]

A small percentage of letter-writers thus urged Ashe to question the status quo vis-à-vis AIDS. Some told him to reject standard treatment in favor of Kemron, a medication developed at the Kenyan Medical Research Institute in Nairobi. Kemron was a form of alpha-interferon, an antiviral substance related to one of the last-ditch treatments that Steve McQueen had received for cancer. At a 1990 conference, Kenyan physicians had reported a "miraculous" response to the medication, with clinical improvement in more than 90 percent of cases. African American media outlets in the United States, such as New York's *Amsterdam News* and radio station WLIB, eagerly broadcast reports about the new wonder drug. When members of the scientific establishment dismissed the value of Kemron, some blacks alleged they were being racist.[59]

Reasoned as always, Ashe neither embraced nor rejected Kemron at first. Instead, he talked with Barbara Justice, an African American physician who was one of the drug's strongest advocates. But when AIDS expert Anthony Fauci and Ashe's trusted infectious diseases physician, Henry F. Murray, informed him that multiple clinical trials conducted by the National Institutes of Health had shown Kemron to be of no medical value, Ashe decided to pass in favor of AZT and ddI. "In this matter as in others," he wrote in *Days of Grace*, "I cannot allow myself to be swayed by arguments based on theories of racial conspiracy and racial genocide."[60]

The Kemron episode was only one example of the complicated interaction of race and AIDS that Ashe confronted. Despite the grave nature of his disease, he continued to stress that his being black in America—not having AIDS—was "the greatest burden I've had to bear." Thus, when Ashe became an AIDS activist after going public with his diagnosis, he did so through the prism of race. As a black man who had long addressed issues of discrimination and poverty, he was even more able than Glaser to fight the idea that some people somehow "deserved" their HIV infection. As he often stated, "The pathologies of the inner city also generate AIDS cases."[61]

Ashe used two specific strategies to foster AIDS education: a foundation and public appearances. The foundation was the Arthur Ashe Foundation for the Defeat of AIDS. Like foundations focusing on other illnesses, Ashe's raised money to support educational programs and research. And, like Glaser, Ashe drew on a group of wealthy, well-known individuals to jumpstart his effort: in this case, the tennis community. In August 1992, at the U.S. Open tennis tournament, an exhibition featuring John McEnroe, Pete Sampras, Andre Agassi, and Martina Navratilova raised $114,000. Over the next decade, donations to the foundation would total more than $5 million. Ashe also lent his name to the funding of the Arthur Ashe chair in pediatric AIDS research at St. Jude's Hospital in Memphis.[62]

Ashe gave speeches at places as diverse as the National Press Club, the National Urban League, and, most notably, the United Nations on World AIDS Day. At many of these appearances Ashe was given awards, including being named the 1992 Sportsman of the Year by *Sports Illustrated* magazine. Ashe also spoke at numerous colleges and other schools, which enabled him to emphasize safe sex and other AIDS-prevention measures. Given that Ashe knew he had so little time left, it is striking that his speeches were not boilerplate at all. They were largely hand-written, specifically geared for the audiences to be addressed.

Throughout these appearances, Ashe consistently underscored the connection of AIDS to larger societal issues. Speaking to the Community Health Centers in Atlanta, he noted that his annual bill for medications, $18,000, was out of the range of most Americans. At the Harvard Medical School commencement in June 1992, he urged the graduates to care less about making money than fighting for lower health care costs and national health care insurance. Ashe also pointedly challenged his audience by calling attention to the continued stigmatization of AIDS patients. "Some of you graduating today," he charged, "wouldn't treat me if I came to you." AIDS as an international issue was crucial to both Ashe and his foundation. In the United Nations World AIDS Day speech, he criticized the fact that 94 percent of funds used to treat AIDS patients were spent in developed nations while 80 percent of new cases were arising in the developing world.[63]

Ashe also tried to spend as much time as he could with Jeanne and Camera. But in early January 1993, he developed *Pneumocystis carinii* pneumonia, a condition that plagued many AIDS patients. Although Ashe re-

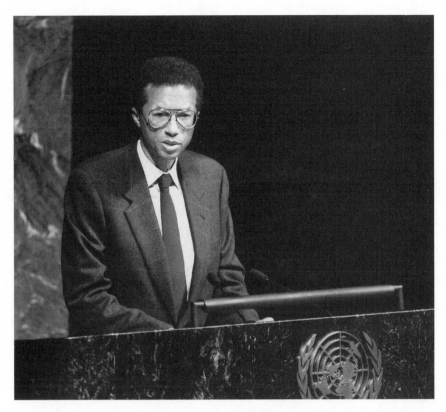

A very thin Arthur Ashe, having publicly disclosed his AIDS diagnosis, addresses the United Nations General Assembly on December 1, 1992, World AIDS Day. He would be dead two months later. UN/DPI photo courtesy of the United Nations Multimedia Resources.

covered from the infection, he suffered a relapse during the first week of February 1993. His body now overwhelmed by the infection, Ashe died at New York Hospital on February 7.

To those following his story closely, Ashe's death could not have been a big surprise. As soon as he went public, he was very candid about the fact that he was dying. "Living with AIDS," he often stated, "is a little like being on death row." Such a frank admission did not have the impact it would have had a few decades earlier, but it still packed a punch. "Hearing you say *death* on *Nightline*," one woman told Ashe, "made me cry." Ashe was preparing himself for death through prayer. He had embraced the teachings of Howard Thurman, an African American theologian who empha-sized the possibility of spiritual growth in the face of racism. If he died from AIDS, Ashe wrote, it was God's will. "I am not afraid of death," he added. Both Jacqueline Kennedy Onassis and former president Richard M. Nixon followed Ashe's footsteps in 1994, declining further aggressive treatment of their serious illnesses. As described in earlier chapters, it was an option that neither Brian Piccolo nor Steve McQueen ever considered.[64]

By educating the public about AIDS and beginning a successful foun-dation that sought to cure the disease, Arthur Ashe followed the formula increasingly expected of an ill celebrity. But by connecting AIDS to broader social issues and by so openly discussing his death, Ashe also became a moral beacon, a true martyr for a secular era. Members of the media, who ten months earlier had debated the ethics of Ashe being outed, shed any appearance of dispassion as they reported on his death. Bryant Gumbel, who had asked Ashe such tough questions after the press conference, cried openly on the *Today* show. ABC sportscaster Dick Schaap described Ashe as a "singular" man: "And as hard as I tried, I couldn't think of a flaw or a weakness. Then I tried to think about anybody else I could say that about and I couldn't come up with one name."[65]

Through her single-minded devotion to her children and other children with AIDS, despite her own deteriorating medical condition, Elizabeth Glaser also served as a moral example. As time went on, Glaser's public statements were less about pediatric AIDS than the larger issue of taking action in the face of adversity or injustice. "The choice and challenge is in how we choose to live," she stated. "People say they care, but actions are what save lives."[66]

One saved life was that of Jake Glaser. "The foundation," Susie Zeegen recently recalled, "was started to save one little boy's life." As of early 2006, Jake is 21 years old and doing well on so-called triple-drug therapy, a com-bination of pills that has dramatically extended the lives of many AIDS patients. Was it the efforts of Elizabeth Glaser and her foundation that actually saved Jake's life? Perhaps, but it doesn't really matter. What is more important is that Jake's mother, Elizabeth, symbolically forged a connec-tion between disease, activism, and survival that served as an example of what other parents, celebrities or not, could also possibly achieve. As one eighth-grade boy said after Glaser died, "She proves that you can do any-thing you want."[67]

Another set of parents who embarked on a mission to save their child's life were Augusto and Michaela Odone. When their 5-year-old son, Lorenzo, developed a rare, fatal neurological disorder, they learned all they could about the disease, raised funds, and urged researchers to work in tandem. Then, when things were still moving too slowly, they pushed the new AIDS-era activism to yet a higher level, attempting by themselves to find a cure for the disease. What the Odones ultimately achieved was nothing short of remarkable. But proving what they had accomplished would not be easy.

Chapter 12

The Last Angry Man and Woman

Lorenzo Odone's Parents Fight the
Medical Establishment

The story of Lorenzo Odone, his parents, Augusto and Michaela, and the home-made remedy, Lorenzo's Oil, contains all the elements of the celebrity illness narratives discussed in this book. First, there was a gravely ill boy who, by dint of his rare disease, adrenoleukodystrophy, became a famous patient of great interest to the media and the public. Second, there were doctors and scientists working to learn about ALD and, if possible, develop successful treatments. Third, there were Lorenzo's parents, who left no stone unturned in their passionate desire to treat, and possibly cure, their son's illness. Finally, there was a powerful Hollywood movie, *Lorenzo's Oil,* which became the definitive version of what was, in reality, a very complicated story.

Was Lorenzo's Oil a remarkable cure that had saved countless lives, a useful preventive measure, or a "sham"? Was the movie the triumphant story of heroic parents succeeding despite the opposition of a stubborn medical profession, or, as some critics argued, was it misleading and manipulative? Part of the inability to definitively answer these questions stems from the familiar problem of inconclusive data. Where some saw answers others continued to see uncertainty.

The story of Lorenzo's Oil represents the apotheosis of the patient-activist movement that emerged at the end of the twentieth century. Like the AIDS activists, the Odones questioned the basic assumptions made by physicians about both scientific evidence and humanity in the face of serious illness. Their efforts engendered tremendous admiration from ill and healthy people across the world. But they also generated a surprising backlash from others who feared the implication of the Odones' story: that sick patients or their families could no longer sit back and trust their doctors but had to engage in some type of personal crusade to make sure they got well.

One would not have pegged Augusto and Michaela Odone as future activists. When they married in 1977, the Italian-born Augusto was an economist working for the World Bank. Michaela Murphy, raised in Yonkers, New York, was an editor working for a Washington, D.C., management company. Their first and only child, Lorenzo, was born in May 1978. In 1980 the family relocated for Augusto's work to the Comoros Islands, off East Africa.[1]

Lorenzo was an exceptionally bright child who knew three languages—English, Italian, and French—by age 5. He was a voracious reader and had a particular love for classical music. Thus, it was especially jarring in September 1983 when Lorenzo, then 5 years old, began having temper tantrums and slurring his words. By this time, the family had moved to Chevy Chase, Maryland, in the suburbs of Washington. Initially, the Odones assumed that Lorenzo's symptoms had something to do with his starting a new school in a new country. But rather than improving he got worse, being disruptive and unkind to other children at school. Then, in December 1983, Lorenzo fell twice, necessitating visits to a local hospital. The results of neurological tests, however, were normal.

The Odones grew increasingly concerned. As so often happens with rare diseases, there was an extensive period of misdiagnosis. Psychologists suspected an emotional disorder or, despite Lorenzo's great intelligence, a developmental delay. But when Lorenzo next developed hearing loss, the organic nature of the problem could no longer be denied. More extensive neurological testing was done, and in April 1984 the doctors arrived at the grim diagnosis of adrenoleukodystrophy. ALD is a rare genetic neurological disorder caused by degeneration of the protective myelin sheath that normally surrounds nerve cells in the brain and the adrenal glands. The disease affects only males, roughly one of every twenty-five thousand born; as of the mid-1980s, between two and three thousand cases had been diagnosed in the United States. In its most severe form, found most commonly in boys between the ages of 5 and 10, ALD causes gradual paralysis, blindness, deafness, and inability to speak and swallow.[2]

The disease is accompanied by the buildup of very-long-chain saturated fatty acids (VLCFAs), which have 24 or 26 carbon atoms, in the blood. As of the mid-1980s, some scientists believed it was the excess VLCFAs that damaged the myelin, but there was no proof for this theory. Only males develop ALD because it, like hemophilia, is X-linked. While females with the defective gene have an extra X chromosome that can produce the enzymes to break down the toxic fatty acids, males do not. Because males inherit their single damaged X chromosome from their mother, Michaela Odone felt especially responsible. It meant that she had unwittingly been the silent carrier of a genetic defect that produced this awful disease in her son.

When it came to discussing prognosis, Lorenzo Odone's doctors did not obfuscate, as had those of Lou Gehrig and Brian Piccolo. The Odones were told that the white matter of Lorenzo's brain would continue to deteriorate at a very rapid rate. He would likely be dead, the doctors said, within two years.

With these words the Odones reached a familiar crossroads, one that Morris Abram and Steve McQueen had experienced and that Elizabeth Glaser would confront in a few years. What do you do when a doctor gives you or your child a death sentence? One can always get second or third opinions, of course, but in Lorenzo's case, as the Odones would soon learn, there was consensus. Research on ALD was ongoing, but the condition was untreatable.

Perhaps the best way to describe the odyssey of the Odones over the next several years is that it was "like a Hollywood movie," full of heroic figures, serendipitous discoveries, remarkable triumphs, and crushing defeats. This is, of course, why it became a Hollywood film. Over time, distinguishing fact from the fictional movie would become increasingly difficult. It is important to remember, therefore, that the Odones were not crusaders from the start, characters following a predestined path. In reality, their mission began more quietly, with a basic unwillingness to be passive in the face of such bad news. The main motivating factor was concern for their son. "We thought," Augusto later remarked, "'We love this kid, and we don't want to lose him.'" "What we did was rise to his needs," Michaela said. "He expected us to do it." Another spur for the Odones was the dismissive reaction of certain members of the medical profession to their desire for more information. Augusto Odone later recalled how one physician responded to his request for scientific articles: "Oh, I wouldn't bother. You wouldn't be able to understand them anyway."[3]

But there were resources available to laypeople wishing to learn more about diseases, especially if one lived in suburban Maryland, home of the National Institutes of Health. Augusto Odone became a constant presence at the NIH library, learning everything he could about ALD. The news was not good. The one existing treatment was a diet low in VLCFAs, devised by the country's expert on ALD, Hugo Moser of Baltimore's John F. Kennedy Institute for handicapped children. The Odones took Lorenzo to see Moser, who placed the boy on the diet in May 1984. Unfortunately, the levels of VLCFAs in Lorenzo's blood did not decrease and he grew progressively less coordinated. A trial of experimental immunosuppression did not help either. By the summer of 1984, Lorenzo was having difficulty speaking and swallowing.

When Michaela was not attending to Lorenzo, she joined her husband in the library. The literature contained far too many mysteries for the Odones, leading Augusto to contact scientists and physicians directly, pushing them for answers. Odone, a courtly man with a thick Italian accent and "old world charm," was invariably polite. But some of his targets were clearly offended that a layperson was fancying himself an expert on such a complicated and obscure disease as ALD. Moreover, Odone noted what he believed was an inherent conflict between his urgency as a parent and the often deliberate nature of scientists. "They were looking at ALD as a route to a Nobel Prize 20 years down the road," Odone stated, "while I was watching my son die." Odone derided the notion that science had to move at its own pace as "baloney."[4]

One thing that particularly bothered the Odones was that ALD researchers across the globe were often working in isolation, unaware of one another's findings. Indeed, it was Michaela's discovery of information in the English abstract of an article in a Polish medical journal that produced the Odones' first "eureka" moment. A scientist reported that rats deprived of VLCFAs simply produced more such fatty acids, thus explaining why Moser's diet had proven ineffective. But feeding the rats a different type of fat, a process known as lipid manipulation, could lower levels of VLCFAs. If such a strategy worked in rats, the Odones wondered, why wouldn't it work in humans?[5]

This was one question the Odones planned to ask at an October 1984 symposium that they organized with the help of Hugo Moser. Thirty-eight doctors from around the world attended, sharing information with one another for the first time. Among the presenters was William B. Rizzo of the Medical College of Virginia, who reported that adding oleic acid, a monounsaturated fat with only 18 carbon atoms, to a test tube with cells from ALD patients halved the production of VLCFAs by those cells. But, Rizzo explained, oleic acid was not available in a form that humans could ingest.[6]

This seemingly closed door was just the impetus that Michaela Odone needed. Over the next several days, she made dozens of phone calls to companies that made medicinal oils, beseeching them to locate—or manufacture—some type of edible oleic acid. After an initial round of apologies and unanswered calls, Michaela succeeded. Capital City Products of Columbus, Ohio, had a product that was 90 percent pure oleic acid and it was willing to send the Odones a sample. There were no guarantees, however, that the fatty acid would be safe for Lorenzo.

Enter Deirdre Murphy, Michaela's sister and herself a carrier of the abnormal ALD gene. Like most carriers, Murphy was healthy but did have elevated VLCFA levels in her blood. In January 1985 she volunteered to be the "family rat," ingesting a series of Italian dishes prepared with the oil by Augusto Odone, an excellent cook. To everyone's joy, Murphy tolerated the oil without difficulty. And when her VLCFA levels were tested one month later, they had fallen by half. The Odones had concurrently put Lorenzo on a special diet containing the oil, similarly lowering his VLCFA levels, although not into the normal range.[7]

How did oleic acid work? The assumption was that patients with ALD had a defective gene that could not produce the enzyme needed to break down the ingested VLCFAs. Yet the body also produces its own VLCFAs by elongating shorter fatty acids from the diet. After yet another night immersed in the ALD literature, Augusto Odone had an epiphany that no scientist had yet had: the same enzyme that produces VLCFAs also elongates unsaturated fatty acids like oleic acid. If animals or patients ingested oleic acid, therefore, the enzymes would be so busy elongating unsaturated fatty acids that they would not make as many VLCFAs. The scientific name for this phenomenon is competitive inhibition.[8]

But the oleic acid diet by itself had not done the trick. Perhaps, Odone hypothesized, there was another monounsaturated fatty acid that could further inhibit the production of VLCFAs. Odone quickly found a candidate: a 22-carbon fatty acid known as erucic acid. But like oleic acid, it was not readily available in an edible form. There is some erucic acid in rapeseed oil, a cooking oil used in Europe that is derived from the seeds of a mustard plant. However, rapeseed oil also contains saturated fats, so it probably would not work. And physicians such as Moser were worried about the possible toxicity of erucic acid, which was known to cause heart damage in laboratory animals.[9]

But these were merely temporary roadblocks for the Odones, whose mottos had become "You never know until you try" and "Fortune favors the brave." Through another round of phone calls, Michaela identified a British biochemist nearing retirement, Don Suddaby, who was willing to try to produce pure erucic acid. It took six months of research, but by December 1986 Suddaby had succeeded. Once again, Deirdre Murphy served as the laboratory rat, now taking a combination of erucic and oleic acids. The results were even more spectacular. After eleven days, Murphy's VLCFA levels were completely normal. Nor had the oils caused any heart problems. Within three weeks, Lorenzo, who had also begun ingesting the oil, had normal VLCFA levels as well. "The bad guys were destroyed," rejoiced Augusto Odone. "Destroyed!"[10]

Unfortunately, Lorenzo was also being destroyed by his disease. As of the end of 1986, he was bed-bound and unable to move his head or arms, swallow his saliva, or talk. Although some people later questioned her assessment, Michaela Odone relentlessly asserted that the mixture of oils, which was named Lorenzo's Oil, had caused significant improvement in Lorenzo's condition. As of early 1990, when Lorenzo was 11, his mother said he was able to kiss her, enjoy hearing stories and classical music, and communicate by blinking his eyes and moving his fingertips. (Augusto Odone reports continued meaningful interactions with his son, who turned 28 in May 2006.) Still, the oil never reversed the ravages of Lorenzo's ALD.[11]

As they tested the oils on Murphy and Lorenzo, the Odones were, by definition, collecting data on blood fatty acid levels. As such, they compiled the results in a series of short unpublished papers that were a curious mix of the complicated science they had mastered and the personal story of Lorenzo. The Odones were careful to couch their findings in the cautious language of science. Their first paper, dated April 30, 1985, characterized the results of the oleic acid testing only as "preliminary observations." The erucic acid data, the Odones wrote in a subsequent, June 1987 report, "would seem to bear out the key hypotheses formulated in our April and June 1985 papers."[12]

The Odones were hardly the only parents devoting their energies to ALD. In 1982, interested families had founded an organization, the United Leukodystrophy Foundation (ULF), that focused on ALD and nine related leukodystrophies, which were other genetic disorders of myelin. As of 1984, when Lorenzo's disease was diagnosed, Ron and Paula Brazeal of Sycamore, Illinois, had assumed leadership of the several-hundred-member organization. The Brazeals had lost their oldest son, Howard, to ALD, and their youngest son, Timmy, was dying of the disease. The ULF was a typical "kitchen table" health organization, run on a shoestring budget out of the Brazeals' basement. Moser worked closely with the ULF, which held annual family meetings and raised funds to support scientists.[13]

The Odones' decision to do their own research led to tension between them and the Brazeals. It was necessary, the Odones had concluded, to constantly challenge the scientific establishment. The ULF was too fatalistic for their taste. "Our message to parents," Michaela Odone stated, "is realize that your interests and the doctors' interests are not parallel." Such a message irked the Brazeals and other ULF members, who saw themselves as facilitating the work of ALD researchers rather than weighing in on the science. "We try to educate parents," Paula Brazeal recently stated, "to do what you have to do to make it easy for the doctor."[14]

In early 1985, when there was suggestive evidence that oleic acid lowered VLCFA levels, conflict emerged over what to do. The Odones, predictably, believed that the entire ALD community was entitled to their findings, however tentative, as soon as possible. On January 18, 1985, shortly after Lorenzo and his aunt had begun the oleic acid, the Odones sent a letter to roughly forty ALD families that summarized both the results of the October 1984 conference and the earliest VLCFA data. As an explanation for their somewhat atypical behavior, the Odones wrote that "motivation can often compensate for a lack of technical background." They were passing on the good reports about Lorenzo "out of a sense of stewardship" and "because we believe they offer some hope." They urged readers to discuss the oil with their children's doctors.[15]

According to Augusto Odone, the report was sent to those families the

Odones had met at the June 1984 ULF conference. It did not go to the larger ULF membership, in large part due to Moser's reservations, which he expressed to Augusto and Michaela Odone in a January 29, 1985, letter. Although the Odones had shown "so vividly what love, motivation, intelligence, enterprise and hard work can do," Moser wrote, he could not associate himself with their anecdotal data. "It goes against my grain," he stated, "and a set of attitudes and understandings of relationships that have grown with me over the 36 years that I have been a physician." That is, Moser's approval of the Odones' report would have blurred the "lay-physician" line in a way that would have made him "uncomfortable." The use of the oil for Lorenzo, he continued, was appropriate, but it needed further, more formal testing.[16]

A version of this interaction was vividly depicted in the 1992 movie *Lorenzo's Oil*, in a scene that, according to Augusto Odone, director George Miller largely let him write. In the scene, Dr. Gus Nikolais, the character meant to represent Moser, asks the Odones to keep the information about oleic acid from the other families. In response, Michaela, played by Susan Sarandon, calls Nikolais "a wretched man." Then Augusto, played by Nick Nolte, urges the Muscatines, the heads of an ALD organization based on the ULF, to alert the entire membership about oleic acid. Other parents, he insists, have "a right to know this." When the Muscatines decline, deferring to Nikolais, Augusto screams at them: "This acquiescence is so disgusting!"[17]

But in the real world, in 1985, Moser could not keep news of this potential magnitude quiet. On May 31, four months after his letter to the Odones, Moser wrote a letter to the ALD membership about "a new nutritional approach to adrenoleukodystrophy." He thanked both the Odones and William Rizzo for their insights, then proposed a ten-patient study of oleic acid that would settle the question of its value "as quickly and as decisively as possible." It was premature to recommend it broadly, Moser believed: "I hesitate to recommend to all families the major change in lifestyle involved in total adherence to the diet before the results of the studies now underway are available."[18]

A similar dynamic occurred when the Odones reached their conclusions about the effectiveness of Lorenzo's Oil, the combination of oleic and erucic acids, in lowering VLCFA levels to normal. By this time, of course, the Odones and their research were well-known in the ALD world. Once again, according to Augusto Odone, Moser was reluctant to recommend the oil widely, especially given the potential cardiac toxicity of the erucic acid. In fact, it was Rizzo—not Moser—who began the first study of Lorenzo's Oil, monitoring the effects of the oil on twelve boys with ALD beginning in August 1987. Rizzo ultimately concluded that the oil was safe, effectively lowered VLCFA levels, and "may prevent further demyelination in some mildly affected boys."[19]

Moser and the Brazeals remember these events differently than does Augusto Odone. Moser has written that within thirty days of the development of Lorenzo's Oil (presumably referring to the date on which he learned of the Odones' data), the Kennedy Institute's institutional review board and the U.S. Food and Drug Administration had approved its use in a trial that Moser planned to organize. At that point, according to Moser, no ALD family was denied the oil, which Moser was given the sole ability to prescribe. Once Moser's trial began in 1989, Ron Brazeal has stated, the ULF contributed "hundreds of thousands of dollars in money and resources" to obtain the oil for families who could not afford it.[20]

On hearing about Lorenzo's Oil, many ALD families desperately wanted to enroll their boys in Moser's trial. By 1987, there was little doubt that the Odones were onto something. They surely had figured out how to lower VLCFA levels and, perhaps, to stem the disease. Only one other treatment for ALD, bone marrow transplantation, showed any promise, and that, too, was experimental.

Contributing to the excitement over Lorenzo's Oil was the media coverage. After all, it wasn't every day that parents went to the library and discovered what their dying child's doctors had not. "They Won't Let Their Son Die," read the headline of a *Newsweek* story on how the Odones "did battle with a fatal disease." "They Had to Find the Cure Themselves," reported *Woman's World*. Lorenzo was alive, according to the London *Times*, "because his parents refused to allow him to die, refused to accept that there was nothing that could be done, absolutely refused to believe the experts." The Odones also received awards, such as honorary degrees from the University of Stirling in Scotland in 1991. Due to their "remarkable standards of dedication and service," according to the Stirling ceremony, the Odones were "held in the greatest esteem, indeed in awe, by many of the foremost authorities in science and medicine."[21]

But it was the movie *Lorenzo's Oil* that made the Odones into full-fledged heroes. In 1990, Australian film director George Miller, after reading a story about the family, approached them about a movie. Miller was best known for the futuristic *Mad Max* films starring Mel Gibson, but he also had another interesting line in his biography. Miller was a physician, although he had practiced medicine only briefly. At first the Odones were skeptical, but they liked the fact that Miller had a medical background. In addition, the money they would receive for the rights to their story could help pay Lorenzo's significant medical costs. Once the Odones agreed, Miller cast Nolte; Sarandon; veteran actor Peter Ustinov to play Nikolais; and an unknown child actor, Zack O'Malley Greenburg, to play Lorenzo.[22]

Miller strove hard to capture the intensity of the Odones. The movie is frenetically paced, full of short scenes that shift between the Odone home, where a demanding Michaela and a series of aides care for Lorenzo, to the library, where Augusto immerses himself in a mountain of medical journals despite near exhaustion. Miller's "propulsive and hyperkinetic" style with close-up shots underscored the Odones' single-minded pursuit of a remedy for their son. Miller chose to highlight Augusto's ethnicity by asking Nolte to speak with an Italian accent. In the film, although the Odones are unified in their mission, there is tension between them as Lorenzo becomes sicker and sicker without hope in sight. There are scenes that did not take place in real life, such as one in which Michaela kicks her sister out of her house when Murphy expresses misgivings over the family's crusade.[23]

As do all Hollywood films depicting actual events, *Lorenzo's Oil* blurs fact and fiction. The real names of the Odones are used. Don Suddaby, the chemist who synthesized the erucic acid, plays himself, giving the film additional verisimilitude. Miller does not shy away from using scientific terminology as the Odones move deeper and deeper into obscure biochemical pathways. But the identities of Moser and the Brazeals are concealed, as are those of other ALD families. Some of the events in the film really "happened," while others are composites of multiple events filtered through Miller and Nick Enright, who co-wrote the screenplay. The Odones get to make many impassioned statements, which they may or may not have really said. "I am a father," Augusto barks when doctors first challenge him about using the oil. "And nobody can tell me what dressing I can put on my kid's salad, O.K.?"

One of the most interesting aspects of *Lorenzo's Oil*, however, is the

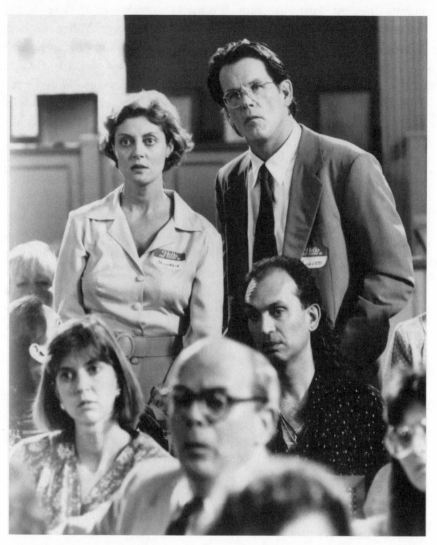

The Odones (Susan Sarandon and Nick Nolte) airing their opinions at a fictional meeting of an adrenoleukodystrophy organization, as depicted in the movie *Lorenzo's Oil*. This scene allowed the film to amplify the conflict between the Odones and the scientific establishment. Courtesy of Universal Studios Licensing LLLP.

degree to which Miller explicitly set out to create a mythical version of the Odones' story. Miller was an aficionado of the work of mythologist Joseph Campbell, author of *The Hero with a Thousand Faces*. Campbell wrote about stories and myths, arguing that they tend to follow a repetitive pattern, in which heroes eventually triumph after suffering many setbacks. Like Campbell, Miller did not criticize this phenomenon but rather celebrated it. When he originally called the Odones, he told them that "I see your child as a mythological figure in the Joseph Campbell tradition."[24]

This outlook informed many of the decisions that Miller made, none more important than that of using the Odones—but not Moser or the Brazeals—as consultants on the film. Miller was not interested in a docudrama presenting Lorenzo's story from multiple angles. Rather, he was thoroughly taken with what the Odones had done and wanted to commemorate their triumph. "As I studied the story in more detail, I discovered that the couple's journey follows the hero's path to a degree I hadn't seen in real life before," he stated. "The purpose in telling this story," he told the *New York Times*, "is to provide a manual of courageous human conduct." To Miller, then, the movie was meant as a triumphant story of human achievement. "I do know that when *I* go to the cinema I want to undergo a transformation," he said. "I want to be drawn up into the screen and feel all the things that people are capable of."[25]

These beliefs help to explain one of the movie's most intense scenes, a conference of the ALD organization at which the earliest results of Lorenzo's Oil are discussed. No such meeting ever took place. In the scene, Nikolais announces the inauguration of a randomized controlled trial of a new therapy for ALD. Family members in the audience demand to know whether this is the Odones' oil. Nikolais admits that it is and says that the preliminary positive results with Lorenzo mandate a randomized scientific trial, in which half of the boys will be untreated. This claim outrages certain parents, who demand to know why all of the boys can't be treated. Nikolais responds as a scientist: "You don't really expect me to endorse a therapy on the basis of one hopeful observation?"

At this point, another parent stands up and announces that her son has been taking the oil as well and that his VLCFA levels are also down to normal. It is a powerful moment. The "n of 1" case has suddenly become an "n of 2," and the argument for delaying availability pending more formal scientific study seems even less justifiable. The Muscatines come to Nikolais's defense, telling the families to trust the doctors, let science take its course, and not be taken in by false hope. But their voices are drowned out by an increasingly angry group of parents, eloquently and desperately demanding the oil for their dying children.

By crafting the scene in this manner, Miller not only further elevated the Odones as heroes but also made a political statement. Miller had enormous respect for the AIDS activists of the 1980s who had fought the medical system for the right to treatments they believed they deserved. To him, the Odones' struggle was equally worthy. By hiring Susan Sarandon to play Michaela Odone, Miller further emphasized the antiestablishment theme. Sarandon was a "self-described Hollywood rebel," very active in progressive political causes. In interviews conducted when the movie was released, she, too, explicitly echoed the language of AIDS activists: "Why shouldn't people who are dying have the right to choose any drug they want? Why is the medical profession slowing down a possible breakthrough with all their red tape? Why are patients treated as things?"[26]

Sarandon was so convincing as Michaela Odone (she would receive an Academy Award nomination for Best Actress) that she even received correspondence from parents wanting information about the oil. In one case, a woman whose child had ALD read about the movie in *People* magazine and got in touch with the actress. "I called her, and it's very humbling," Sarandon stated. As has so often happened in the world of celebrity patients, the movies had become real life.[27]

Critics largely praised *Lorenzo's Oil*, which opened in theaters in December 1992. Terrence Rafferty of the *New Yorker* termed it "an inspirational drama that's genuinely inspiring." Janet Maslin of the *New York Times* found the movie to be "tough-minded and completely gripping." To *USA Today*, it was a "cinematic wonder." Small publications were equally effusive. "*Lorenzo's Oil*," wrote Jeffrey Westhoff of the Illinois *Northwest Herald*, "is as inspiring a portrayal of the human spirit as you are likely to see for many years."[28]

At times it seemed as if critics were less interested in praising the film than praising the real-life Odones. Maslin, for example, noted that the Odones had "responded magnificently" to the horrible news about Lorenzo. In the middle of her review, Joanna Connors of the *Cleveland Plain Dealer* suddenly spoke in her own voice about what the Odones had accomplished. "This, to my mind, is nothing less than a miracle," she wrote, "a miracle created by the profoundest of loves, that of a parent for a child." She told her readers she cried throughout the second half of the movie.[29]

Given that *Lorenzo's Oil* was a well-made and well-acted film that embodied the new zeitgeist, in which patients and families became empowered medical consumers, the positive reception of the film was not surprising. Yet at the same time, a series of criticisms emerged, some quite hostile, that revealed a more complicated public take on issues of science, activism, and even parenting.

Among the earliest and most persistent critics of the movie was Moser, who wrote a series of articles explaining his objections to the film, which he at one point called an "abomination." First, he identified what he believed were several historical inaccuracies, most notably the ALD conference described above, which he termed a "preposterous and totally invented scene in which parents demand the availability of the oil from the unsympathetic leadership [of the ULF], analogous to the French public demanding bread before the Bastille." Second, Moser argued that the depicted conflicts between the immediate needs of the patients and the demands of scientific rigor had been significantly exaggerated. Here Moser pointed to the trial of Lorenzo's Oil that he began once Rizzo had shown it to be safe. Moser had not conducted a placebo experiment that left half the boys untreated but rather an "open trial" giving the oil to all comers. Finally, Moser claimed that the movie had given an overly optimistic assessment of the value of Lorenzo's Oil.[30]

What Moser did not say, but surely felt, was that the character of Nikolais made him look like an uncaring doctor concerned only with his own reputation and prestige. After all, Moser had chosen to specialize in a remote corner of medicine—genetic diseases of children—that was gloomy and far from lucrative. But others came rapidly to Moser's defense. Moser "is one of the most caring and honest individuals I know," geneticist Reuben Matalon wrote to the Brazeals. "They made him out to be sort of a bumbling, not very caring person," wrote geneticist and ULF board member John A. Barranger. "It's unfortunate because it kind of broke his heart."[31]

Ron and Paula Brazeal shared Moser's displeasure with the film, which they believed had disgracefully portrayed the scientific community as "bumbling idiots" and used the ULF membership as foils for the heroic Odones. Noting that many boys had worsened or died despite using Lorenzo's Oil, the Brazeals agreed with Moser that the movie had made false claims about its effectiveness. Particularly disquieting was the film's implication that the ULF was somehow more interested in comforting parents than in trying to save dying children. (The real-life Odones had once described a ULF conference as "kind of like a wake.") To the Brazeals, who continued to devote dozens of hours each week to running the ULF even though both of their sons had died, such a suggestion must have been almost unbearable.[32]

People active in the ULF also took exception to how the Brazeals had been portrayed. "We are not complacent parents who take everything the doctors say as final," wrote Cheryl K. Danner of Huntley, Illinois. "The movie portrays the . . . Foundation as a superficial group whose focus seems to be parental coping," wrote a Baltimore nurse, Susan O'Donnell O'Toole, who had worked with the ULF. "Nothing could be further from the truth." Johns Hopkins University psychologist David Edwin was "saddened and angered" at the suggestion that the Odones were the only strong and loving parents in the movie. "The movie seemed to say," he stated, "that caring for the parents is a betrayal of the children and that, too, is wrong."[33]

But these attempts by real-life participants to correct the record were mild compared with some of the hostile comments made by certain movie critics, journalists, and scientists. One such piece was a film review by Boston scientist Fred S. Rosen that appeared in the prestigious scientific journal *Nature*. Rosen was especially upset at the portrayal of the medical establishment. "We learn in the course of two hours that nurses are heartless, physicians pompous fools and patient support groups as mindless as a herd of sheep," he wrote. "Michaela and Augusto Odone to the rescue!" Rosen would not even consider the possibility that the Odones, despite their irregular methods, had actually made a valuable medical contribution, something Moser himself readily admitted. To Rosen, Michaela Odone was "monomaniacal" and the film celebrating her achievements "pernicious."[34]

And these were not even the angriest comments. Writing in *L.A. Weekly*, a Los Angeles magazine, reviewer Ella Taylor accused Miller of having "eradicate[d] the fine line between parental love and cruelty, between perseverance and utter lunacy, between the love of life and the blind terror of death." She was especially critical of the Odones' decision to "torture their helpless son" with experimental treatments. Given Lorenzo's largely irreversible deterioration, it was fair game to raise the touchy issue of whether, in retrospect, his life had been worth saving. But doing so in such a nasty manner seemed much more disquieting than the movie itself.[35]

Taylor had a compatriot in a Macalester College student who posted her reflections on the Internet. Going so far as to invoke the grisly experiments that the Nazis had performed in concentration camps, the author remarked that in the case of Lorenzo, "Ethics were thrown aside, tossed to the wind; the Odones were allowed to medically experiment on their son." The Odones, she concluded, were vigilantes, "abusing their rights as parents." Such comments are all the more disturbing when one recalls just what the Odones did, with little help from the medical profession: elucidate the cause of their son's neurological deterioration and develop a remedy that possibly slowed or prevented progression of the disease.[36]

Putting matters of taste aside, why did *Lorenzo's Oil* and, by extension, the Odones' story generate such contempt? There are no easy answers. One explanation is a societal backlash against the bold activism typified by both the Odones and AIDS patients who chained themselves to the trucks of pharmaceutical companies and traded pills to avoid getting placebos in clinical trials. As Rosen said in his review, the movie was "an antiestablishment diatribe."[37]

But beyond this was the issue of just how high the Odones had set the bar. As consumerism emerged in medicine in the 1970s and 1980s, Talcott Parsons's "sick role"—in which ill patients passively put faith in their doctors—had become passé, but the Odones had completely upended it. No longer could patients and their families sit back, expecting competent medical care. They had to become active participants, even scouring the globe for experts and possible treatments. "The real value of the movie," Augusto Odone said, "has been to show people that in cases where you have a disease in the family or yourself, you have to be proactive—don't wait for doctors to tell you what the remedies are." It was the duty of parents with a sick child "to go beyond conventional wisdom."[38]

But this concept, however empowering in theory, remained daunting and unrealistic in the face of illness and other constraints of ordinary life. Jerry Adler of *Newsweek* captured this quandary in a 1987 article on the Odones. "Who among us could do what Augusto and Michaela Odone did?" he asked. "We would all jump into an icy river to save a drowning child, but would we spend months in libraries tracking down an article on fatty-acid metabolism in a Polish medical journal? The one is an act of courage; the other of faith, which is rarer."[39]

In addition to being praised by correspondents who had seen *Lorenzo's Oil*, Susan Sarandon recalls getting critical letters that called her naive or told her to "shut up." These letters, she believes, stemmed from the uncomfortable issue of whether one should become a protagonist in one's own life. "Sick people want someone to take care of them," she added. "People don't want to be told they have to ask questions and be involved. This takes a lot of courage and time." Or, as Sidney Zion has stated, "People can't not believe in doctors."[40]

One criterion for judging what the Odones had done, of course, was whether the oil "worked." If it was "snake oil," as some critics charged, then their claims would hold less weight. But if they had, indeed, developed a valuable remedy in the face of indifference and opposition from the medical profession, then it would be hard to dismiss both the oil and the Odones' philosophy.[41]

Unfortunately, as with many of the other "miraculous" treatments discussed in this book, the effectiveness of Lorenzo's Oil is itself a matter of contention. One need look no further than the case of Lorenzo to see this. According to the Odones, Lorenzo's condition improved after he began the oil, leading them to conclude that it had had a positive—if limited—effect. Moreover, the Odones believed that the oil was the major factor allowing Lorenzo to live for so long with ALD. As of 1992, when *Lorenzo's Oil* was released, he was 14 years old and had been sick for more than nine years. Most boys with ALD died within a few years of their diagnosis. But to Moser, Lorenzo's survival was not proof of the oil's value; other boys had lived that long without the oil. He speculated that the excellent care that Lorenzo received was a more likely explanation. As was so often the case, what one could conclude from an "n of 1" case was limited.[42]

But what about the more interesting issue? Was there evidence that Lorenzo's Oil had helped any of the hundreds of boys who had undergone the therapy as part of Moser's 1989 trial? To Augusto Odone, the answer was surely yes. As he often stated, a large number of anecdotes builds toward proof. Moser, of course, was extremely uncomfortable with such a claim, preferring randomized controlled data that would have compared the oil with placebo. Such a trial, however, was never done. Given the lack of alternative therapies for ALD, it would have been unethical to deprive any boys of the oil. Thus, Moser was forced to compare his subjects with how earlier boys at risk for ALD, not taking the oil, had done. This type of research was fraught with peril. No good data existed on ALD risk in the era before Lorenzo's Oil. And because the two comparison groups were not equally matched, it would be difficult to prove that the oil, as opposed to some other factor, had caused any different outcomes that resulted.[43]

It was this uncertainty that led to Moser's extreme frustration with the ending of *Lorenzo's Oil*. In this scene, dozens of healthy boys are shown running, swimming, and playing baseball. Several introduce themselves and announce how long they have been taking the oil. Then contact information appears on the screen for the Myelin Project, an organization begun by the Odones in 1990 that funds research aimed at regenerating the defective myelin of boys with ALD and other leukodystrophies.

The closing of *Lorenzo's Oil* is indubitably affecting, suggesting a real-life happy ending that is better than any that Hollywood could have invented. Even though the Odones had not discovered the oil in time to cure Lorenzo, other boys with ALD were living seemingly normal lives because they had taken it. And because the boys were "real," it seemed that the film's conclusion had to be true. Audiences who had been weeping at Lorenzo's cruel fate could now cry tears of joy.

But according to Moser and the Brazeals, despite the "proof" displayed on the screen, Hollywood had invented the ending. Just because there were healthy boys who had taken the oil, it did not necessarily mean that the oil had helped them. For one thing, as had long been known, between 40 and 50 percent of boys with the ALD gene do not develop the disease as children; most of them come down with a milder form, known as adreno-myeloneuropathy (AMN), as adults. In addition, a small number of them might remain asymptomatic for their whole lives. Since it was possible that the boys shown in the film fell into one of these last two categories, their good health may have had nothing to do with the oil.[44]

It was also not clear from the movie whether the boys who ostensibly benefited from Lorenzo's Oil had recovered from early ALD or had taken the oil purely as a preventive measure. The film ambiguously stated that "if a diagnosis is made early enough, the treatment stops the disease." The implication that the oil somehow cured symptomatic boys especially infuriated ULF parents, many of whose sons had worsened or died despite using it religiously. One such parent was New Jersey mother Debora Gail, who began giving Lorenzo's Oil to her son, Anthony, just after he was diagnosed with ALD in 1991. But Anthony got worse, leaving Gail with feelings of anger and guilt. "I'm asking myself what I did wrong, why Anthony did not get better," she stated. "Should I have done something differently?" The Brazeals, who collected dozens of these stories from distraught parents, were particularly incensed. "It's cruel what they have done," Ron Brazeal said. "[The film] purports the oil to be a cure, when it's not proven as such." Another problem was that symptomatic boys who were potentially candidates for bone marrow transplantation might miss this opportunity because of overconfidence in the value of the oil.[45]

As Moser's data began to accumulate, it seemed that the Brazeals were correct on this point. As of December 1992, just before the release of the film, Moser had studied 240 patients for up to three years. For the boys with advanced ALD, he reported, the oil did not seem to be of benefit. Later data would corroborate this finding. Once a boy had significant symptoms, lowering the VLCFA levels had no effect. Thus, as Moser and others had charged, references to Lorenzo's Oil as a "cure" were misleading. The only symptomatic subjects who seemed to benefit from the oil were adults with AMN, the milder form of ALD, whom Moser had also enrolled in the study.[46]

But what about asymptomatic boys with the ALD gene, many of whom had been identified because they had a sibling with active disease? Did Lorenzo's Oil prevent them from developing the crippling, devastating disease that was killing their brothers? As Moser noted, "This is the most important question." He had enrolled sixty-one such boys, all under age 6, in his trial, roughly one-third to one-half of whom would have been expected to develop the severe childhood form of ALD without the oil. As of December 1992, Moser reported, one of the boys had developed symptoms and seven others had ominous findings on their brain imaging studies suggesting that they might soon develop symptoms of the disease. But this left between ten and twenty boys for whom the oil might have prevented the disease. "It is highly encouraging," Moser wrote, "that most of the boys who have been treated have *not* developed symptoms of the rapidly progressive form of the disease."[47]

Moser was understandably reluctant to draw any final conclusions at this time. Not only was the trial still ongoing, but it would be important to do long-term follow-up to see, for example, whether the oil was only delaying the onset of—but not actually preventing—the disease. And possible statistical biases would always be possible because the data were not randomized and controlled.

Finally, in September 2002, Moser was willing to go public with the conclusion that Lorenzo's Oil and the accompanying low VLCFA diet seemed to prevent ALD. Moser had wound up pooling his results with other data collected in Europe; all in all, 104 previously asymptomatic boys were being studied. Among boys who had been very compliant with the therapy regimen, Moser estimated, the oil had lowered their chance of developing ALD by 66 percent.[48]

By the time Moser published his data in July 2005, his study group consisted of eighty-nine children followed up for thirteen years. Sixty-six (74%) of the boys had normal findings on neurological examinations and brain scans. Only twenty-one boys (24%) had abnormal scans and eight (9%) had abnormal neurological findings. The oil and diet had lowered the risk of ALD by roughly 50 percent. These results were strengthened by the fact that Moser had been able to correlate lower VLCFA levels with absence of abnormalities. The data, Moser concluded, were "strongly suggestive, albeit not fully definitive, evidence of a preventive effect." Lorenzo's Oil, he underscored, prevented ALD in some—but not all—the asymptomatic boys who took it.[49]

Moser reported his findings dispassionately, but for Augusto Odone, they represented a definitive vindication of what he had been arguing all along. Unfortunately, his triumph was bittersweet. Michaela Odone had died in 2001 of lung cancer, which Augusto attributed to the exhaustion of caring so dutifully for Lorenzo for so many years. Augusto unabashedly pushed the media to cover the story of Moser's results, in large part, he said, to raise funding for the Myelin Project, which had not yet achieved a success of the magnitude of Lorenzo's Oil. Even Moser had to admire this strategy. "People used to say it doesn't help to throw money at things," he stated, "but it does."[50]

The press once again responded with enormous enthusiasm. "After all the doubts and ridicule," London's *Guardian* wrote, the Odones' homemade treatment "really does work." "Up until now the oil's success was anecdotal," CNN reported. "Now it is scientific." Talk show host Montel

Williams told his guest Susan Sarandon that "it's really one of those things where Hollywood preceded science," almost as if it were Sarandon and Nolte who had done the conclusive experiments. And once again there were plenty of boys available to provide "n of 1" examples. One was Michael Benton, a 22-year-old who had been taking the oil for fifteen years and had recently graduated college. "I feel great," he told ABC News. "I'm very active. I like to ride my bike, go down to the beach, play volleyball, go surfing." If seeing is believing, Benton was probably as much proof as most viewers needed to be convinced that Lorenzo's Oil was the real deal.[51]

Beyond the actual value of Lorenzo's Oil, however, the case of Lorenzo Odone has had a more enduring legacy: its demonstration of the enormous chasm that exists between defenders of the scientific method and desperate patients and parents. Hugo Moser was indisputably a compassionate doctor willing to do whatever he could for children afflicted with horrifying genetic diseases. Indeed, despite their quarrels over the years, the Odones consistently maintained great respect for Moser. Yet perhaps because Moser was used to such dire circumstances, which promoted false hopes, he remained a passionate advocate of good science, particularly randomized trials. The movie *Lorenzo's Oil*, he wrote, "may well be the ultimate antithesis of controlled clinical trials" and "depicts a totally uncontrolled clinical trial for all the world to see."[52]

Others agreed with Moser. For example, pediatrician William A. Silverman reported that readers of the medical journal *Controlled Clinical Trials* "were unhappy about the anti-trial message of this very successful movie." In an insightful article by Gina Kolata in the *New York Times*, Boston University lawyer and ethicist George J. Annas argued that "Americans love a personal story" but "cannot identify with a randomized clinical trial." Reliance on the potentially misleading lessons of such stories, he concluded, was "scary." Elsewhere in her article, Kolata said that both the Odones and the movie *Lorenzo's Oil* were critical of scientific studies.[53]

But such a claim was not really fair. The Odones did not oppose science. It was their mastery of the scientific literature that had enabled them to generate insights about VLCFAs. If there had been time to investigate Lorenzo's Oil in a more formal study, the Odones surely would have agreed. But their son was dying. Their passion for trying to save Lorenzo rendered Moser's passion for randomized trials incomprehensible to them.

As demonstrated both by the Odone case and by its depiction in *Lorenzo's Oil*, the idea of waiting for definitive scientific proof before venturing into uncharted waters made no sense for a growing number of patients and families. As long as they trusted their instincts and caregivers, they forged ahead. The possibility of making the wrong choice always existed, but it was a chance that many of them were willing to take. As the Odones had said in defending their decision to give Lorenzo potentially toxic erucic acid, "As the parents of an ALD child, we would not mind taking this order of risk."[54]

The case of Lorenzo Odone highlighted a series of questions that would only become more commonplace in the coming decades. What medical interventions, both last-ditch and more routine, are too risky to outweigh any possible benefits? Who should decide whether to proceed with such tests or treatments? How should the effectiveness of such interventions best be evaluated? And who is entitled to the final word on whether, in retrospect, it has all been worth it: doctors, patients and their families, or biostatisticians?

Throughout his two best-selling books, Lance Armstrong interweaves the two most important stories of his life: his 1996 bout with far-advanced testicular cancer and his subsequent series of triumphs in the Tour de France. Either challenge by itself might have warranted a book, but Armstrong took advantage of the logical opportunity to tell both stories simultaneously. Still, he struggles mightily to find the proper way to connect the two.

Armstrong is careful to state that beating cancer is not the same as beating opponents in a bike race. As an athlete, he augmented his basic talent for bike riding with a furious training schedule that ultimately made him one of the best cyclists in history. "I wouldn't be able to win a Tour de France until I had enough iron in my legs, and lungs, and heart, and brain," he once told himself. "Until I was a man." But surviving cancer, he writes, "was more a matter of blind luck." "Good, strong people get cancer," he adds, "and they do all the right things to beat it, and they still die."[1]

At the same time, however, Armstrong has trouble *not* equating his two triumphs. "Cancer," he states, is the "Tour de France of illnesses." At the close of the second book, Armstrong summarizes his history with cancer succinctly: "I got treated, I fought like hell, and I got better." On the Lance Armstrong Foundation website (www.laf.org), Armstrong writes: "When I was sick, I didn't want to die. When I race I don't want to lose. Dying and losing, it's the same thing." The program begun by the foundation to provide cancer survivors with physical, emotional, and practical advice is known simply as "Live Strong." The same optimism and confidence Armstrong brought to cycling, therefore, need to be marshaled against cancer.[2]

The Internet is teeming with tributes to Armstrong—from cancer survivors to athletes to others who have simply heard and felt a connection to his story. These comments freely blur his lessons about illness, sports, and life. "Lance refused to become a statistic and instead rallied and became cancer's worst enemy," wrote Judith E. Pavluvcik in a review of Armstrong's first book. "He refused to give in and chose to fight the disease with all he had." Armstrong's toughness and his unwillingness to give up "has saved so many lives," wrote a college student who herself had had cancer. To some people, Armstrong has become a symbol for the notion that anything is possible. "Lance beat cancer and then he went on to win 5 Tour de Frances," a computer programmer wrote on his blog in 2003. "That pretty much means I can overcome whatever ills I have in my life so I can keep going after that."[3]

Armstrong's story is thus utterly emblematic of the other stories in this book. In all of these cases, a celebrity, or someone fated to become a celebrity due to illness, became sick and confronted a complicated series of choices. Because of their notoriety, the patients themselves, their families, and their caregivers needed to manage not only the disease in question but how it was being spun. From the very start, therefore, what really happened and what was reported began to diverge. The press, which covered such stories more aggressively as the twentieth century proceeded, provided the next layer of spin. Even when journalists were willing and able to distinguish fact from fiction, their editors and headline writers showed less fealty to this ideal. Thus, definitive language was often used— "triumph," "breakthrough," "cure," "tragedy," and, in the Libby Zion case, even "murder"—when more nuanced assessments were appropriate. Attracting and keeping readers and viewers through oversimplifications remained the usual practice for media outlets wishing to stay in business.[4]

Enter Hollywood, which made movies about a number of the celebrity patients in this book. Even though filmmakers were under no obligation to tell the "truth," the fact that their movies were based on true stories further conflated actual and fictional events. Like the famous patients, their families, and the press, Hollywood directors and writers were also historical actors, telling stories based on who they were and the times in which they were living. At times, such as in *Fear Strikes Out*, with its emphasis on father-son conflict as the sole cause of Jimmy Piersall's mental illness, the film contradicted the story told by its hero. At other times, as with *Lorenzo's Oil*, the movie was an unabashed vindication of a family's desired narrative.

It is a tribute to the mythmaking power of Hollywood that the films in question—which, unlike press reports, were not obliged to be truthful—in effect became the definitive accounts of the stories in question. This phenomenon is perhaps best exemplified by Susan Sarandon fielding questions and letters about Lorenzo's Oil and becoming a spokesperson for Augusto Odone's Myelin Project. But even for celebrity patients whose lives were not portrayed by Hollywood, slanted versions of their stories became the accepted accounts of what had "actually" happened. The stories were like historian Daniel Boorstin's "pseudo-events," assuming a real significance even though they had not really occurred.[5]

So what should be done with this type of information? To the degree that historians are supposed to discover the truth about the past, such findings can disprove long-standing myths: Jimmy Piersall did not cure himself simply by learning to fight his fears; Brian Piccolo did not die a serene and somehow redemptive death; Morris Abram did not beat leukemia by insisting on an obscure immunological treatment; and Rita Hayworth's perpetual problems could not just be attributed to undiagnosed Alzheimer's disease.[6]

But the more interesting task for the historian is to ask why certain stories, and not others, have been so enduring. Overwhelmingly, the stories that became fixed were those that had a particular cultural resonance, those that somehow provided meaning to the public. Just as celebrities could define popular tastes in clothes, food, and style, so, too, could they demonstrate how to be a successful patient and, increasingly over time, a successful disease activist.

What were the themes that repeatedly stood out among these celebrity illnesses? As early as the case of Lou Gehrig, there was the notion that seeking cutting-edge treatment, at least in the face of ominous illness, was both admirable and necessary. So was the establishment of some type of network—formal or informal—among fellow sufferers of a given disease. The importance of "fighting" one's illness, or, more exactly, the perception that one was fighting one's illness, was crucial. This might be achieved by volunteering for experimental treatments or valiantly enduring major surgery or toxic chemotherapy.

Beginning in the 1970s, the stories evolved to incorporate some element of opposition to, or at least questioning of, the medical profession, the Food and Drug Administration, and other representatives of the "establishment." The implication was that even celebrity patients could not assume that everything possible was being done to cure them. The media could often be an ally in such battles, although as Elizabeth Glaser and Arthur Ashe learned, such assistance could come at the price of sacrificing one's privacy. Finally, the positive energy displayed by these patients needed to be perpetuated, either during their lifetimes or posthumously, generally in the form of a charitable foundation. These organizations provided an upbeat message about the possibilities that science offered for their particular malady and, as in the cases of the Myelin Project and the Michael J. Fox Foundation for Parkinson's Research, closely scrutinized and managed the research projects they funded.

To some degree, of course, the stories told drew on the facts of the cases. But what is more striking is the degree to which the stories increasingly conformed to predictable patterns. This book has recounted the illness narratives of thirteen famous patients since the 1930s; the details of thirteen other stories would have been different, but the overall trajectory would have been quite similar. That is, during the years in question, celebrities who became ill were increasingly "supposed" to act in a certain manner, going public with their sicknesses, sharing details of their treatments, and then becoming visible and optimistic spokespeople. By the 1990s, organizations representing still-stigmatized diseases, such as lung cancer, actively sought celebrities who could provide needed cachet and attention. One article even made this process into a game, challenging readers to match a list of celebrities with their diseases. Illness, it could be argued, was becoming fetishized.[7]

By corollary, "ordinary" patients were now supposed to act like ill celebrities—not starting foundations, necessarily, but becoming knowledgeable about their conditions and fighting their diseases. "By fight," Armstrong told his readership, "I mean arm yourself with all the available information, get second opinions, third opinions, and fourth opinions." Playing the warrior rather than the victim, Armstrong proudly displayed his bald scalp and urged fellow cancer sufferers to do the same. If illness could destroy the more traditional type of beauty, it could create another.[8]

Another role of the historian is to judge what has happened. To what degree should we be alarmed that celebrity patients have often become the reference point for members of the public with serious illnesses? One concern is that important decisions about funding may be driven by the ability of a given celebrity to generate concern about his or her disease. As did Yasmin Aga Khan and Elizabeth Glaser, celebrities routinely appear in front of Congress, lobbying for greater NIH appropriations. These spokespeople carefully state that they are not attempting to take away funds from other good causes, merely promoting their own. But in reality, funding is a zero-sum game that, other political considerations notwithstanding, can largely be won by those who scream and argue loudest.[9]

Moreover, any expectation that it is possible to emulate the "illness career" of a sick celebrity is worrisome. For example, there is surely disappointment ahead for many people with cancer who think they can survive if they force themselves to try as hard as Lance Armstrong did. Or, for that matter, take the same medications that he did. Many cancer patients who contact him, Armstrong writes, want to know "everything I did, every drug I took, every morsel I digested." Referring to actor and Parkinson's spokesperson Michael J. Fox, one woman wrote: "I just tried to follow right behind him and step in the footprints and do as much as I knew how to in terms of keeping a positive attitude." Such people may be no less misguided than those who followed Steve McQueen to Mexican cancer clinics or begged their doctors for a dubious "miracle cure," boldly touted on the cover of the March 29, 2004, *Star*, that had supposedly healed Fox.[10]

In this sense, the veneration of sick celebrities is as perilous as—or even more perilous than—the veneration of celebrities in general. Celebrity worship, according to Daniel Boorstin's landmark book *The Image*, has contributed to America's self-deception, "how we hide reality from ourselves." In *Intimate Strangers*, critic Richard Schickel agreed, charging that celebrities "are used to simplify complex matters of the mind and spirit; they are used to subvert rationalism in politics, in every realm of public life; and, most important, they are both deliberately and accidentally employed to enhance in the individual audience member a confusion of the realms between public life and private life." The result of all of this, Schickel forcefully concluded, was "a corruption of that process of rational communication on which a democratic political system and reasonable social order must be based."[11]

Finally, the ulterior motives of sick celebrities must be considered. Because of the clout of famous individuals, industry and health organizations often generously pay them to become spokespeople for given products or philosophies. One obvious example of this phenomenon occurred in 2002 when Earvin "Magic" Johnson began appearing on billboards advertising Combivir, an HIV medication made by pharmaceutical giant Glaxo-SmithKline. The drug seemed to be working for Johnson, which is something that the public deserved to know. But while the intelligent consumer could figure out that Johnson was likely being paid for his endorsement, the advertisement nevertheless played on the vulnerabilities of sick, HIV-positive patients, especially those in African American communities where the advertisements were prominently displayed.[12]

A scandal eventually emerged when a series of celebrities began booking themselves on television talk shows to describe positive experiences that they or others had had with particular medical products. Some companies, such as Celebrity Connection, even existed to match up Hollywood stars with pharmaceutical companies. When the media discovered that such individuals, who included Kathleen Turner (rheumatoid arthritis), Lynda Carter (irritable bowel syndrome), Rob Lowe (febrile neutropenia, a combination of fever and insufficient white blood cells in cancer patients), and Olympia Dukakis (shingles), were being highly compensated for these seemingly altruistic testimonials, ethical questions about conflicts of interest were rightly raised.[13]

Despite these concerns and transgressions, however, the stories of sick celebrities have resulted in far more benefits than drawbacks. Most notably, they have democratized the subject of illness. Because television, radio, newspapers, and tabloids reach all classes and races in society, information about celebrity illnesses is readily available. Thus, it is reasonable to assume that a man newly diagnosed with testicular cancer, or an acquaintance, or his doctor will be familiar with Lance Armstrong's story. Information about Armstrong and, more importantly, testicular cancer is then only a phone call or a few computer clicks away. The same goes for any number of diseases now championed by various celebrities.[14]

In addition, someone perusing Armstrong's website or books can also learn that all doctors, hospitals, and treatments are not equal, an important lesson that patient-activists have been preaching since the 1970s. There is nothing wrong, Armstrong writes, "with seeking a cure from a combination of people and sources" and insisting that "the patient [is] as

The stories of celebrity illness discussed in this book have not run entirely counter to this trend. When Rose Kushner and her peers became breast cancer activists in the 1970s, they were pushing for better scientific trials, believing that physicians were overly reliant on their anecdotal clinical experiences. Advocates following in Kushner's footsteps, such as Elizabeth Glaser and Augusto Odone, have always favored statistically sophisticated research.[20]

Yet such data did not always provide definitive answers. For one thing, as we have seen, it sometimes took too long to generate results when the disease in question, like AIDS or ALD, was uniformly fatal. But even when there was time to conduct adequate research, large-scale studies often provided contradictory information. A perusal of newspaper articles from the 1980s and 1990s reveals a seemingly endless list of topics in which each new study seemingly conflicted with the previous one. Did oat bran lower cholesterol levels and save lives? Did estrogen replacement therapy prevent heart disease? Did a low-fat diet prevent breast cancer? Did exposure to environmental waste increase the risk of breast and other cancers? Did an unknown toxic exposure during the Gulf War cause severe illness in thousands of soldiers?

Perhaps the most vivid example of the difficulties in obtaining definitive statistical knowledge occurred in the case of screening mammography. As of 2001, there were eight randomized controlled trials—a quite substantial number—that sought to determine whether the test prolonged survival and saved lives from breast cancer. A meta-analysis of these trials, performed by some of the top statisticians in the field, came to the remarkable conclusion that mammograms in healthy women were not only of no value but might do more harm than good. But when other experts did their own meta-analysis using the same data, they came to the diametrically opposed result: mammograms clearly saved lives, as had been assumed for decades.[21]

The denouement of this controversy was instructive. Although certain women and physicians may have changed their minds about mammography as a result of the new data, most simply appropriated whichever arguments were available to defend their preexisting beliefs. This point was well demonstrated at U.S. Senate hearings held on the subject of mammography during February 2002. Iowa Senator Tom Harkin, who had lost two sisters to breast cancer, voiced his continued strong support for the test, which might have picked up their cancers earlier. "I am personally convinced," Harkin stated, "that had my two sisters had access to mammography that they would not have died so young because of this terrible disease." It is worth noting that no professional advocates of mammography would likely have made such a definitive statement. At best, mammograms save only a small percentage of lives among women who have them regularly. Yet Harkin's personal story rang true, both to the families of women who had died from breast cancer and to survivors of the disease whose cancers were detected through mammography. Suffice it to say, the pro-mammography forces won the day among the senators.[22]

The enduring lessons drawn from reassuring and powerful stories, such as those of Harkin's sisters (we can prevent future deaths from breast cancer), Morris Abram (he willed his way to a cure), Steve McQueen (he almost had the cancer beaten), Barney Clark (he did not die in vain), and Elizabeth Glaser (she saved her son's life), raise some legitimate epistemological questions about how we determine the efficacy of specific medical and public health interventions. Why, for example, have randomized studies and meta-analyses become a mandatory way station on the road to proof? A majority of evidence-based medicine experts would argue that the results of such studies get us closer to the "truth." But the claims that such data truly provide definitive answers or that patients and health professionals necessarily base their choices on a "rational" assessment of these statistics are as mythical as many of the stories recounted in this book.

That is, the notion that patients use only statistical knowledge to guide their clinical decisions is spurious. Those people who take the time to "learn the data" will still use their own personal calculus for evaluating the available scientific evidence. An individual's particular reference points come from what we might call narrative knowledge: the story of a celebrity patient, one's own past bouts with illness, the experiences of a relative, or personal beliefs about risk, prognosis, and particular treatment options. As a result, if a given therapy has a 5 percent chance of working, different patients, provided with the same statistics, may make opposite choices about trying it.[23]

Such a calculus applies to scientists, too. When famed evolutionary biologist and author Stephen Jay Gould developed abdominal mesothelioma in 1982, he conceived of himself as being not in the middle of the bell curve for the disease, where survival was eight months, but at the far end, where a small percentage of people managed to live for years, even decades. He subsequently underwent intensive therapy and survived for twenty years. It had become a "bit too trendy," Gould warned, "to regard the acceptance of death as something tantamount to intrinsic dignity."[24]

The inclination to choose interventions not fully supported by the existing data is strongest, it would seem, in desperate circumstances. As the examples of AZT and Lorenzo's Oil show, there are times when demanding treatments before the availability of definitive scientific proof turns out, in retrospect, to have been the right decision. To put it another way, while it is true that many seemingly successful anecdotal remedies, like Lou Gehrig's vitamin E injections and Morris Abram's immunotherapy, ultimately prove worthless, others do prove to prolong or save lives. While the "pure" scientific approach would argue against treating any such preliminary data as meaningful, sick people often feel otherwise. If members of society conclude that they value different criteria of proof in different circumstances, are they necessarily wrong? Can't certain types of anecdotal data, in certain situations, be accepted as reasonable, pending additional studies?[25]

The fact is that some, although not all, of the boys shown celebrating at the end of Lorenzo's Oil were probably doing so because they had been taking the oil. Their parents were right to have demanded it as early as possible, and Hugo Moser was right to have made it available to them. So, too, was Katie Couric right to use her Today show pulpit to ardently advocate screening colonoscopy after her husband, Jay Monahan, died from colon cancer in 1998. Subsequent studies have shown that the test almost surely saves lives. So, too, was actor Christopher Reeve, paralyzed as a result of a 1995 equestrian accident, right to engineer an "exotic" rehabilitation program that produced a limited but remarkable physical recovery. Referring to his fellow advocates, Reeve stated that "if we push, that's our prerogative." In other words, it is wrong to simply dismiss as irrelevant the fact that certain past anecdotal data have been validated and that many future anecdotes are also likely to be correct. Rather, we need to ask how to deal with this reality.[26]

One can make an even more provocative argument—that our inclination to judge past therapeutic efforts by our modern knowledge of science is misguided. That is, assuming that something did not "work" because subsequent testing did not demonstrate its efficacy is ahistorical. "What works in medicine is not an abstract, universal quality that transcends when and where," historian Jack D. Pressman argued in *Last Resort*, his book on the history of surgery for psychiatric disorders. "Rather, it is contingent upon the local circumstances in which physicians practice, characteristics that vary in place as well as time." By this criterion, an intervention could have benefited a given patient even if later sophisticated statistical studies suggest that it could not have "worked."[27]

Having said this, reliance on the results of individual cases is quite perilous turf—from the perspective of both the historian and the scientist. First, for the historian, looking back from the vantage point of a seeming therapeutic triumph risks the writing of teleological or "great man" history, in which heroic patients or families were simply correct all along. Conversely, looking back from a bad outcome may wrongly imply that the efforts were simply misguided from the start. What remains crucial for the historian is to understand how the historical actors made decisions based on the knowledge and options they had at the time.

Second, physicians, researchers, and health policy experts who deal with real-life patients must also be wary of such "n of 1" stories. For them, the idea of making treatment decisions, developing policy recommendations, and allocating scarce resources based on individual cases would be foolhardy. By this criterion, any test or therapy shown to be of value in a small, uncontrolled study would become the gold standard, pending further research. In such a scenario, moreover, it would be patients fighting the most terrifying diseases who would be the most vulnerable and susceptible to false hopes.

It remains crucial, then, to keep existing safeguards in place. The Food and Drug Administration should not be bullied into approving inadequately tested drugs. Institutional review boards should fastidiously monitor research projects to make sure that they have a legitimate scientific basis and that potential subjects are truly informed. Researchers should adhere to ethical standards and fastidiously avoid conflicts of interest that compromise their objectivity. Policy makers should not recommend tests, and funding for testing, without reasonable evidence that they are effective. Patient autonomy should not be considered an absolute, despite its welcome appearance over the past few decades. The public, via the media, must constantly be warned about the so-called therapeutic misconception, the idea that any medical intervention is necessarily better than doing nothing. It surely may not be, even for those who are dying. Patients need to be reminded of the limits of anecdotes. And they should be encouraged to enter randomized controlled trials if the best therapy is truly not known. As bioethicist Rebecca Dresser argues, disease advocates can play a crucial educational role in communicating the complex nature of therapeutic research to potential participants.[28]

But just because stories of patients who unexpectedly defy death may raise overly high expectations, the scientific community should no longer disdainfully dismiss anecdotal cases as worthless or unscientific. At the same time, bioethicists, who have tended to characterize cases such as those of Barney Clark and Lorenzo Odone as cautionary tales about unrealistic expectations, might profitably ask why such warnings have often had so little impact on sick people and their families. In other words, we should not reflexively assume that a hopeful choice that bucks the odds is necessarily the wrong one or that people who volunteer for a long-shot or unconventional therapy have necessarily been coerced to participate. After all, if these assertions were true, no one would go to Las Vegas or play the lottery. If we live in a culture that values information and the right to act upon it, such a right should be respected. As the journalist Chuck Klosterman recently wrote, "Culture can't be wrong. That doesn't mean it's always 'right,' nor does it mean you always have to agree with it. But culture is never wrong. People can be wrong. Movements can be wrong. But culture—as a whole—cannot be wrong. Culture is just *there*."[29]

On April 13, 1997, Charlie Tolchin, a 29-year-old man dying from cystic fibrosis, underwent an experimental bilateral lung transplant. Four years later, as the result of the immunosuppressive drugs that he had to take, he developed lymphoma. The chemotherapy he received scarred his lungs. By 2003, Tolchin's lung capacity was back down to 28 percent of normal, the same as before his transplant. A second lung transplant was being contemplated.

But the four years following his transplant, Tolchin explained, had been a gift. "I had the opportunity to live life as a truly healthy person," he stated, "with 100 percent healthy lungs." Shortly after his transplant, Tolchin wrote a book, *Blow the House Down*, documenting his experiences, which included skiing and playing ice hockey. He subsequently received hundreds of letters and e-mail messages from people with cystic fibrosis, health professionals, and the general public. Tolchin became a highly sought-after speaker at medical centers and other educational institutions. On January 14, 2003, he was the subject of a lengthy feature in the Science Times section of the *New York Times*. For fifteen minutes or so, in Andy Warhol fashion, Charlie Tolchin had become a celebrity patient.[30]

Tolchin's main message was simple and straightforward. "Don't believe there's nothing you can do," he told Jane E. Brody of the *Times*. "I tell doctors to think twice before they tell a patient that nothing can be done." Did this mean that all other patients with serious cystic fibrosis should receive lung transplants? Did this mean that if they did, they would do as well as Tolchin had? Did this mean that a second transplant, gene therapy, or some other intervention would restore Tolchin's lung function again? The answer to all of these questions was no. But that didn't matter. Tolchin had quite a story to tell.[31]

Introduction

1. Lance Armstrong with Sally Jenkins, *It's Not About the Bike: My Journey Back to Life* (New York: Penguin Putnam, 2000). The second book is Lance Armstrong with Sally Jenkins, *Every Second Counts* (New York: Broadway Books, 2003).

2. The only other book dealing with this subject is Dennis L. Breo, *Extraordinary Care* (New York: Ivy Books, 1986), a nonscholarly account of the illnesses of several famous people.

3. "Young Roosevelt Saved by New Drug," *New York Times*, December 17, 1936, pp. 1, 10.

4. This importance of "extraordinary" stories is well argued in Susan Ware, *Letter to the World: Seven Women Who Shaped the American Century* (New York: W. W. Norton, 1998), especially p. xvii. On the turn from "great man" history to social history, discussed in the next paragraph, see Richard J. Evans, *In Defense of History* (New York: W. W. Norton, 2000), pp. 139–63.

5. Jim Cullen, *The Civil War in Popular Culture: A Reusable Past* (Washington, DC: Smithsonian Institution Press, 1995); Ron Rosenbaum, *Explaining Hitler: The Search for the Origins of His Evil* (New York: Random House, 1998); David Greenberg, *Nixon's Shadow: The History of an Image* (New York: W. W. Norton, 2003).

6. For an overview of the history of medicine, see Jacalyn Duffin, *History of Medicine: A Scandalously Short Introduction* (Toronto: University of Toronto Press, 1999). On the history of medical technology, see Joel D. Howell, *Technology in the Hospital: Transforming Patient Care in the Early Twentieth Century* (Baltimore: Johns Hopkins University Press, 1996).

7. "Prontosil," *Time*, December 28, 1936, p. 21.

8. Perrin H. Long and Eleanor A. Bliss, "Para-amino-benzene-sulfonamide and Its Derivatives," *Journal of the American Medical Association* 108 (1937): 32–37.

9. "Young Roosevelt Saved," p. 10.

10. Eleanor Roosevelt to Anna Roosevelt Halsted, December 10, 1936, Anna Roosevelt Halsted papers, Franklin D. Roosevelt Library, Hyde Park, NY, box 56, folder 14.

11. Victoria Harden, *Inventing the N.I.H.: Federal Biomedical Research Policy, 1887–1937* (Baltimore: Johns Hopkins University Press, 1986).

12. Baruch quoted by Secretary of Health and Human Services Tommy G. Thompson, Society for Women's Health Services, May 1, 2001, www.hhs.gov/news/speech/2001/010501a.html (accessed December 20, 2004). See also Allan M. Brandt, "Risk, Behavior, and Disease: Who Is Responsible for Keeping Americans Healthy?" in John Harley Warner and Janet A. Tighe, eds., *Major Problems in the History of American Medicine and Public Health* (New York: Houghton Mifflin, 2000), pp. 532–37. The term *courage to fail* was coined by sociologist Renee M. Fox.

13. Renee Sentilles, *Performing Menken: Adah Isaacs Menken and the Birth of American Celebrity* (Cambridge: Cambridge University Press, 2003), p. 5.

14. Richard Schickel, *Intimate Strangers: The Culture of Celebrity in America* (Chicago: Ivan R. Dee, 2000), p. 29.

15. Ibid., p. 52; Leo Braudy, *The Frenzy of Renown: Fame and Its History* (New York: Oxford University Press, 1986), p. 571.

16. Daniel J. Boorstin, *The Image: A Guide to Pseudo-Events in America*, 25th anniv. ed. (New York: Vintage Books, 1987), p. 59.

17. Warren Susman, *Culture as History* (New York: Pantheon, 1984).

18. Schickel, *Intimate Strangers*, pp. 255, 256, 259; Neal Gabler, *Life: The Movie. How Entertainment Conquered Reality* (New York: Vintage Books, 1998), p. 7; Braudy, *Frenzy of Renown*, p. 506.

19. Jules Tygiel, *Past Time: Baseball as History* (New York: Oxford University Press, 2000), p. 84.

20. Larry Tye, *The Father of Spin: Edward L. Bernays and the Birth of Public Relations* (New York: Henry Holt, 1998), p. 249.

21. On framing, see Elizabeth Atwood Gailey, *Write to Death: News Framing of the Right to Die Conflict, from Quinlan's Coma to Kevorkian's Conviction* (Westport, CT: Praeger, 2003), pp. 2–8. See also Michael Schudson, *Discovering the News: A Social History of American Newspapers* (New York: Basic Books, 1980).

22. Kenneth R. Crispell and Carlos F. Gomez, *Hidden Illness in the White House* (Durham, NC: Duke University Press, 1988), pp. 13–74.

23. "Young Roosevelt Saved," p. 1.

24. Braudy, *Frenzy of Renown*, pp. 16, 17; Terra Ziporyn, *Disease in the Popular American Press: The Case of Diphtheria, Typhoid Fever, and Syphilis, 1870–1920* (Westport, CT: Greenwood Press, 1988), pp. 153–55.

25. "Fiancee to Visit Young Roosevelt," *New York Times*, December 25, 1936, p. 21.

26. Frank J. Digney, Jr., to Franklin Roosevelt, December 28, 1936, Roosevelt papers, President's Personal File (PPF) 5, folder: Franklin Roosevelt, Jr., 1937; Gilbert

Price to Franklin Roosevelt, December 31, 1936, Roosevelt papers, PPF 4260, folder: Justice Gilbert Price.

27. C. R. Fisher to Franklin D. Roosevelt, August 30, 1937, and Mrs. J. H. Melvin to Franklin Roosevelt, January 2, 1937, Roosevelt papers, PPF 5, folder: Franklin Roosevelt, Jr., 1937.

28. Ziporyn, *Disease*, p. 24; Bert Hansen, "New Images of a New Medicine: Visual Evidence for the Widespread Popularity of Therapeutic Discoveries in America after 1885," *Bulletin of the History of Medicine* 73 (1999): 629–78.

29. Mark Roseman, *A Past in Hiding: Memory and Survival in Nazi Germany* (New York: Picador, 2000), pp. 111, 368–73.

30. Edwin M. Yoder, Jr., *The Historical Present: Uses and Abuses of the Past* (Jackson: University Press of Mississippi, 1997), pp. 7, 56; Marita Sturken, *Tangled Memories: The Vietnam War, the AIDS Epidemic, and the Politics of Remembering* (Berkeley: University of California Press, 1997), p. 22.

31. "Cheats Death from Throat," *Boston American*, December 17, 1936, p. 3; Waldemar Kaempffert, "The Week in Science: New Control for Infections," *New York Times*, December 20, 1936, p. xx4.

32. James Harvey Young, *The Medical Messiahs: A Social History of Health Quackery in Twentieth-Century America* (Princeton, NJ: Princeton University Press), p. 261.

33. Sturken, *Tangled Memories*, p. 2.

34. Schickel, *Intimate Strangers*, p. 129; Joseph J. Ellis, *Founding Brothers: The Revolutionary Generation* (New York: Alfred A. Knopf, 2000), p. 216; Joy S. Kasson, *Buffalo Bill's Wild West: Celebrity, Memory, and Popular History* (New York: Hill and Wang, 2000), p. 158.

35. Gabler, *Life: The Movie*; Ellis, *Founding Brothers*, p. 216; Robert B. Toplin, *History by Hollywood: The Use and the Abuse of the American Past* (Urbana: University of Illinois Press, 1996), p. 4.

36. Information on the cases in this book comes not only from standard print sources, such as newspapers and magazines, but also from television programs, thanks in large part to the Television News Archive at Vanderbilt University.

37. Sentilles, *Performing Menken*, p. 6.

38. Evidence-Based Medicine Working Group, "Evidence-Based Medicine: A New Approach to Teaching the Practice of Medicine," *Journal of the American Medical Association* 268 (1992): 2420–25.

39. Schachtel quoted in Alex Kuczynski, "Treating Disease with a Famous Face," *New York Times*, December 15, 2002, sect. 9, pp. 1, 15.

Chapter 1. The First Modern Patient

1. Richard Hubler, *Lou Gehrig: Iron Horse of Baseball* (Boston: Houghton Mifflin, 1941); Frank Graham, *A Quiet Hero* (New York: G. P. Putnam's Sons, 1942); Ray Robinson, *Iron Horse: Lou Gehrig in His Time* (New York: Harper Perennial, 1990);

Richard Bak, *Lou Gehrig: An American Classic* (Dallas, TX: Taylor, 1995); William C. Kashatus, *Lou Gehrig: A Biography* (Westport, CT: Greenwood Press, 2004).

2. Stanley W. Carlson, *Lou Gehrig: Baseball's Iron Man* (Minneapolis: S. W. Carlson, 1941), p. 97.

3. Edward J. Kasarskis and Mary Winslow, "When Did Lou Gehrig's Personal Illness Begin?" *Neurology* 39 (1989): 1243–45.

4. Kashatus, *Lou Gehrig*, pp. 85, 86. See also Richard J. Tofel, *A Legend in the Making: The New York Yankees in 1939* (Chicago: Ivan R. Dee, 2002), p. 133.

5. Eleanor Gehrig and Joseph Durso, *My Luke and I* (New York: Thomas Y. Crowell, 1976). It is possible, of course, that Eleanor Gehrig simply fixed an unreliable version of events in her head in 1939 and eventually came to believe that they really happened.

6. Ibid., p. 4.

7. On the ways diseases can be understood differently in different eras, see Robert A. Aronowitz, *Making Sense of Illness: Science, Society and Disease* (Cambridge: Cambridge University Press, 1998).

8. DiMaggio quoted in Al Hirshberg, "The Lingering Shadow of the Iron Man," *Pageant*, October 1963, pp. 117–19; Rud Rennie, "DiMaggio Clouts Two Homers as Yankees Rout Newark, 11–6," *New York Herald-Tribune*, March 24, 1939, p. 27; Joe Williams, "About Lou Gehrig and Father Time in the Field of Sports," *New York World Telegram*, April 6, 1939, p. 28.

9. Jonathan Eig, *Luckiest Man: The Life and Death of Lou Gehrig* (New York: Simon and Schuster, 2005), p. 269; Leo Braudy, *The Frenzy of Renown: Fame and Its History* (New York: Oxford University Press, 1986), p. 20.

10. Williams, "About Lou Gehrig," p. 28; James M. Kahn, "Marse Joe Analyzes Strength," *New York Sun*, April 6, 1939, p. 27; Sid Mercer, "Leader of Yanks Retains His Faith in 'Iron Horse,'" *New York Journal American*, April 7, 1939, p. 18.

11. Vincent X. Flaherty, "Straight from the Shoulder," *Orlando Morning Sentinel*, June 22, 1939, Lou Gehrig file, National Baseball Hall of Fame (HOF), Cooperstown, NY.

12. James M. Kahn, "Old Iron Horse Wrestling with Himself," *New York Sun*, April 3, 1939, p. 35.

13. Tofel, *Legend*, p. 63; Eig, *Luckiest Man*, p. 288.

14. Edward T. Murphy, "Yankees Part Company with Puzzled Gehrig," *New York Sun*, June 12, 1939, p. 24.

15. Harold C. Habein to the author, March 19, 2002.

16. Donald Mulder, M.D., interview by the author, January 9, 2003.

17. Letter reprinted in Robinson, *Iron Horse*, p. 258.

18. Gehrig quoted in Edward T. Murphy, "Gehrig Proves Real Iron Man as He Fights to Overcome Ailment," *New York Sun*, June 22, 1939, p. 26; Dickey and Kauff quoted in "Mates, Fans Are Shocked," *New York Post*, June 21, 1939, p. 17.

19. Eig, *Luckiest Man*, p. 305; Habein quoted in "Doctor Explains: Gehrig Ailment Progressive," *New York Journal American*, June 22, 1939, p. 22.

20. Eleanor Gehrig to Mrs. Kanab, October 1, 1939, courtesy of Ellyn C. Phillips.

21. Eig, *Luckiest Man*, p. 324; "Gehrig Cheered over Condition," *New York Times*, January 10, 1940, p. 24.

22. "Vitamin B Gives Aid in Nerve Disease," *New York Times*, November 29, 1939, p. 25.

23. I. S. Wechsler, "Recovery in Amyotrophic Lateral Sclerosis," *Journal of the American Medical Association* 114 (1940): 948–50. See also Eig, *Luckiest Man*, p. 235.

24. I. S. Wechsler, "The Treatment of Amyotrophic Lateral Sclerosis with Vitamin E (Tocopherols)," *American Journal of Medical Sciences* 200 (1940), 765–78. See also Eig, *Luckiest Man*, p. 343.

25. Louis Linn, M.D., interview by the author, December 24, 2002.

26. "Vitamins E and B6 in the Treatment of Neuromuscular Diseases," *Proceedings of the Staff Meetings of the Mayo Clinic* 16 (1943): 523–27.

27. Harry M. Marks, *The Progress of Experiment: Science and Therapeutic Reform in the United States, 1900–1990* (Cambridge: Cambridge University Press, 1997).

28. Robert M. Pascuzzi, "Blinded and Seeing the Light: John Noseworthy, Lou Gehrig and Other Tales of Enlightenment," *Seminars in Neurology* 18 (1998): 415–18. See also Eig, *Luckiest Man*, p. 235.

29. Russell M. DeJong, "Vitamin E and Alpha Tocopherol Therapy of Neuromuscular and Muscular Disorders," *Archives of Neurology and Psychiatry* 46 (1941): 1068–75.

30. Gehrig and Durso, *My Luke and I*, p. 13.

31. Ibid., pp. 13, 14; David Noonan, "Double Legacy of the Iron Horse," *Sports Illustrated*, April 4, 1988, pp. 112–24.

32. On what patients did and did not know about their diseases, see Susan E. Lederer, "Medical Ethics and the Media: Oaths, Codes and Popular Culture," in Robert B. Baker et al., eds., *The American Medical Ethics Revolution* (Baltimore: Johns Hopkins University Press, 1999), pp. 91–103.

33. Rud Rennie, "Gehrig Has Infantile Paralysis; Can Never Play Baseball Again," *New York Herald-Tribune*, June 22, 1939, pp. 1, 25; Jimmy Powers, "Paralysis Ends Gehrig's Career," *New York Daily News*, June 22, 1939, pp. 54, 56.

34. Joe Williams, "Get Health Back, Win Dugout Job, Gehrig's Aim Now," *New York World Telegram*, June 22, 1939, p. 24. See also Bak, *Lou Gehrig*, p. 161; Tofel, *Legend*, p. 137; Eig, *Luckiest Man*, pp. 310, 311.

35. On the clubby nature of journalism in this era, see John F. Stacks, *Scotty: James B. Reston and the Rise and Fall of American Journalism* (Boston: Little, Brown, 2002).

36. Bill Corum, "Lou Gehrig," *New York Journal American*, June 3, 1941, p. 17; Max Kase, "Lou Fought Game Battle with Death," *New York Journal American*, June 3, 1941, p. 17.

37. Gehrig and Durso, *My Luke and I*, p. 17; Graham, *Quiet Hero*, p. 210.

38. Frank Graham, "He Knew It All the Time," *New York Sun*, June 3, 1941, p. 27; Robinson, *Iron Horse*, p. 261.

39. Eig, *Luckiest Man*, pp. 332, 343.

40. Ibid., pp. 344, 345.

41. Harold Weissman, "Doctor Reveals How Lou Fought Gamely to Finish," *New York Daily Mirror,* June 4, 1941, p. 31.

42. Robinson, *Iron Horse,* p. 272.

43. James Kieran, M.D., interview by the author, December 17, 2002.

44. Joe Williams, "Baseball's Iron Man Still Lives in the Hearts of Fans," *New York World Telegram,* June 3, 1941, pp. 23, 24.

45. Philippe Aries, *Western Attitudes toward Death: From the Middle Ages to the Present* (Baltimore: Johns Hopkins University Press, 1975), p. 11. See also Sherwin B. Nuland, *How We Die: Reflections on Life's Final Chapter* (New York: Alfred A. Knopf, 1994); Peter G. Filene, *In the Arms of Others: A Cultural History of the Right-to-Die in America* (Chicago: Ivan R. Dee, 1999).

46. Weissman, "Doctor Reveals," p. 31.

47. Gehrig and Durso, *My Luke and I,* pp. 226, 228.

48. Kase, "Lou Fought Game Battle," p. 17; Hubler, *Lou Gehrig,* p. 196; Gehrig and Durso, *My Luke and I,* p. 228.

49. Jack Sher, "Lou Gehrig: The Man and the Legend," *Sport,* October 1948, reprinted in David Gallen, ed., *The Baseball Chronicles* (New York: Carroll and Graf, 1991), pp. 2–22, quotations from pp. 4, 21; Earle W. Moss, "Lou Gehrig and Baseball," Heilbroner Baseball Bureau, Fort Wayne, Indiana, n.d., Gehrig file, HOF. Until the very end, Gehrig told visitors he would recover. See Kashatus, *Lou Gehrig,* p. 99.

50. Kase, "Lou Fought Game Battle," p. 17.

51. Hubler, *Lou Gehrig,* p. 197.

52. Ibid., p. 195.

53. Gary E. Dickerson, *The Cinema of Baseball: Images of America, 1929–1989* (Westport, CT: Meckler, 1991), pp. 44, 52.

54. Paul Gallico, *Lou Gehrig: Pride of the Yankees* (New York: Grosset and Dunlap, 1942); "The Pride of the Yankees," *Pacific Coast Musician,* July 18, 1942.

55. Edwin Schallert, "'Pride of the Yankees' Appealing, Human Saga," *Los Angeles Times,* August 19, 1942, p. 14; Bosley Crowther, "Play Ball!" *New York Times,* July 19, 1942, p. X3.

56. Kashatus, *Lou Gehrig,* p. 108; David J. Walsh, "Cooper More Gehrig Than Himself as Yank's Pride," *Variety,* July 16, 1942, p. 3; "The Pride of the Yankees," *Variety,* July 16, 1942, pp. 3, 8.

57. Larry King, "Suggestion for Ripken: Just Tie Gehrig's Record," *USA Today,* August 21, 1995, p. D2.

58. Florence King, "Baseball Immortality, Fair and Square," *New York Times,* August 21, 1995, p. A15.

59. Jeane Hoffman, "'Gehrig Foundation' Dream of Widow of Ex-Yankee Ballplayer," *Los Angeles Times,* December 8, 1953, p. C3.

60. Bak, *Lou Gehrig,* pp. 165, 181.

Chapter 2. Crazy or Just High-Strung?

1. Jimmy Piersall as told to Al Hirshberg, "They Called Me Crazy—and I Was!" *Saturday Evening Post*, January 29, 1955, pp. 17–19, 42, 46, 47. The subsequent chronology of events until Piersall's breakdown is from this article.

2. Ibid.; Jimmy Piersall as told to Al Hirshberg, "They Called Me Crazy—and I Was!" *Saturday Evening Post*, February 5, 1955, pp. 27, 70–72; Jim Piersall and Al Hirshberg, *Fear Strikes Out: The Jim Piersall Story* (Boston: Little, Brown, 1955).

3. Piersall, "They Called Me Crazy," January 29, 1955, p. 46.

4. Ibid.

5. Ibid., p. 47.

6. Piersall, "They Called Me Crazy," February 5, 1955, p. 70.

7. Ibid., p. 71.

8. Ibid.

9. Al Hirshberg, "The Strange Case of Jim Piersall," *Sport*, April 1953, pp. 51, 89; Leo Braudy, *The Frenzy of Renown: Fame and Its History* (New York: Oxford University Press, 1986), p. 20.

10. Bernie Sherwill, interview for ESPN *Sports Classics* documentary "Jimmy Piersall," 2001, courtesy of ESPN; Danny Peary, ed., *We Played the Game* (New York: Black Dog and Leventhal, 1994), pp. 202, 203.

11. Jerry Nason, "Piersall Sent to Minors," *Boston Globe*, June 28, 1952, pp. 1, 6, quotation from p. 1; Arthur Daley, "The Optimistic Mr. Boudreau," *New York Times*, July 1, 1952, p. 28.

12. Harold Kaese, "If Piersall Could Hit Like Ted Did as Rookie He'd Still Be with Sox," *Boston Globe*, June 30, 1952, pp. 1, 9.

13. Austen Lake, "Queer Case of Piersall: Cute or Quaint?" *Boston American*, June 30, 1952, p. 14; Al Hirshberg to Harry Paxton, June 10, 1952, from the Al Hirshberg Collection in the Howard Gotlieb Archival Research Center at Boston University, Boston (hereafter cited as Hirshberg papers), box 43, folder 7.

14. "Piersall in Hospital," *Boston American*, July 22, 1952, p. 36; Hy Hurwitz, "Piersall, Gene Stephens Sign; Right Field Battle Looms," *Boston Globe*, January 25, 1953, p. 58; Hirshberg, "Strange Case," p. 51; Piersall, "They Called Me Crazy," January 29, 1955, p. 17; Piersall and Hirshberg, *Fear Strikes Out*, p. 3.

15. Joel Braslow, *Mental Ills and Bodily Cures: Psychiatric Treatment in the First Half of the Twentieth Century* (Berkeley: University of California Press, 1997); Jack D. Pressman, *Last Resort: Psychosurgery and the Limits of Medicine* (Cambridge: Cambridge University Press, 1998).

16. Morris L. Sharp to Al Hirshberg, June 21, 1954, Hirshberg papers, box 5, folder e.

17. Piersall and Hirshberg, *Fear Strikes Out*, p. 213.

18. A.H. to Jimmy Piersall, October 13, 1954, Hirshberg papers, box 44, folder 4.

19. T.D.R. to Jimmy Piersall, May 14, 1954, Hirshberg papers, box 44, folder 3.

20. Al Hirshberg to Harry Paxson, July 23, 1953, Hirshberg papers, box 44, folder 2.

21. Harry Paxson to Al Hirshberg, July 28, 1953, Hirshberg papers, box 44, folder 2; Harry Paxson to Al Hirshberg, February 26, 1954, Hirshberg papers, box 5, folder e.

22. Sharp to Hirshberg, June 21, 1954; Harry Paxson to Al Hirshberg, June 15, 1954, Hirshberg papers, box 5, folder e.

23. Al Hirshberg to Sterling Lord, July 3, 1954, Hirshberg papers, box 5, folder e; Al Hirshberg to Frank Lane, March 22, 1955, Hirshberg papers, box 44, folder 5.

24. Nancy Reynolds to Al Hirshberg, November 24, 1954, Hirshberg papers, box 44, folder 4; Mary Piersall, "Why Do They Keep Calling My Husband Crazy?" draft of manuscript, 1962, Hirshberg papers, box 37, folder 3.

25. John N. Makris, "Jimmy Piersall Tells Tale of Faith, Hope," *Boston Herald*, May 22, 1955, Hirshberg papers, box 42, folder 3.

26. Piersall and Hirshberg, *Fear Strikes Out*, p. 128.

27. Braslow, *Mental Ills and Bodily Cures*.

28. Gerald N. Grob, *From Asylum to Community: Mental Health Policy in Modern America* (Princeton, NJ: Princeton University Press, 1991), pp. 134–39.

29. "The New Pictures," *Time*, March 18, 1957, *Fear Strikes Out* production code file, Margaret Herrick Library, Los Angeles.

30. I obtained a video copy of the *Climax!* version through the generosity of Allan Glaser and Tab Hunter.

31. James Powers, "'Fear Strikes Out' Tops with Perkins as New Star," *Hollywood Reporter*, February 4, 1957, *Fear Strikes Out* production code file, and Paramount Press Sheets for *Fear Strikes Out*, Herrick Library.

32. Robert B. Toplin, *History by Hollywood: The Use and Abuse of the American Past* (Urbana: University of Illinois Press, 1996).

33. H.J.S., "Fear Strikes Out," unpublished memorandum, May 7, 1956, Herrick Library, included with *Fear Strikes Out* script.

34. Jimmy Piersall, *The Truth Hurts* (Chicago: Contemporary Books, 1984), p. 30. Of course, Piersall's recollections of his father are themselves susceptible to selective recall.

35. Don Slovin to Jimmy Piersall, May 22, 1954, and M.R.H. to Jimmy Piersall, May 25, 1954, Hirshberg papers, box 44, folder 2; "Piersall Now Works to Help Mentally Ill," United Press International (UPI) wire story, September 5, 1976, Jimmy Piersall file, National Baseball Hall of Fame (HOF).

36. Edward Shorter, "The History of ECT: Unsolved Mystery," *Psychiatric Times*, February 2004, www.psychiatrictimes.com/p040293.html (accessed January 11, 2005).

37. Tim Cohane, "Jimmy Piersall: Baseball's Greatest Outfielder," *Look*, May 18, 1954, pp. 57–60; Piersall, *Truth Hurts*, p. 16.

38. Ed Linn, "Jimmy Piersall's Second Fight with Fear," *Sport*, March 1961, pp. 12, 81–86; Mary Piersall as told to Al Hirshberg, "Why Do They Call My Husband Crazy?" *Saturday Evening Post*, March 31, 1962, pp. 52–54.

39. Mary Piersall, "Why Do They Call My Husband Crazy?" p. 52. See also Dave Brady, "Piersall Turns Author, Raps Cleveland Writers," *Washington Post*, February 22, 1962, p. C2.

40. "Baseball: Indian Chiefs," *Newsweek*, June 19, 1961, p. 86; Dave Anderson, "The Problem with Piersall: Putting on an Act—Or Really Sick?" *Dell Sports*, spring 1961, pp. 4–6, 92; Linn, "Jimmy Piersall's Second Fight," p. 81.

41. Piersall, *Fear Strikes Out*, p. 128; Jimmy Piersall as told to Al Hirshberg, "Sure I'm a Pest, But . . . ," *Sport*, February 1963, pp. 38–40, 92, 93.

42. Daniel M. Fox, *Power and Illness: The Failure and Future of American Health Policy* (Berkeley: University of California Press, 1993).

43. Piersall, *Truth Hurts*, p. 2; Al Hirshberg, "An Interview with Jimmy Piersall," unpublished manuscript, n.d., Hirshberg papers, box 34, folder 4.

44. Mary Piersall, "Why Do They Call My Husband Crazy?" p. 54.

45. Compare ibid. with Mary Piersall, "Why Do They Keep Calling My Husband Crazy?" draft of manuscript, 1962.

46. Mary Piersall, "Why Do They Call My Husband Crazy?" pp. 52, 54. The second draft of the article is also in Hirshberg papers, box 37, folder 3.

47. Mary Piersall, "Why Do They Call My Husband Crazy?" p. 54.

48. Murray Robinson, "The New Piersall," *New York Journal American*, May 17, 1961, Piersall file, HOF.

49. Quoted in Peary, *We Played the Game*, p. 517.

50. Piersall, *Truth Hurts*, pp. 107–9.

51. Ibid., pp. 119–20.

52. Ibid., p. 143.

53. Ibid., pp. 147–51.

54. Ibid., pp. 151, 155.

55. Ibid., p. 151; Linn, "Jimmy Piersall's Second Fight," p. 81.

56. Al Hirshberg, "Jimmy Piersall's Greatest Day," *Pageant*, October 1957, pp. 154–57; Bill Madden, "Has Fear Struck Back?" *New York Daily News*, July 27, 1980, p. 31C; Kay Redfield Jamison, *An Unquiet Mind: A Memoir of Moods and Madness* (New York: Vintage, 1996), p. 215.

57. Ken Rosenberg, "Jim Piersall Aids Mental Patients," UPI wire story, September 3, 1976, Piersall file, HOF; Phillip Lee, "Classic Catches Up with Jimmy Piersall," June 22, 2001, www.espn.go.com/classic/s/Where_now_piersall_jimmy.html (accessed June 28, 2001).

58. Rosenberg, "Jim Piersall Aids Mental Patients"; Lee, "Classic Catches Up."

59. "Breakdown in Ball Park," *Life*, April 1, 1957, *Fear Strikes Out* production code file.

1. Robert S. Schwab to Margaret Bourke-White, September 6, 1967, Margaret Bourke-White papers, Syracuse University Library, Syracuse, NY (hereafter cited as B-W papers), box 37, folder: 1967.

2. Biographical material about Bourke-White is available in Margaret Bourke-White, *Portrait of Myself* (New York: Simon and Schuster, 1963); Vicki Goldberg, *Margaret Bourke-White: A Biography* (New York: HarperCollins, 1986); and Susan Goldman Rubin, *Margaret Bourke-White: Her Pictures Were Her Life* (New York: Harry N. Abrams, 1999).

3. Margaret Bourke-White, "Famous Lady's Indomitable Fight," *Life*, June 22, 1959, pp. 102–9; Rubin, *Margaret Bourke-White*, pp. 64–85.

4. Bourke-White, *Portrait*, p. 358.

5. Ibid., p. 359.

6. Margaret Bourke-White to Howard Rusk, January 15, 1954, B-W papers, box 35, folder: Parkinson's 1954–8; Bourke-White, *Portrait*, p. 358.

7. On the sick role, see Renee C. Fox, *The Sociology of Medicine: A Participant Observer's View* (Englewood Cliffs, NJ: Prentice Hall, 1989), pp. 22, 23.

8. Bourke-White, *Portrait*, pp. 359, 360.

9. Margaret Bourke-White to Dr. Prutting, June 29, 1955, B-W papers, box 35, folder: Parkinson's 1954–8.

10. Richard Stolley, interview by the author, December 12, 2003.

11. Goldberg, *Margaret Bourke-White*, p. 364; Bourke-White, *Portrait*, p. 345.

12. Bourke-White, *Portrait*, pp. 366, 367.

13. Lewis J. Doshey, *Parkinson's Disease: Its Meaning and Management* (Philadelphia: J. B. Lippincott, 1960), pp. 94–97; Barron H. Lerner, *The Breast Cancer Wars: Hope, Fear and the Pursuit of a Cure in Twentieth-Century America* (New York: Oxford University Press, 2001), pp. 69–79.

14. Kaushik Das et al., "Irving S. Cooper (1922–1985): A Pioneer in Functional Neurosurgery," *Journal of Neurosurgery* 89 (1998): 865–73.

15. Robert W. Gentry, "The Medical Profession and Network Television," 1956, American Medical Association Archives, Chicago, Communications Division, folder 3349. There is not as yet a history of the media's coverage of medicine, but for an overview, see Susan E. Lederer and Naomi Rogers, "Media," in Roger Cooter and John Pickstone, eds., *Medicine in the Twentieth Century* (Amsterdam: Harwood Academic, 2000), pp. 487–502.

16. Delos Smith, "Parkinsonism Aid Found," United Press International wire story, 1954, B-W papers, box 38, folder: Parkinson's Disease—Printed Materials; Earl Ubell, "Brain Blood Vessel Surgery Called Aid in Shaking Palsy," *New York Herald-Tribune*, November 13, 1954, B-W papers, box 38, folder: Parkinson's Disease—Printed Materials.

17. Walter C. Alvarez, "Parkinson Disease Relief Found in New Operation," *New*

York *Herald-Tribune*, October 25, 1954, B-W papers, box 38, folder: Parkinson's Disease—Printed Materials.

18. William L. Laurence, "Chemical 'Knife' Used on Brain," *New York Times*, March 5, 1955, p. 17.

19. Margaret Bourke-White to Paul [Sanger], July 4, 1957, B-W papers, box 35, folder: Parkinson's 1954–8.

20. Margaret Bourke-White to Paul [Sanger], November 19, 1958, B-W papers, box 35, folder: Parkinson's 1954–8.

21. Bourke-White, *Portrait*, p. 369; Margaret Bourke-White to Irving S. Cooper, November 5, 1958, B-W papers, box 35, folder: Parkinson's 1954–8; Bourke-White to Sanger, November 19, 1958. See also Bert Hansen, "How *Life* Looked at Medicine: Magazine Photography and the American Public's Image of Medical Progress," talk given at the annual meeting of the American Association for the History of Medicine, Madison, WI, April 30, 2004.

22. Bourke-White, *Portrait*, p. 368.

23. Ibid., p. 370. See also Margaret Bourke-White to H.D., July 30, 1959, B-W papers, box 36, folder: Late July 1959.

24. Lerner, *Breast Cancer Wars*, pp. 268–74; Susan Sontag, *Illness as Metaphor* (New York: Farrar, Straus and Giroux, 1978).

25. R.H. to Margaret Bourke-White, July 4, 1959, B-W papers, box 36, folder: Early July 1959; M.L. to Margaret Bourke-White, August 6, 1959, B-W papers, box 36, folder: August 1959.

26. E.H. to Margaret Bourke-White, January 12, 1960, B-W papers, box 36, folder: January 1960.

27. Bourke-White, "Famous Lady's Indomitable Fight," pp. 102–9.

28. Ibid., p. 106.

29. Ibid., p. 105.

30. Ibid., pp. 107, 108.

31. "A Brave Story Retold," *Life*, January 11, 1960, pp. 78, 79; "When TV Needs an MD," *Roche Medical Image*, April 1960, pp. 32–34; Jack Gould, "Margaret Bourke-White's Struggle with Parkinson's Disease Told Effectively," *New York Times*, January 4, 1960, p. 59; Goldberg, *Margaret Bourke-White*, pp. 348–51.

32. Bourke-White, "Famous Lady's Indomitable Fight," p. 105; Bourke-White, *Portrait*, p. 369.

33. W.C. to Margaret Bourke-White, June 28, 1959, B-W papers, box 36, folder: June 1959; M.L. to Margaret Bourke-White, January 3, 1960, B-W papers, box 36, folder: January 1960.

34. C.D. to Margaret Bourke-White, November 2, 1959, B-W papers, box 36, folder: November–December 1959; J.C. to Margaret Bourke-White, September 7, 1959, B-W papers, box 36, folder: September 1959.

35. H.B. to Margaret Bourke-White, July 1, 1959, B-W papers, box 36, folder: Early July 1959; T.W. to Margaret Bourke-White, January 17, 1960, B-W papers, box 36, folder: January 1960.

36. M.D. to Margaret Bourke-White, September 18, 1959, B-W papers, box 36, folder: September 1959; Margaret Bourke-White to M.D., January 15, 1961, B-W papers, box 37, folder: 1961; D.D. to Margaret Bourke-White, June 11, 1964, B-W papers, box 37, folder: May–December 1964.

37. Goldberg, *Margaret Bourke-White*, p. 357; Margaret Bourke-White to S.C., August 19, 1959, B-W papers, box 36, folder: August 1959.

38. Margaret Bourke-White to M.D., August 1, 1959, B-W papers, box 36, folder: August 1959.

39. Bourke-White, "Famous Lady's Indomitable Fight"; Bourke-White to S.C., August 19, 1959.

40. Margaret Bourke-White to R.W., November 17, 1959, B-W papers, box 36, folder: November–December 1959; Bourke-White to S.C., August 19, 1959; Goldberg, *Margaret Bourke-White*, p. 359.

41. Unnamed author to Margaret Bourke-White, June 16, 1959, B-W papers, box 36, folder: June 1959.

42. R.P. to Margaret Bourke-White, December 17, 1959, B-W papers, box 36, folder: November–December 1959; A.M. to Margaret Bourke-White, January 11, 1960, B-W papers, box 36, folder: January 1960; [Mrs.] E.M. to Margaret Bourke-White, October 23, 1959, B-W papers, box 36, folder: October 1959; M.K. to Margaret Bourke-White, July 2, 1959, B-W papers, box 36, folder: Early July 1959.

43. A.S. to Margaret Bourke-White, June 25, 1959, and A.L. to Margaret Bourke-White, June 22, 1959, B-W papers, box 36, folder: June 1959.

44. Mabel Foust, "Summary of Mail Received about LIFE, June 22 as of July 2," unpublished ms., B-W papers, box 36, folder: Early July 1959. The remaining 18 percent of the correspondence was miscellaneous.

45. A.L. to Bourke-White, June 22, 1959; Jeanne Levey to Margaret Bourke-White, June 27, 1959, B-W papers, box 36, folder: June 1959.

46. Bourke-White, "Famous Lady's Indomitable Fight," p. 108.

47. Bourke-White to M.D., January 15, 1961; Goldberg, *Margaret Bourke-White*, p. 356.

48. Bourke-White, *Portrait*, p. 382; Bourke-White to M.D., January 15, 1961; Goldberg, *Margaret Bourke-White*, p. 356.

49. Margaret Bourke-White to H.E., November 15, 1967, B-W papers, box 37, folder: 1967; Robert S. Schwab to Margaret Bourke-White, October 15, 1966, B-W papers, box 37, folder: 1966.

50. Goldberg, *Margaret Bourke-White*, p. 360; Robert S. Schwab to Margaret Bourke-White, December 4, 1970, B-W papers, box 37, folder: 1969–71.

51. Robert S. Schwab to Margaret Bourke-White, May 6, 1968, B-W papers, box 37, folder: 1968.

52. Simone A. Betchen and Michael Kaplitt, "Future and Current Surgical Therapies in Parkinson's Disease," *Current Opinions in Neurology* 16 (2003): 487–93.

53. C.C. to Margaret Bourke-White, February 24, 1964, and C.A. to Margaret Bourke-White, February 14, 1964, B-W papers, box 37, folder: January–April 1964.

54. Jean Bradfield to Margaret Bourke-White, July 13, 1962, B-W papers, box 37, folder: 1962; Schwab to Bourke-White, December 4, 1970; Margaret Bourke-White to Robert S. Schwab, December 16, 1970, B-W papers, box 37, folder: 1969–71.

Chapter 4. Politician as Patient

1. "Patient's Progress," *Newsweek*, March 30, 1959, p. 60.

2. Deane Heller and David Heller, *John Foster Dulles: Soldier for Peace* (New York: Holt, Rinehart and Winston, 1960); Richard Goold-Adams, *John Foster Dulles: A Reappraisal* (Westport, CT: Greenwood Press, 1962); Townsend Hoopes, *The Devil and John Foster Dulles* (Boston: Little, Brown, 1973).

3. Heller and Heller, *John Foster Dulles*, p. 8.

4. Ibid., pp. 12, 13.

5. Donald Oken, "What to Tell Cancer Patients: A Study of Medical Attitudes," *Journal of the American Medical Association* 175 (1961): 1120–28.

6. James T. Patterson, *The Dread Disease: Cancer and Modern American Culture* (Cambridge, MA: Harvard University Press, 1987); Kenneth R. Crispell and Carlos F. Gomez, *Hidden Illness in the White House* (Durham, NC: Duke University Press, 1988); Robert H. Ferrell, *Ill-Advised: Presidential Health and Public Trust* (Columbia: University of Missouri Press, 1992), pp. 53–150; Alvin Shuster, "Dulles' Surgery Removed Cancer," *New York Times*, November 5, 1956, pp. 1, 26.

7. Heller and Heller, *John Foster Dulles*, pp. 296–98.

8. Ibid., p. 300. See also Eleanor Lansing Dulles, *John Foster Dulles: The Last Year* (New York: Harcourt, Brace and World, 1963), pp. 225–27.

9. Barron H. Lerner, *The Breast Cancer Wars: Hope, Fear and the Pursuit of a Cure in Twentieth-Century America* (New York: Oxford University Press, 2001), pp. 17–23.

10. Harold J. Wanebo, ed., *Colorectal Cancer* (St. Louis, MO: C. V. Mosby, 1993), pp. 62, 69.

11. General Leonard D. Heaton, interview by Philip A. Crowl, August 19, 1966, John Foster Dulles Oral History Project, John Foster Dulles papers, Princeton University Library, Princeton, NJ (hereafter cited as JFD papers), p. 3.

12. Dennis Connaughton, *Warren Cole, MD and the Ascent of Scientific Surgery* (Chicago: Warren and Clara Cole Foundation, 1991), pp. 149–54.

13. Goold-Adams, *John Foster Dulles*, p. 282; Heaton interview, p. 4.

14. Shuster, "Dulles' Surgery," p. 1; "'Take Care of My Boy,'" *Time*, November 12, 1956, www.time.com/time/archive/preview/0,10987,824556,00.html (accessed February 23, 2005); Carl McCardle, "Boundless Trust and Faith," *Washington Daily News*, May 25, 1959, Allen Dulles papers, Princeton University, Princeton, NJ (hereafter cited as AD papers), box 22, folder 5.

15. "Eisenhower Visits Dulles in the Hospital," *New York Times*, December 9, 1958, p. 11

16. Marguerite Higgins, "How Secretary Dulles Faced Death: Battled Disease as

Job Intruder," *New York Herald-Tribune*, July 26, 1959, JFD papers, box 139, folder: Mrs. John Foster Dulles. The other articles appeared on July 27 and 28.

17. Transcripts of Press and Radio Briefings, February 14 and 20, 1959, JFD papers, box 139, folder: JFD health.

18. Frank Carey, "Cancer of 'Highly Malignant' Type," *Washington Post and Times Herald*, February 15, 1959, p. A15; Benjamin Bradlee, "The Dulles Team at Work . . . And the Secretary's Struggle to Return to Duty," *Newsweek*, March 2, 1959, pp. 20–22.

19. E. W. Kenworthy, "Dulles Found to Have Cancer; Treatment Set," *New York Times*, February 15, 1959, pp. 1, 3; "Dulles—The Cruel Facts of His Future," *Newsweek*, February 23, 1959, p. 25.

20. United Press International (UPI) wire, February 20, 1959, AD papers, box 21, folder 1; "Dulles—The Cruel Facts," p. 25; Bradlee, "Dulles Team," p. 21.

21. "Humphrey Wants Dulles Replaced," *New York Times*, February 23, 1959, pp. 1, 17; teletype from Hamburg DPA, April 17, 1959, AD papers, box 21, folder 1.

22. Dorothy McCardle, "The Secretary of State's Staunchest Ally," *Stars and Stripes*, March 8, 1959, p. 11, JFD papers, box 618, folder: 1956–1959.

23. "Dulles' Status Is 'Gratifying,'" *Philadelphia Inquirer*, March 1, 1959, I. S. Ravdin papers, University of Pennsylvania Archives, Philadelphia, box 13, folder 30; "Patient's Progress," p. 60.

24. "Patient's Progress," p. 60.

25. Olivia and Robert French to John Foster Dulles, November 12, 1956, JFD papers, box 215, folder: Fr–Fz.

26. Blanche Craig to John Foster Dulles, November 14, 1956, JFD papers, box 214, folder: Cos–Cz; Ernest R. Duff to John Foster Dulles, November 22, 1956, JFD papers, box 214, folder: Dr–Dz.

27. Russell Luerssen to John Foster Dulles, February 10, 1959, JFD papers, box 250, folder: 10–15 Feb.; Charles H. Hempler to John Foster Dulles, February 15, 1959, JFD papers, box 258, folder: 26 February 1959 (1).

28. Walter H. Dubard to John Foster Dulles, February 15, 1959, JFD papers, box 258, folder: 26 February 1959 (1); Sadie C. Wilson to John Foster Dulles, February 15, 1959, JFD papers, box 258, folder: 26 February (3).

29. Catharine F. McLaughlin to John Foster Dulles, February 17, 1959, JFD papers, box 258, folder: 26 February (3).

30. George W. Crane to John Foster Dulles, November 7, 1956, and Jasper E. Crane to John Foster Dulles, November 13, 1956, JFD papers, box 214, folder: Cos–Cz.

31. Paul Starr, *The Social Transformation of American Medicine* (New York: Basic Books, 1982), pp. 93–112; James C. Whorton, *Nature Cures: The History of Alternative Medicine in America* (New York: Oxford University Press, 2002).

32. James Harvey Young, *The Medical Messiahs: A Social History of Health Quackery in Twentieth-Century America* (Princeton, NJ: Princeton University Press, 1967); Jerome I. Rodale, *Cancer: Facts and Fallacies* (Emmaus, PA: Rodale Books, 1969); David Cantor, "Cancer, Quackery and Vernacular Meanings of Hope in 1950s America,"

unpublished ms., courtesy of David Cantor; Fishbein quoted in Barbara Clow, *Negotiating Disease: Power and Cancer Care, 1900–1950* (Montreal: McGill-Queen's University Press, 2001), p. 61.

33. Clow, *Negotiating Disease*, pp. 60–88; Howard Cady to Allen Dulles, February 17, 1959, AD papers, box 21, folder 3; J. Elmer Fairchild to John Foster Dulles, December 1, 1956, JFD papers, box 215, folder: Fa–Fio.

34. Helen M. Harris to Isidor S. Ravdin, February 22, 1959, Ravdin papers, box 13, folder 30.

35. Kay Fager to John Foster Dulles, November 10, 1956, JFD papers, box 215, folder: Fa–Fio.

36. Fanny to Allen Dulles, April 13, 1959, AD papers, box 21, folder 6.

37. Ernesta Barton to Allen Dulles, May 1, 1959, AD papers, box 21, folder 2.

38. Ibid.

39. Frank M. Chapin to Allen Dulles, February 25, 1959, AD papers, box 21, folder 5.

40. Note written by Allen Dulles, February 25, 1959, AD papers, box 21, folder 5.

41. C. Gordon Zubrod, "Historic Milestones in Cancer Chemotherapy," *Seminars in Oncology* 6 (1979): 490–505.

42. Ibid., p. 495.

43. Cantor, "Cancer, Quackery and Vernacular Meanings"; Howard A. Rusk, "Cancer, Dulles and Hope," *New York Times*, February 22, 1959, p. 43.

44. Leonard D. Heaton to Howard A. Rusk, February 24, 1959, and I. S. Ravdin to Howard A. Rusk, March 12, 1959, Ravdin papers, box 13, folder 30.

45. Robert Crater, "Juggler of World Crises Finds Fountain of Youth?" *Columbus (Ohio) Citizen*, November 30, 1958, JFD papers, box 467, folder: 1958 (4).

46. Arthur Peckham, M.D., interview by Philip A. Crowl, July 7, 1965, John Foster Dulles Oral History Project, p. 2, JFD papers; Heller and Heller, *John Foster Dulles*, p. 10.

47. Norman Armour to Allen Dulles, February 17, 1959, and J. M. Barker to Allen Dulles, February 17, 1959, AD papers, box 21, folder 2; *Congressional Record* (Senate), February 16, 1959, pp. 2063, 2064.

48. Clover Dulles to John Foster Dulles, November 1957, JFD papers, box 115, folder: Mrs. Allen W. Dulles; "The Administration: Doctors' Verdict," *Time*, February 23, 1959, pp. 16–18.

49. Allen W. Dulles, interview by Philip A. Crowl, May 17 to June 3, 1965, John Foster Dulles Oral History Project, p. 79, JFD papers.

50. "Dulles Chose a Lesser Cancer," *Los Angeles Tidings*, April 17, 1959, p. 10; Joseph Grazier to Allen Dulles, June 3, 1959, quoting Mrs. Heinrich Albert, AD papers, box 21, folder 5; Eddy and Anita von Selzam to Allen Dulles, June 1, 1959, AD papers, box 22, folder 2.

51. UPI wire story, June 3, 1959, AD papers, box 22, folder 5; Higgins, "How Secretary Dulles Faced Death," July 26, 1959; "Heroes: Freedom's Missionary," *Time*, June 1, 1959, pp. 12, 13.

52. Higgins, "How Secretary Dulles Faced Death," July 28, 1959.

53. Ibid.

54. Barton to Dulles, May 1, 1959.

55. Arthur S. Flemming to Nelson Mills, n.d., AD papers, box 19, folder 10; "Target—A Cure," *Newsweek*, June 8, 1959, pp. 28, 29.

Chapter 5. No Stone Unturned

1. Jeannie Morris, *Brian Piccolo: A Short Season*, 25th anniv. ed. (Chicago: Bonus Books, 1995), pp. 39–49.

2. Ibid., pp. 47, 49.

3. Ibid., pp. 70–92.

4. William Blinn, *Brian's Song* (New York: Bantam Books, 1972).

5. Gale Sayers with Al Silverman, *I Am Third* (New York: Viking Press, 1970); Gale Sayers with Al Silverman, *I Am Third* (New York: Penguin Books, 2001).

6. Blinn, *Brian's Song*, pp. 25–29.

7. Jeannie Morris, interview by the author, April 9, 2004; Sayers, *I Am Third* (2001), p. 62; Don Page, "Delicate Beauty in 'Brian's Song,'" *Los Angeles Times*, November 30, 1971, pt. IV, p. 19.

8. Quoted in Sayers, *I Am Third* (2001), pp. vi, 62, 67.

9. Douglas Gomery, "*Brian's Song:* Televison, Hollywood, and the Evolution of the Movie Made for TV," in Alan Rosenthal, ed., *Why Docudrama? Fact-Fiction on Film and TV* (Carbondale: Southern Illinois University Press, 1999), pp. 78–100, quotation from p. 93.

10. Blinn, *Brian's Song*, pp. 82–84.

11. Ibid., pp. 86–90.

12. Ibid., p. 86.

13. Morris, *Short Season*, p. 19.

14. Blinn, *Brian's Song*, p. 102. On stiff upper lips and cancer, see Barron H. Lerner, "*First, You Cry,* 25 Years Later," *Journal of Clinical Oncology* 19 (2001): 2967–69.

15. Blinn, *Brian's Song*, p. 106.

16. Ibid., p. 115.

17. Ibid., p. 117.

18. Morris, *Short Season*, intro.

19. Morris interview.

20. Morris, *Short Season*, pp. 15, 16.

21. Ibid., p. 14.

22. Ibid.

23. Ibid., p. 28.

24. Ibid., p. 22.

25. Ibid.

26. Ibid., pp. 27, 30.

27. Ibid., p. 28.

28. Ibid., pp. 49, 65.

29. Ibid., pp. 68, 69.

30. Joy and Kristi Piccolo, interview by the author, October 7, 2003. See also Joy Piccolo, interview for ESPN *Sports Century* documentary "Brian Piccolo," November 2, 2001, courtesy of ESPN.

31. Morris, *Short Season*, p. 135.

32. Ibid., p. 138.

33. Ibid., p. 135; see also Ralph Kurek, interview for ESPN, "Brian Piccolo."

34. Morris, *Short Season*, p. 140. The version in *Brian's Song* was similar. See Blinn, *Brian's Song*, pp. 111, 112.

35. Morris, *Short Season*, pp. 141, 142; Gale Sayers, interview for ESPN, "Brian Piccolo."

36. Morris, *Short Season*, pp. 143, 149.

37. Ibid., p. 145.

38. Ibid.

39. Ibid., p. 150.

40. Ibid., p. 151.

41. Ibid., p. 67.

42. Ibid., pp. 22, 144; Joy and Kristi Piccolo interview.

43. Morris, *Short Season*, p. 147.

44. Joy and Kristi Piccolo interview.

45. Ibid.; Joy Piccolo, interview for ESPN, "Brian Piccolo."

46. David M. Lubin, *Shooting Kennedy: JFK and the Culture of Images* (Berkeley: University of California Press, 2003), p. 153.

47. Dan Arnold, interview for ESPN, "Brian Piccolo"; Lubin, *Shooting Kennedy*, p. 141.

48. John J. O'Connor, "'Brian's Song' Is Proving to Be a Film Phenomenon," *New York Times*, January 28, 1972, p. 91.

49. John J. O'Connor, "TV: Love Was Link for Tuesday and Wednesday," *New York Times*, December 3, 1971, p. 83; Sayers, *I Am Third* (2001), p. ix; Joy and Kristi Piccolo interview.

50. Traci Piccolo, interview for ESPN, "Brian Piccolo."

51. See www.geocities.com/dipiccolo41/research.html. The remake, while faithful to the original, did depict Piccolo's illness more realistically.

52. Sue Silver, "Larry Einhorn—President of ASCO, 2000–2001," *Lancet Oncology* 2 (2001): 316–20.

53. Lance Armstrong with Sally Jenkins, *It's Not About the Bike: My Journey Back to Life* (New York: Berkley, 2001), p. 83; Arthur Allen, "Triumph of the Cure," Salon.com, July 29, 1999, www.salon.com/health/feature/1999/07/29/lance/print.html (accessed January 18, 2005). See also http://tcrc.acor.org/celeb.html.

54. See www.findagrave.com/cgi-bin/fg.cgi?page=flf&Grid=810&Flgrid=810&; Joe Piccolo, interview for ESPN, "Brian Piccolo."

Chapter 6. Persistent Patient

1. Marian Christy, "How Morris Abram Said No to Death," *Boston Globe*, July 21, 1982, pp. 21, 23.

2. William Honan, "Morris Abram Is Dead at 81; Rights Advocate Led Brandeis," *New York Times*, March 17, 2000, p. C19.

3. Ibid.

4. Morris B. Abram, "Living with Leukemia," in *1979 Medical and Health Annual* (Chicago: Encyclopaedia Britannica, 1978), pp. 158–70.

5. Ibid., pp. 160–66.

6. Steven Teitelbaum, M.D., interview by the author, January 3, 2003; Ruth Abram, interview by the author, May 18, 2004.

7. Joseph Letkoff to Morris Abram, July 21, 1982, Morris Abram papers, Robert W. Woodruff Library, Emory University, Atlanta (hereafter cited as Abram papers), box 7, loose letters; Morris B. Abram, *The Day Is Short: An Autobiography* (New York: Harcourt Brace Jovanovich, 1982); David Margolick, "Books of the Times," *New York Times*, September 8, 1982, p. C25. See also Ann Abram, interview by the author, August 30, 2002.

8. Barbara Seaman, *The Doctors' Case against the Pill* (New York: Peter H. Wyden, 1969); Judy Klemesrud, "New Voice in Debate on Breast Surgery," *New York Times*, December 12, 1972, p. 56; Jean Heller, "Syphilis Victims in U.S. Study Went Untreated for 40 Years," *New York Times*, July 26, 1972, pp. 1, 8; Ivan Illich, *Medical Nemesis: The Expropriation of Health* (New York: Pantheon, 1976).

9. "Chapter 12," notes on yellow legal pads, n.d., Abram papers, box 7; notes on yellow legal pads, 1977, Abram papers, box 67, folder: The Day Is Short.

10. Morris B. Abram to Pranay Gupte, March 17, 1977, Abram papers, box 57, folder: correspondence, GU.

11. Morris Abram, interview, unpublished manuscript, June 25, 1982, Abram papers, box 7, folder: newspaper clips; "Chapter 12" (see n. 9); Abram, *Day Is Short*, p. 206. Abram embodied the new type of patient who actively sought experimental treatment. But the history of human experimentation for much of the twentieth century had often consisted of overzealous researchers experimenting on disadvantaged populations, generally without consent. See David J. Rothman, *Strangers at the Bedside: A History of How Law and Bioethics Transformed Medical Decision Making* (New York: Basic Books, 1991); Susan E. Lederer, *Subjected to Science: Human Experimentation in America before the Second World War* (Baltimore: Johns Hopkins University Press, 1994).

12. "Prince of Darkness," notes on yellow legal pads, n.d., Abram papers, box 7.

13. Untitled notes on yellow legal pads, 1977, Abram papers, box 67, folder: The Day Is Short. In the published version of *The Day Is Short*, p. 200, Abram presented this event as nonconfrontational.

14. Untitled notes on yellow legal pads (see n. 13).

15. Ibid.

16. Abram, *Day Is Short*, p. 205.

17. Ibid., pp. 205, 206; Morris B. Abram to Janet Cuttner, September 12, 1977, Abram papers, box 55, folder: correspondence, CPR–CUTT.

18. Abram, "Living with Leukemia," pp. 160, 161.

19. James F. Holland, M.D., interview by the author, January 9, 2003.

20. Abram, *Day Is Short*, p. 217.

21. Ibid., p. 217. Holland recalls these events somewhat differently, stating that he was quite familiar with MER and did not need the intervention of Goodman or Jackson to obtain it for Abram. See Holland interview.

22. Morris B. Abram to Janet Cuttner, March 1, 1974, Abram papers, box 104, folder: personal/family correspondence.

23. Abram to Cuttner, September 12, 1977.

24. Ibid. See also Janet Cuttner, interview by the author, November 6, 2003.

25. Abram to Cuttner, March 1, 1974.

26. Abram, *Day Is Short*, p. 219.

27. Ibid., pp. 219, 220; Holland interview.

28. Morris B. Abram to David Weiss, September 10, 1976, and David Weiss to Morris B. Abram, September 16, 1976, Abram papers, box 64, folder: correspondence, WEIS–WEY.

29. Abram to Cuttner, September 12, 1977.

30. Janet Cuttner to James Holland, George Bekesi, and Louis Wasserman, April 10, 1978, Abram papers, box 104, folder: personal/family correspondence.

31. Abram, *Day Is Short*, p. 222.

32. Pranay Gupte, "Noted Lawyer Free of Symptoms 4 Years after Getting Leukemia," *New York Times*, August 15, 1977, pp. 1, 23.

33. *The Day Is Short* drew heavily on an oral history of Abram begun by the historian Eli Evans shortly after Abram was diagnosed with leukemia. This document surely increased the accuracy of Abram's recollections.

34. Gupte, "Noted Lawyer," p. 23.

35. H.U. to Morris B. Abram, January 18, 1978, Abram papers, box 1, folder: NYT Article, 8/15/77; D.J., Jr., to Morris B. Abram, August 30, 1977, and S.E. to Morris B. Abram, August 16, 1977, Abram papers, box 1, accordion folder, A–K.

36. A.S. to Morris B. Abram, August 30, 1977, Abram papers, box 1, folder: NYT Article, 8/15/77; B.C. to Morris B. Abram, August 16, 1977, Abram papers, box 1, accordion folder, A–K; A.S. to Mr. Benthold [*sic*], August 17, 1977, Abram papers, box 1, accordion folder, L–Z; E.S., Jr., to Morris B. Abram, August 15, 1977, Abram papers, box 1, folder: NYT Article, 8/15/77.

37. Barry Coller to Morris B. Abram, August 19, 1977, and R.S. to Morris B. Abram, August 19, 1977, Abram papers, box 1, folder: NYT Article, 8/15/77.

38. Abram, "Living with Leukemia," p. 160.

39. Ibid.; Abram, *Day Is Short*, p. 5.

40. Ruth Abram interview; Diane Ravitch, review of *The Day Is Short*, unpublished manuscript, 1982, Abram papers, box 7, folder: newspaper clippings, etc.

41. Teitelbaum interview. See also Morris B. Abram to Larry Smith, February 12, 1980, Abram papers, box 7, loose letters.

42. Holland interview; Cuttner interview.

43. David Spiegel et al., "Effect of Psychosocial Treatment on Survival of Patients with Metastatic Breast Cancer," *Lancet* 2 (1989): 888–91; A. G. K. Edwards et al., "Psychological Interventions for Women with Metastatic Breast Cancer," *Cochrane Database of Systematic Reviews* 4 (2) (2004).

44. Morris B. Abram to David Weiss, December 27, 1974, Abram papers, folder: correspondence, WEIS–WEY.

45. Matthew Smith et al., "Acute Adult Myeloid Leukaemia," *Critical Reviews in Oncology/Hematology* 50 (2004): 197–222.

46. Abram, "Living with Leukemia," pp. 158, 164.

47. Christy, "How Morris Abram Said No." The article was considerably more nuanced than the headline.

48. D.B. to Morris B. Abram, August 16, 1977, Abram papers, box 1, folder: NYT article, 8/15/77; E.B. to Morris B. Abram, August 15, 1977, Abram papers, box 1, accordion folder, L–Z; D.J., Jr., to Abram, August 30, 1977.

49. B.C. to Abram, August 16, 1977; J.S. to Morris B. Abram, August 18, 1977, Abram papers, box 1, folder: NYT article, 8/15/77. Hubert Humphrey was diagnosed with bladder cancer in the early 1970s and died in 1978.

50. Irving Rimer to Morris B. Abram, November 16, 1978, Abram papers, box 12, folder: American Cancer Society.

51. Morris B. Abram to Alexander Capron, January 20, 1981, Abram papers, box 9, folder: The Day Is Short, 1981.

52. Ibid.; Morris B. Abram, "The Patient's Eyeview of Investigative Research (At What Price to the Individual Do We Buy Medical Progress?)," talk given at American Cancer Society conference, Washington, DC, April 23–25, 1981, Abram papers, box 12, folder: American Cancer Society.

53. Untitled notes on yellow legal pads (see n. 13); Morris B. Abram to F.B., August 25, 1977, Abram papers, box 1, folder: NYT Article, 8/15/77; Abram, "Living with Leukemia," p. 168.

54. Abram, "Patient's Eyeview." See also Abram, *Day Is Short*, p. 274.

Chapter 7. Unconventional Healing

1. P. Brook, "Dr. Kelley's Cure" (letter to the editor), *Newsweek*, November 17, 1980, pp. 13, 14.

2. "Steve McQueen," segment of the television show *Biography*, A&E, October 30, 2004.

3. Peter B. Flint, "Steve McQueen, 50, Is Dead of a Heart Attack after Surgery for Cancer," *New York Times*, November 8, 1980. Biographies of McQueen include Malachy McCoy, *Steve McQueen: The Unauthorized Biography* (New York: Signet, 1974);

Grady Ragsdale, Jr., *Steve McQueen: The Final Chapter* (Ventura, CA: Vision House, 1983); William F. Nolan, *McQueen* (New York: Berkley Books, 1985); Neile McQueen Toffel, *My Husband, My Friend* (New York: Atheneum, 1986); Penina Spiegel, *McQueen: The Untold Story of a Bad Boy in Hollywood* (New York: Berkley Books, 1987); Marshall Terrill, *Steve McQueen: Portrait of an American Hero* (London: Plexus, 1993); Christopher Sandford, *McQueen: The Biography* (New York: Taylor Trade, 2003).

4. Nolan, *McQueen*, back cover; Spiegel, *McQueen*, back cover; Rydell quoted in "McQueen," *Biography* A&E; Steve McQueen, untitled document, Associated Press (AP) wire, November 8, 1980; Toffel [Adams], *My Husband*.

5. Toffel [Adams], *My Husband*, p. 288.

6. Spiegel, *McQueen*, p. 365.

7. Geoffrey Tweedale, "Asbestos and Its Lethal Legacy," *Nature Reviews Cancer* 2 (2002): 311–15.

8. "Steve McQueen's Love of Racing Cars May Have Triggered His Cancer Crisis," *Star*, October 21, 1980, p. 5.

9. Tony Brenna and Donna Rosenthal, "Steve McQueen's Heroic Battle against Terminal Cancer," *National Enquirer*, March 11, 1980, p. 28.

10. Ragsdale, *Steve McQueen*, p. 77; "Courageous Steve McQueen Meets Death as He Lived Life—Defiantly and Rebelliously," *Star*, December 27, 1983, courtesy of American Media, Inc., Boca Raton, FL.

11. Nolan, *McQueen*, p. 375; Spiegel, *McQueen*, pp. 378–80; Toffel [Adams], *My Husband*, pp. 298, 302, 303. It is likely that Terry and Chad were soon told, or figured out, the truth.

12. Spiegel, *McQueen*, p. 376; Toffel [Adams], *My Husband*, p. 298. On the *Enquirer*, see Iain Calder, *The Untold Story: My 20 Years Running the National Enquirer* (New York: Miramax, 2004).

13. Brenna and Rosenthal, "Heroic Battle," p. 28.

14. Liz Smith, "The Terminal Man," *Los Angeles Herald-Examiner*, March 18, 1980, Steve McQueen clips file, Margaret Herrick Library, Los Angeles; "McQueen Surfaces," *People*, March 24, 1980, Steve McQueen clips; Ted Mutch, "McQueen Says Cancer Reports Are Ridiculous," *Globe*, April 8, 1980, courtesy of American Media, Inc.

15. Toffel [Adams], *My Husband*, p. 298.

16. Ibid., p. 306; Ragsdale, *Steve McQueen*, pp. 111, 119.

17. Sara Davidson, "The Court of Last Hope," *New Times*, January 25, 1974, pp. 48–59. See also Peter Barry Chowka, "Alternative Medicine and the War on Cancer," *Better Nutrition*, August 1999, http://members.aol.com/naturmedia/pioneers.html (accessed November 29, 2002).

18. Sharon Watson and Kathy Mackay, "McQueen's Holistic Medicine Man Claims He Cured His Own Cancer with His Unorthodox Treatments," *People*, October 20, 1980, p. 56; William D. Kelley, "The REAL Cancer Outlaw," www.drkelley.info/articles/archive.php?artid=269 (accessed March 31, 2003). See also William D. Kelley,

"One Answer to Cancer," updated version, 1998, www.drkelley.com/CANLIVER55 .html (accessed September 2, 2003).

19. Kelley, "REAL Cancer Outlaw."

20. Richard Walters, "Kelley's Nutritional-Metabolic Therapy," www.drkelley .info/index.php?section=A+View+From+The+Outside (accessed March 31, 2003).

21. Ibid.; Nolan, *McQueen*, p. 205; Sandford, *McQueen*, pp. 422–24; Harold C. Habein, Jr., to the American Medical Association, July 25, 1974, Historical Health Fraud and Alternative Medicine Collection, AMA Archives, Chicago, box 16, folder: William Donald Kelley, D.D.S.

22. Spiegel, *McQueen*, p. 382; Sandford, *McQueen*, p. 427; "McQueen Treatment: Laetrile, Megavitamins, Animal Cells," AP wire story, October 10, 1980.

23. F. J. Inglefinger, "Laetrilomania," *New England Journal of Medicine* 296 (1977): 1167–68; Philip M. Boffey, "Laetrile and the Law," *New York Times*, August 2, 1978, p. 20; Marjorie Sun, "Laetrile Brush Fire Is Out, Scientists Hope," *Science* 212 (1981): 758–59.

24. Terrill, *Steve McQueen*, p. 371; Ragsdale, *Steve McQueen*, p. 121.

25. Terrill, *Steve McQueen*, p. 377.

26. Toffel [Adams], *My Husband*, p. 298.

27. Spiegel, *McQueen*, p. 383.

28. McQueen quoted in Jerry Buck, "Tough-Guy Actor's Terminal Cancer Reported in Remission," AP wire story, October 2, 1980; Richard West and Paul Jacobs, "Steve McQueen Has Rare Form of Lung Cancer," *Los Angeles Times*, October 3, 1980, pp. 3, 28.

29. Rodriguez quoted in Buck, "Tough-Guy Actor's Terminal Cancer." See also Robert Locke, "Doctors Reveal McQueen Treatment," AP wire story, October 9, 1980.

30. Ragsdale, *Steve McQueen*, p. 124; "Steve McQueen Thanks Mexico 'For Saving My Life,'" AP wire story, October 8, 1980.

31. "McQueen Treatment," October 10, 1980; Joan Sweeney, "M'Queen's Doctors Extol Treatment, Ignore Queries," *Los Angeles Times*, October 10, 1980, pp. 1, 7.

32. Dave Palermo and Ann Salisbury, "New Cancer Therapy Used by McQueen," *Los Angeles Herald-Examiner*, October 3, 1980, pp. A1, A12; Thorson quoted in "McQueen Vows from Hospital Bed to Fight Cancer 'Every Inch of the Way,'" *Star*, October 28, 1980, McQueen clips; Selikoff quoted in Matt Clark with Ronald Henkoff, "A Strange Sort of Therapy," *Newsweek*, October 20, 1980, pp. 65, 66; Terrill, *Steve McQueen*, p. 384.

33. Watson and Mackay, "McQueen's Holistic Medicine Man"; Nolan, *McQueen*, pp. 207, 211; Ragsdale, *Steve McQueen*, p. 125.

34. Ragsdale, *Steve McQueen*, pp. 145, 149, 150.

35. Ibid., pp. 169–75.

36. Nolan, *McQueen*, p. 214; Toffel [Adams], *My Husband*, p. 318; Spiegel, *McQueen*, p. 389; Terrill, *Steve McQueen*, p. 394; Ragsdale, *Steve McQueen*, p. 172; Sandford, *McQueen*, p. 440.

37. Ragsdale, *Steve McQueen*, pp. 182–85.

38. Terrill, *Steve McQueen*, p. 403; Sandford, *McQueen*, p. 445.

39. Terrill, *Steve McQueen*, p. 385; Ragsdale, *Steve McQueen*, p. 189; Nolan, *McQueen*, p. 213.

40. Spiegel, *McQueen*, p. 386; Nolan, *McQueen*, p. 217.

41. Terrill, *Steve McQueen*, p. 390; "Actor Steve McQueen Dies after Cancer Surgery," AP wire story, November 8, 1980. One of McQueen's biographers, Marshall Terrill, obtained a CT scan done before the operation, which he said also showed severe disease. See Terrill, *Steve McQueen*, p. 398.

42. Claudia Cohen, "The Final $25G Agony of McQueen," *Daily News Tonight*, November 10, 1980, p. M5; Toffel [Adams], *My Husband*, p. 323; Ron Rosenbaum, "Tales from the Cancer Care Underground," in Rosenbaum, *The Secret Parts of Fortune* (New York: Perennial, 2000), pp. 298–329. Kelley's later diatribes were laced with anti-Semitism. See Sandford, *McQueen*, p. 423.

43. Liz Smith, "Casting Doubt and Peddling Influence," *New York Daily News*, November 18, 2000, p. 6; Landers's column cited by Smith.

44. "Desperate Cancer Patients Are Flocking to Mexican Hospitals Seeking McQueen's Therapy," *Star*, November 11, 1980, p. 17; *CBS Evening News* with Dan Rather, January 11, 1981.

45. Quoted in Sandford, *McQueen*, p. 446.

46. Michael Specter, "The Outlaw Doctor," *New Yorker*, February 5, 2001, pp. 48–61; Nicholas Gonzalez, M.D., interview by the author, November 19, 2003.

47. "Evolution of Intensive Pancreatic Proteolytic Enzyme Therapy with Ancillary Nutritional Support in the Treatment of Inoperable Pancreatic Adenocarcinoma," grant application, February 28, 2000, courtesy of John Chabot, M.D.

48. Ken Adachi, "Biological Weapons in the Cancer War," http://educate-yourself .org/cn/2001/bioweaponscancerwars01oct01.shtml (accessed December 30, 2004).

Chapter 8. Medicine's Blind Spots

1. Bert Barnes, "'Love Goddess' Rita Hayworth Dies," *Washington Post*, May 16, 1987, p. B6. Caren Roberts-Frenzel, president of the Rita Hayworth Fan Club, has established a remarkably comprehensive website dedicated to the actress. See http:// members.tripod.com/~claudia79/fanclub.html.

2. Barbara Leaming, *If This Was Happiness: A Biography of Rita Hayworth* (New York: Viking, 1989), pp. 17–27. On the "Gilda" comment, see Adrienne L. McLean, *Being Rita Hayworth: Labor, Identity, and Hollywood Stardom* (New Brunswick, NJ: Rutgers University Press, 2004), pp. 1–3.

3. Leaming, *If This Was Happiness*, pp. 336, 337, 348–51.

4. "Rita Hayworth's Sad and Shocking Final Days," *Globe*, March 17, 1987, p. 5.

5. David Shenk, *The Forgetting. Alzheimer's: Portrait of an Epidemic* (New York: Anchor Books, 2003), p. 13.

6. Ibid., p. 15.

7. Ibid., p. 25.

8. Ibid., pp. 74–78.

9. Ibid., pp. 132, 133; Robert Katzman and Katherine Bick, *Alzheimer Disease: The Changing View* (San Diego: Academic Press, 2000), pp. 266, 270.

10. Katzman and Bick, *Alzheimer Disease*, p. 266.

11. On culture and disease, see Robert A. Aronowitz, *Making Sense of Illness: Science, Society, and Disease* (Cambridge: Cambridge University Press, 1998); Charles E. Rosenberg and Janet Golden, eds., *Framing Disease: Studies in Cultural History* (New Brunswick, NJ: Rutgers University Press, 1992).

12. Leaming, *If This Was Happiness*, p. 182.

13. Ibid., pp. 270, 281, 286.

14. Ibid., p. 333, and see also pp. 119, 120; James Hill, *Rita Hayworth: A Memoir* (New York: Simon and Schuster, 1983).

15. Sam Zolotow, "Nancy Kelly Set for New Drama," *New York Times*, August 24, 1962, p. 13; Joe Morella and Edward Z. Epstein, *Rita* (New York: Delacorte Press, 1983), p. 227.

16. Leaming, *If This Was Happiness*, p. 336; Gene Ringgold, *The Complete Films of Rita Hayworth* (New York: Citadel Press, 1991), p. 231.

17. Jack Gould, "Honesty and Ad Libs Liven Ceremony," *New York Times*, April 15, 1964, p. 79; Ringgold, *Complete Films*, p. 234.

18. Morella and Epstein, *Rita*, p. 240; Leaming, *If This Was Happiness*, p. 337.

19. Leaming, *If This Was Happiness*, p. 338.

20. Ibid., p. 347.

21. Ibid., pp. 348–50; Bud Moss, interview for *Rita: The Real Story of Hollywood's Love Goddess*, *Rita Hayworth*, September 19, 2002, Playboy Films, 2004, courtesy of Elaina Archer.

22. Rosemary Santini and Katherine Barrett, "The Tragedy of Rita Hayworth," *Ladies' Home Journal*, January 1983, pp. 84, 85, 139–42; "Rita Hayworth Ill, Needs Help Deplaning," *Los Angeles Herald-Examiner*, January 20, 1976, and "Newsmakers," *Newsweek*, January 21, 1976, Rita Hayworth clips file, Margaret Herrick Library, Los Angeles.

23. Morella and Epstein, *Rita*, p. 245; Dennis D'Antonio, "Friends of Former Screen Goddess Tell of . . . The Sad, Lonely Life of Rita Hayworth," *National Enquirer*, February 1, 1977, p. 4.

24. Leaming, *If This Was Happiness*, p. 354.

25. Morella and Epstein, *Rita*, p. 246.

26. Ibid., pp. 246, 247; Leaming, *If This Was Happiness*, p. 356. See also Ruta Lee, interview for *Rita*, October 15, 2002, courtesy of Elaina Archer.

27. Yasmin Aga Khan, interview by the author, October 6, 2003.

28. Ronald Fieve to Yasmin Aga Khan, April 23, 1979, courtesy of Ronald Fieve. See also Ronald Fieve, M.D., interview by the author, November 12, 2003.

29. Cyril B. Courville, *Effects of Alcohol on the Nervous System in Man* (Los Angeles: San Lucas Press, 1955).

30. Aga Khan interview; Marian Christy, "The Princess and the Movie Star," *Boston Globe*, March 26, 1989, p. 43.

31. Leaming, *If This Was Happiness*, p. 355.

32. Lee interview.

33. Leaming, *If This Was Happiness*, p. 348. See also Moss interview.

34. Ringgold, *Complete Films*, p. 250; Neal Gabler, *Life: The Movie. How Entertainment Conquered Reality* (New York: Vintage Books, 1998). The *Carol Burnett Show* episode is available at the University of California, Los Angeles, Film and Television Archive.

35. Shearlean Duke, "Rita: A 'Love Goddess' at 58," *Los Angeles Times*, March 10, 1977, pp. 1, 13; "Gilda Goes to Oxford," *Los Angeles Herald-Examiner*, June 23, 1978, and John Francis Lane, "In Camera," *Films and Filming*, September 1978, Hayworth clips; Neil Blincow, "Rita Hayworth Swears off Bottle for Good," *National Enquirer*, April 15, 1980, courtesy of American Media, Inc., Boca Raton, FL.

36. Duke, "Rita: 'Love Goddess,'" p. 13.

37. Dorothy Manners, "Friends Back Rita Hayworth," *Los Angeles Herald-Examiner*, March 21, 1977, Hayworth clips; Dorothy Manners, "Rita Not in Hiding," *Los Angeles Herald-Examiner*, May 9, 1977, p. B1; Moss interview.

38. Daniel A. Pollen, *Hannah's Heirs: The Quest for the Genetic Origins of Alzheimer's Disease* (New York: Oxford University Press, 1993), pp. 79–85.

39. Abigail Van Buren, "Dear Abby," *Denver Rocky Mountain News*, October 23, 1980, p. 86.

40. Santini and Barrett, "Tragedy of Rita Hayworth"; Yasmin Aga Khan, "Remembering Rita," *People*, June 1, 1987, pp. 72–80.

41. Christy, "Princess and the Movie Star," p. 43; Princess Yasmin Aga Khan, "My Mother, Rita Hayworth," *Star*, June 3, 1986, p. 37. See also Pia Lindstrom, "Yasmin Aga Khan: Alzheimer's Fight in Her Mother's Name," *New York Times*, February 23, 1997, sect. 13, pp. LI1, LI2.

42. The headline comes from a syndicated version of the Santini and Barrett article originally published in *Ladies' Home Journal*, Hayworth clips; Todd McCarthy, "Rita Hayworth, 68, Dies in N.Y.: Col's Shining Light of the '40s," *Variety*, May 20, 1987, and Stefan Kanfer, "Rita Hayworth: The Pin-Up Who Became a Princess," *Memories*, April–May 1989, Hayworth clips; Leaming, *If This Was Happiness*, p. 336.

43. Leaming, *If This Was Happiness*, p. 335; Santini and Barrett, "Tragedy of Rita Hayworth," p. 141; Paul Hendrickson, "Rita Hayworth's Fade to Black: In Memory of the Star, Daughter Yasmin's Crusade against Alzheimer's Disease," *Washington Post*, April 6, 1989, p. B1.

44. Richard Cansino, interview for *Rita*, September 16, 2002, courtesy of Elaina Archer; Santini and Barrett, "Tragedy of Rita Hayworth," p. 139.

45. Lonnie Wollin, interview by the author, June 5, 2003; Jerome Stone, interview by the author, July 8, 2003.

46. Wollin interview; Aga Khan interview.

47. See www.alz.org/Events/RHG.asp.

48. See www.alz.org/Advocacy/successes/overview.asp.

49. Wollin interview; Stone interview; Abigail Van Buren, "Alzheimer's Disease Puts Strain on Family," *Los Angeles Times*, June 6, 1983, pt. II, p. 6.

50. Patricia A. Sprague, "Rita Hayworth," *People*, June 22, 1987, p. 6, in response to Yasmin, "Remembering Rita."

Chapter 9. Hero or Victim?

1. William C. DeVries, Institutional Review Board Proposal, June 1980, Barney Clark papers, University of Utah, Salt Lake City (hereafter cited as Clark papers), box 21, folder 38.

2. William C. DeVries et al., "Clinical Use of the Artificial Heart," *New England Journal of Medicine* 310 (1984): 273–78; Gregory E. Pence, *Classic Cases in Medical Ethics*, 2nd ed. (New York: McGraw-Hill, 1995), pp. 274–76.

3. William DeVries, M.D., interview by Earl and Miriam Selby, April 15, 1983, Clark papers, box 13, folder 5.

4. William J. Broad, "Dr. Clark's Heart: A Story of Modern Marketing as Well as Modern Medicine," *New York Times*, March 20, 1983, p. 2; Lawrence K. Altman, "Reflections of a Reporter on Unresolved Issues," in Margery W. Shaw, ed., *After Barney Clark: Reflections on the Utah Heart Program* (Austin: University of Texas Press, 1984), pp. 113–28.

5. Cristine Russell, "Recipient of Plastic Heart Weathers a 2nd Operation," *Washington Post*, December 5, 1982, p. A1.

6. Peter G. Filene, *In the Arms of Others: A Cultural History of the Right-to-Die in America* (Chicago: Ivan R. Dee, 1999).

7. Cristine Russell, "In the Pink: Patient with Artificial Heart Speaks for the First Time since his Surgery," *Washington Post*, December 4, 1982, pp. A1, A10.

8. Scott Herold, "Surgeons Stand in Awe as Implant Defies Death," *Portland Oregonian*, December 3, 1982, p. A1; "Taking Heart," *Wall Street Journal*, December 14, 1982, p. 30.

9. See, e.g., Twila Van Leer, "Clark Suffers Seizures as He Begins Sixth Day on the Artificial Heart," *Deseret (Utah) News*, December 7, 1982, pp. A1, A10; Cristine Russell, "Clark's Case Impels FDA to Review Heart Program," *Washington Post*, December 18, 1982, p. A2; Fred L. Anderson, M.D., interview by Earl and Miriam Selby, May 23, 1983, Clark papers, box 8, folder 10.

10. Denton A. Cooley, "Reservations Voiced on the Utah Artificial Heart," *American Medical News*, December 10, 1982, p. 4; Renee C. Fox and Judith P. Swazey, *Spare Parts: Organ Replacement in American Society* (New York: Oxford University Press, 1992), pp. 156, 157; Ronald and Nancy Reagan to Barney Clark, December 8, 1982, Clark papers, box 1, folder 9.

11. Broad, "Dr. Clark's Heart," p. 2; Lawrence K. Altman, "The Old Heart That

Failed," *New York Times*, December 14, 1982, pp. C1, C2; William C. DeVries, M.D., interview by Earl and Miriam Selby, May 28, 1983, Clark Papers, box 13, folder 12.

12. George Raine, "A Patient with Leading Credentials," *New York Times*, December 4, 1982, p. 14.

13. Jay Mathews, "Clark's Heart: Old Values Remain Vital in Modern Medicine," *Washington Post*, December 25, 1982, pp. A1, A8.

14. "Artificial Heart Recipients Will Have Choice on Life," *New York Times*, December 5, 1982, p. 48.

15. Van Leer, "Clark Suffers Seizures," p. A10.

16. Jay Mathews, "In the End, Barney Clark's Heart Was Still Beating," *Washington Post*, March 25, 1983, p. A1.

17. Renee C. Fox, "'It's the Same, but Different': A Sociological Perspective on the Case of the Utah Artificial Heart," in Shaw, *After Barney Clark*, pp. 68–90.

18. DeVries interview, April 15, 1983. See also Dennis L. Breo, "In the Wait for Artificial Heart, All Is Ready but the Patient," *American Medical News*, November 5, 1982, pp. 3, 36–41.

19. DeVries interview, April 15, 1983. The consent form is replicated in Appendix A in Shaw, *After Barney Clark*, pp. 195–201.

20. Una Loy Clark to Lucy Kroll, n.d., Clark papers, box 2, folder 6; Terence Block, M.D., interview by Earl and Miriam Selby, June 24, 1983, Clark papers, box 8, folder 36.

21. Block interview; speech given by Una Loy Clark in honor of Peggy Miller, October 1983, Clark papers, box 1, folder 2; Una Loy Clark to Robert H. Ruby, March 4, 1987, Clark papers, box 1, folder 30.

22. Albert R. Jonsen, "The Selection of Patients," and Denise Grady, "Summary of Discussion on Ethical Perspectives," in Shaw, *After Barney Clark*, pp. 5–10, 42–52.

23. From an unpublished draft of Earl and Miriam Selby, "True Valor: Barney Clark and the Artificial Heart," p. 7, Clark papers, box 21, folder 1. See also Pence, *Classic Cases*, p. 290.

24. Altman, "Reflections," p. 120.

25. Appendix A, in Shaw, *After Barney Clark*, p. 195. See also Fox and Swazey, *Spare Parts*, pp. 108, 109.

26. Fox and Swazey, *Spare Parts*; Renee C. Fox and Judith P. Swazey, "Leaving the Field," *Hastings Center Report*, September–October 1992, pp. 9–15; Renee C. Fox, "Experiment Perilous: Forty-Five Years as a Participant Observer of Patient-Oriented Clinical Research," *Perspectives in Biology and Medicine* 39 (1996): 206–26.

27. Fox and Swazey, *Spare Parts*, pp. 105–8, 172, 173; William C. DeVries, M.D., interview by Earl and Miriam Selby, March 10, 1984, Clark papers, box 13, folder 13. See also Pierre M. Galletti, "Replacement of the Heart with a Mechanical Device: The Case of Dr. Barney Clark," *New England Journal of Medicine* 310 (1984): 312–14.

28. Fox and Swazey, *Spare Parts*, pp. 108, 156, 180, 181; Fox, "Experiment Perilous," p. 223.

29. Clinical notes on Barney Clark by Terry Rogers, M.D., Clark papers, box 5, folder 1; Fox and Swazey, *Spare Parts*, pp. 110, 114.

30. Fox, "It's the Same,'" pp. 80, 81; Lawrence K. Altman, "The Artificial Heart: Mired in Delay and Uncertainty," *New York Times*, October 25, 1983, p. C1.

31. Fox, "It's the Same,'" pp. 80, 81.

32. Ibid., p. 82.

33. Ibid., pp. 84–87, 164.

34. Fox and Swazey, *Spare Parts*, p. 193, and "Leaving the Field," p. 11; Fox, "Experiment Perilous," p. 224.

35. Caplan in Russell, "Clark's Case," p. A2; Pence, *Classic Cases*, p. 284; George J. Annas, "Consent to the Artificial Heart: The Lion and the Crocodiles," *Hastings Center Report*, April 1983, pp. 20–22.

36. Thomas A. Preston, "The Case against the Artificial Heart," *Utah Holiday*, July 1983, pp. 39–49; Barton J. Bernstein, "Is It a Boon or a High-Tech Fix?" *Nation*, January 22, 1983, pp. 71, 72.

37. "Prolonging Death Is No Triumph," *New York Times*, December 16, 1982, p. A26; "More than Just a Pump," *New York Times*, September 12, 1985, p. 34; "The Dracula of Medical Technology," *New York Times*, May 16, 1988, p. A16.

38. "Transcript of Interview with Barney Clark," Associated Press news story, March 2, 1983.

39. Erik Barnouw, *Documentary: A History of the Non-Fiction Film*, 2nd rev. ed. (New York: Oxford University Press, 1993); Joe Morgenstern, "Taking Heart from Barney Clark," *Los Angeles Herald-Examiner*, March 27, 1983, p. 3.

40. Claudia K. Berenson and Bernard I. Grosser, "Total Artificial Heart Implantation," *Archives of General Psychiatry* 41 (1984): 910–16. For more on the controversy, see Willem Kolff to Chase Peterson, September 21, 1984, and Chase Peterson to Willem Kolff, October 19, 1984, Willem Kolff papers, University of Utah, Salt Lake City, box 353, folder 3.

41. Dennis L. Breo, "Historic Surgery Was Worth It," *American Medical News*, March 25, 1983, pp. 1, 40–43; Berenson and Grosser, "Total Artificial Heart Implantation," p. 915; Claudia K. Berenson, M.D., interview by Earl and Miriam Selby, June 10, 1983, Clark papers, box 8, folder 34.

42. Gregory Pence used this strategy in his excellent summary of the Clark case.

43. Lawrence K. Altman, "Heart Patient Sits in Chair on His Best Day in Months," *New York Times*, December 19, 1982, p. 22; George Raine, "Heart Patient's Family Marks a Special Holiday," *New York Times*, December 26, 1982, p. 22.

44. Note written by Una Loy Clark, March 7, 1983, Clark papers, box 1, folder 14; Claudia Wallis, "Feeling Much Better, Thank You," *Time*, March 14, 1983, p. 74; Fox and Swazey, *Spare Parts*, pp. 160, 188; Dennis L. Breo, "Barney Clark's MD-Son: 'I'm Ambivalent,'" *American Medical News*, April 22–29, 1983, pp. 1, 15, 18–20.

45. Una Loy Clark to the author, July 11, 2003.

46. Una Loy Clark, interview by Earl and Miriam Selby, June 1983, Clark papers, box 10, folder 21; Breo, "Barney Clark's MD-Son," p. 1.

47. Claudia K. Berenson, M.D., interview by Earl and Miriam Selby, June 20, 1983, Clark papers, box 8, folder 35; Una Loy Clark to Birdie and Erie, January 17, 1983, Clark papers, box 2, folder 1; Una Loy Clark interview.

48. Peggy Miller, interview by Earl and Miriam Selby, n.d., Clark papers, box 17, folder 30; Twila Van Leer, "Doctors Look Back on Drama of Clark Heart Experiment," *Deseret (Utah) News*, November 29, 1992; Beth Ann Cole, interview by Earl and Miriam Selby, May 17, 1983, Clark papers, box 12, folder 30.

49. Dorothy Gilliam, "What If . . . ?" *Washington Post*, December 13, 1982, p. D1; Howard S. Miller, "A Man-Made Heart Well Worth Trying," *New York Times*, December 23, 1982, p. A14; William Safire, "Fighting for Life," *New York Times*, December 20, 1982, p. A19.

50. Morgenstern, "Taking Heart," p. 3; Ellison Rodgers cited in Grady, "Summary of Discussion," p. 47.

51. Jon Nelson to Una Loy Clark, May 2, 1986, Clark papers, box 1, folder 23; Bruce Jeannot to Una Loy Clark, March 29, 1983, Clark papers, box 1, folder 18.

52. Cristine Russell, "Widow Blames 25 Years of Smoking for Barney Clark's Death," *Washington Post*, May 4, 1983, p. A2.

53. Transcript of press conference with Una Loy Clark, June 17, 1983, Clark papers, box 22, folder 18; Una Loy Clark to Willem Kolff, September 4, 1983, Kolff papers, box 353, folder 6.

54. Fox and Swazey, *Spare Parts*, pp. 149–53; Fox, "Experiment Perilous," p. 224; Michael E. DeBakey, "The Odyssey of the Artificial Heart," *Artificial Organs* 24 (2000): 405–11.

55. See www.abiomed.com/products/heart_replacement/index.cfm.

56. Sheryl Gay Stolberg, "On Medicine's Frontier: The Last Journey of James Quinn," *New York Times*, October 8, 2002, pp. F1, F4.

57. Fox and Swazey, "Leaving the Field," p. 10.

58. DeVries quoted in Dennis L. Breo, "Two Surgeons Who Dared Are Still Chasing Their Dreams," *Journal of the American Medical Association* 262 (1989): 2904, 2910, 2911, 2916; Shaffer quoted in Carol M. Ostrom, "No Regrets: Clark's Family Remembers the Good Times," *Seattle Times*, March 27, 2003, pp. A1, A4.

Chapter 10. *"You Murdered My Daughter"*

1. Itamar Kubovy to Theodore H. Friedman, April 1993, in the Sidney Zion Collection, the Howard Gotlieb Archival Research Center, Boston University, Boston (hereafter cited as Zion papers), box 14, folder 7.

2. This account comes from Natalie Robins, *The Girl Who Died Twice: The Libby Zion Case and the Hidden Hazards of Hospitals* (New York: Dell, 1995); and "Report Concerning the Care and Treatment of a Patient and the Supervision of Interns and Junior Residents at a Hospital in New York County," Grand Jury Report, Supreme Court of the State of New York, December 31, 1986, Zion papers, box 12, folder 4.

3. Robins, *Girl Who Died Twice*, p. 390.

4. "Report Concerning the Care and Treatment," pp. 21, 23.

5. Robins, *Girl Who Died Twice*, pp. 144–47.

6. Charles L. Bosk, *Forgive and Remember: Managing Medical Failure* (Chicago: University of Chicago Press, 1979).

7. Robins, *Girl Who Died Twice*, p. 35.

8. Ibid.

9. Ibid., pp. 45, 171, 173.

10. Ibid., pp. 48, 49.

11. David M. Studdert et al., "Medical Malpractice," *New England Journal of Medicine* 350 (2004): 283–92.

12. Steven Roose to Jethro Eisenstein, July 2, 1984, and Harvey J. Makadon to Jethro Eisenstein, August 31, 1984, Zion papers, box 11, folder: correspondence 3; untitled document by Jonathan M. Alexander, July 22, 1986, Zion papers, box 17, folder 3; Timothy B. McCall to Itamar Kubovy, August 23, 1993, Zion papers, box 14, folder 2.

13. "Docs Killed My Daughter—N.Y. Writer," *New York Post*, August 26, 1985, p. 4; Robins, *Girl Who Died Twice*, pp. 236, 237.

14. M. L. Millenson, "Pushing the Profession: How the News Media Turned Patient Safety into a Priority," *Quality and Safety in Health Care* 11 (2002): 57–63; Louis J. Regan, *Doctor and Patient and the Law* (St. Louis, MO: C. V. Mosby, 1956); intern quoted in Richard C. Friedman et al., "The Intern and Sleep Loss," *New England Journal of Medicine* 285 (1971): 201–3. See also Mark Green, "How Hospitals Still Violate the 'Bell' Regulations Governing Resident Working Conditions," unpublished report, December 1997, pp. 31–36.

15. Doctor X, *Intern* (New York: Harper and Row, 1965), p. 5; Terry Mizrahi, *Getting Rid of Patients: Contradictions in the Socialization of Doctors* (New Brunswick, NJ: Rutgers University Press, 1986).

16. N. R. Kleinfeld, "Doctor's Criticism in '84 Case Strains Hospitals' Bond," *New York Times*, August 5, 1991, pp. B1, B4; Sidney Zion, "Doctors Know Best?" *New York Times*, May 13, 1989, p. 25.

17. Theodore H. Friedman to Helen Thorpe, August 11, 1993, Zion papers, box 11, folder: correspondence 4.

18. Tom Wicker, "Doctors in the Dock?" *New York Times*, December 23, 1985, p. A17, and "Blaming the System," *New York Times*, February 4, 1987, p. A27; Warren Hinckle, "Hospital Smear Tactic Worsens Dad's Agony," *San Francisco Examiner*, January 27, 1987, pp. A1, B4.

19. Mike Wallace, "The Problems of Medical People Working Very Long Hours," *60 Minutes*, June 3, 1990, CBS News Transcripts, Burrelle's Information Services; this was a rebroadcast of the 1987 show "The 36-Hour Day."

20. Robins, *Girl Who Died Twice*, p. 174; Stephen Brill, "Curing Doctors," *American Lawyer*, September 1985, pp. 1, 12–17; Robins, *Girl Who Died Twice*, p. 233.

21. "Report Concerning the Care and Treatment of a Patient."

22. Bertrand M. Bell, "Evolutionary Imperatives and Quiet Revolutions," unpublished manuscript, 1988, courtesy of Bertrand Bell.

23. Bertrand M. Bell, untitled letter [to Theodore H. Friedman], 1991, courtesy of Bertrand Bell. On Bell, see "A Personal History of Work Hours Reform—An Interview with Dr. Bert Bell," November 6, 2003, www.hourswatch.org/48breakingnewsstory.htm (accessed February 10, 2004).

24. Georgia Mihalakis to Sidney Zion, January 28, 1987, Zion papers, box 11, folder: correspondence 2; Antonia New to Bertrand Bell, May 6, 1989, courtesy of Bertrand Bell; Toby Moore to Sidney Zion, January 20, 1987, Zion papers, box 15, folder: correspondence 6; A.K. and I.K. to Sidney Zion, April 7, 1988, Zion papers, box 11, folder: correspondence 5.

25. Robins, *Girl Who Died Twice*, pp. 185–87.

26. Brill, "Curing Doctors," p. 12; William Shawcross, *The Shah's Last Ride: The Fate of an Ally* (New York: Simon and Schuster, 1998).

27. Adele Lubell, "Libby Zion Case Prompts Nationwide Debate on House Staff Training," April 22, 1988, draft of two-part article published in *American Medical News*, June 24 and July 1, 1988, courtesy of Bertrand Bell.

28. Robins, *Girl Who Died Twice*, pp. 266, 345; Michael Stone, "New York Hospital on the Spot," *New York*, June 22, 1987, pp. 40–47.

29. M. A. Farber and Lawrence K. Altman, "A Great Hospital in Crisis," *New York Times Magazine*, January 24, 1988, pp. 18, 20, 21, 38, 40, 50, 57, quotation from p. 40. According to journalist Warren Hinckle, the press release was written by Diana Golden, wife of New York City controller Harrison J. Golden. See Hinckle, "Hospital Smear Tactic," p. B4.

30. Robins, *Girl Who Died Twice*, pp. 312–15.

31. Skinner quoted in Farber and Altman, "A Great Hospital," p. 40; Dennis Murphy, "A Father's Story," *Dateline NBC*, May 25, 1997, NBC News Transcripts. Natalie Robins argued that New York Hospital was planning its cocaine defense as early as 1984. See Robins, *Girl Who Died Twice*, p. 229.

32. Theodore H. Friedman to R. Gordon Douglas, March 31, 1988, Zion papers, box 11, folder: correspondence 4.

33. Francis P. Bensel to Andrew Stein, January 15, 1986, Zion papers, box 11, folder: correspondence 4; Court TV documentary "Deadly Dosage: Who's at Fault?" May 1995.

34. Sidney Zion to undisclosed recipient, n.d., Zion papers, box 11, folder: correspondence 3; Theodore H. Friedman to Jeffrey H. Daichman, December 1, 1987, Zion papers, box 15, folder: correspondence 6; Theodore H. Friedman to Sidney Zion, September 25, 1989, Zion papers, box 11, folder 15; Hinckle, "Hospital Smear Tactic," pp. A1, B4.

35. Richard J. Evans, *In Defense of History* (New York: W. W. Norton, 1999), pp. 217–20; Guenter B. Risse and John Harley Warner, "Reconstructing Clinical Activities: Patient Records in Medical History," *Social History of Medicine* 5 (1992): 183–205.

36. Murphy, "Father's Story"; Robins, *Girl Who Died Twice*, pp. 323, 324. It should

be noted that by preventing his lawyers from conceding that Libby Zion used cocaine, Sidney Zion interfered with a potential argument that might have helped the plaintiffs: that the New York Hospital doctors, confronted with an agitated patient, should have strongly considered surreptitious cocaine use. See David J. Rothman, "What Doctors Don't Tell Us," *New York Review of Books*, February 29, 1996, pp. 30–34.

37. Joan McGettigan, "Troubled Teen or Troubled System? TV Interprets the Zion Malpractice Case," *Literature and Medicine* 18 (1999): 192–209.

38. Robins, *Girl Who Died Twice*, p. 323. Similarly, see Eugene D. Robin, untitled manuscript submitted to Committee on Ethical Scientific Performance of Stanford University Medical Center, August 1988, Zion papers, box 15, folder 10.

39. Andrew Blum, "A Father's Crusade Finally Gets to Court," *National Law Journal*, December 12, 1994, p. A12; *Zion v. New York Hospital*, trial transcript, p. 6097. I thank Cheryl Bulbach for pointing out this interaction.

40. *Zion v. New York Hospital*, p. 6097.

41. Ibid., pp. 6486, 6487.

42. Ibid., p. 6489.

43. Ibid., p. 6492.

44. One of the six jurors, Loretta Andrews, later stated that she had several misgivings about the verdict. One of these was the jury's conclusion that the training system at New York Hospital was not a proximate cause of Libby Zion's death. See Robins, *Girl Who Died Twice*, pp. 335–43, 398–413. See also Loretta Andrews, "I Was Juror No. 6, the Lone Dissenter in the Libby Zion Case," *New York Times*, February 21, 1995, p. A18.

45. There may be yet another way to frame the story of Libby Zion, focusing on the physician-nurse relationship. It seems as if the nurses were truly alarmed at Zion's condition but were unable to get the doctors to share their concern. In this sense, hospital hierarchies may have played a role in Zion's death.

46. Susana Morales, M.D., interview by the author, June 12, 2004; McCall to Kubovy, August 23, 1993. See also Robin, untitled manuscript.

47. Timothy B. McCall, "No Turning Back: A Blueprint for Residency Reform," *Journal of the American Medical Association* 261 (1989): 909–10.

48. "Residency Work Hours: New Rules, Fresh Vigilance," *American Medical News*, June 23, 2003, www.ama-assn.org/amednews/2003/06/23/edsa0623.htm (accessed February 13, 2005). See also Bertrand Bell, M.D., interview by the author, June 13, 2003.

49. Murphy, "Father's Story"; "Deadly Dosage," *Court TV.*

50. Ira A. Hoffman, quoted in Kleinfeld, "Doctor's Criticism," p. B4; William Dement, quoted in Green, "How Hospitals Still Violate," p. 34.

51. Priscilla to Natalie Robins, January 27, 1996, and Eileen King to Natalie Robins, March 20, 1996, courtesy of Natalie Robins.

52. Anne Roiphe, "A Tough Father, a Lost Child and a Scary Culture," *New York Observer*, February 20, 1995, p. 5.

53. Lubell, "Libby Zion Case"; Willard Gaylin, "Who Killed Libby Zion?" *Nation*, October 9, 1995, pp. 394–97.

54. Kenneth R. Manning to Sidney Zion, April 18, 1995, Zion papers, box 18, folder 2; Judith Oliver-Grimm to Sidney Zion, November 4, 1985, Zion papers, box 11, folder: correspondence 1.

55. Maureen Hurley to Sidney Zion, June 23, 1987, Zion papers, box 11, folder: correspondence 3; Mrs. George J. Campo to Sidney Zion, 1987, Zion papers, box 15, folder 8; H. Tramontano to Sidney Zion, February 1987, Zion papers, box 11, folder: correspondence 2.

56. David A. Asch and Ruth M. Parker, "The Libby Zion Case: One Step Forward or Two Steps Backward?" *New England Journal of Medicine* 318 (1988): 771–75; Sidney Zion, "Arrogant Docs Keep Violating My Libby's Law," *New York Daily News*, November 18, 1999, p. 51. Recent data have suggested a correlation between sleep deprivation and poor clinical performance. See Jeffrey M. Drazen, "Awake and Informed," *New England Journal of Medicine* 351 (2004): 1884.

57. D.H. to Sidney Zion, n.d., Zion papers, box 11, folder: correspondence 2; Francine to Sidney Zion, December 28, 1985, Zion papers, box 11, folder: correspondence 5; Judy Rubin to Sidney Zion, November 6, 1994, Zion papers, box 18, folder 2.

58. Sidney Zion, "Stop the Killing in Hospitals," *New York Daily News*, December 2, 1999, www.nydailynews.com/1999–11–30/News_and_Views/Beyond_the_City/a-48809.asp (accessed March 27, 2000); Sidney Zion, "Docs Still Get Away with Murder," *New York Daily News*, February 29, 2000, p. 12.

59. Sue Black to Craig Anderson and Wendy Kram, March 20, 2000, courtesy of Sidney Zion.

60. Quoted in Warren Hinckle, "A Father's Day," *San Francisco Examiner*, n.d., courtesy of Sidney Zion.

Chapter 11. Patient Activism Goes Hollywood

1. Elizabeth Glaser and Laura Palmer, *In the Absence of Angels* (New York: Berkley Books, 1991), pp. 5–8.

2. Ibid., p. 3.

3. Randy Shilts, *And the Band Played On: Politics, People and the AIDS Epidemic* (New York: Penguin Books, 1987), p. 171; Glaser and Palmer, *In the Absence*, p. 4.

4. Glaser and Palmer, *In the Absence*, pp. 25–33.

5. Ibid., p. 36; George Lewis, *NBC Nightly News*, December 3, 1994.

6. Glaser and Palmer, *In the Absence*, p. 37.

7. Arthur Ashe and Arnold Rampersad, *Days of Grace: A Memoir* (New York: Ballantine Books, 1993), pp. 66, 152.

8. Ibid., pp. 44, 117; *NBC Nightly News* with Tom Brokaw, February 8, 1993.

9. Ashe and Rampersad, *Days of Grace*, p. 57.

10. Ibid., pp. 57–59.

11. Kenny Moore, "The Eternal Example," *Sports Illustrated*, December 21, 1992, pp. 16–27. See also Ashe and Rampersad, *Days of Grace*, pp. 122, 210, 215.

12. Ashe and Rampersad, *Days of Grace*, pp. 218–29.

13. Ibid., p. 226.

14. Shilts, *And the Band Played On*, p. 575.

15. Gretchen M. Krueger,"'A Cure Is Near': Children, Families and Cancer in America, 1945–1980," Ph.D. diss., Yale University, 2003.

16. Catherine Woodard, "When a Child Dies of AIDS," *Newsday (Long Island)*, February 3, 1991, p. 25; Glaser and Palmer, *In the Absence*, p. 75.

17. Glaser and Palmer, *In the Absence*, p. 75.

18. Larry Kramer, *Reports from the Holocaust: The Story of an AIDS Activist* (New York: St. Martin's Press, 1994); Steven Epstein, *Impure Science: AIDS, Activism, and the Politics of Knowledge* (Berkeley: University of California Press, 1996).

19. Thomas C. Merigan, "You Can Teach an Old Dog New Tricks: How AIDS Trials Are Pioneering New Strategies," *New England Journal of Medicine* 323 (1990): 1341–43.

20. Glaser and Palmer, *In the Absence*, p. 75.

21. Ibid., pp. 91, 98.

22. Ibid., p. 99.

23. Ibid., p. 103.

24. Ibid., pp. 103, 112.

25. Patricia McCormick, "Living with AIDS," *Parents*, November 1993, pp. 40–49.

26. Glaser and Palmer, *In the Absence*, pp. 105, 113.

27. Joy Horowitz, "The Plague and the Players," *Lear's*, September 1992, pp. 66–69, 110.

28. Glaser and Palmer, *In the Absence*, p. 115.

29. Ibid., pp. 118, 119.

30. Michael Dorris, "When the World Falls Apart," *Los Angeles Times*, February 3, 1991, book review sect., pp. 1, 9.

31. Glaser and Palmer, *In the Absence*, pp. 121, 123.

32. Ibid., p. 131.

33. Ibid., p. 150.

34. "For a Star-Studded Gala against AIDS, Some Politicians Will Even Cross Party Lines," *People*, July 10, 1989, pp. 104, 105.

35. Glaser and Palmer, *In the Absence*, pp. 227–41; Janet Huck, "Breaking a Silence: 'Starsky' Star, Wife Share Their Family's Painful Battle against AIDS," *Los Angeles Times*, August 25, 1989, home edition sect., www.aegis.com/news/It/1989/LT890811 .html (accessed March 22, 2004).

36. Glaser and Palmer, *In the Absence*, p. 231.

37. Ibid., p. 278. See also Lois Romano, "The Glasers' Grim Plea: Actor and Wife Testify on Pediatric AIDS," *Washington Post*, March 14, 1990, pp. C1, C6. There were roughly 2,400 known cases of pediatric AIDS in the United States at this time.

38. Betty Goodwin, "Star-Studded Picnic for AIDS Research," *Los Angeles Times*, June 12, 1991, p. E3.

39. Glaser and Palmer, *In the Absence*, p. xi.

40. Ibid.

41. Lewis, *NBC Nightly News*, December 3, 1994.

42. Jeanne Moutoussamy-Ashe, interview by the author, October 29, 2004.

43. Ashe and Rampersad, *Days of Grace*, p. 7.

44. Ibid., pp. 7, 18.

45. Ibid., p. 7.

46. Ibid., p. 8.

47. Ibid., pp. 12–18.

48. Peter Prichard, "Arthur Ashe's Pain Is Shared by Public and Press," *USA Today*, April 13, 1992, p. A11; Debra Gersh, "Unclear Boundaries," *Editor and Publisher*, April 18, 1992, pp. 7–9.

49. Transcript of *Today* show, NBC, April 9, 1992.

50. Lance Morrow, "Fair Game?" *Time*, April 20, 1992, pp. 74, 75; Charen quoted in Gersh, "Unclear Boundaries," p. 9; Jonathan Yardley, "Arthur Ashe and the Cruel Volleys of the Media," *Washington Post*, April 13, 1992, p. C2; Anna Quindlen, "Journalism 2001," *New York Times*, April 12, 1992, sect. 4, p. 21.

51. Acel Moore appearing on *First Person* with Maria Shriver, NBC, October 8, 1992; Garrick Utley, *NBC Nightly News*, April 11, 1992.

52. Gersh, "Unclear Boundaries," p. 8; *First Person with Maria Shriver*, October 8, 1992; Steve Denton to Arthur Ashe, September 12, 1992, Arthur Ashe papers, Schomburg Center for Research in Black Culture, New York, box 2, folder: general correspondence, 1–9/92; Ruth McCreary to Arthur Ashe, October 27, 1992, Ashe papers, box 2, folder: general correspondence, 10–11/92.

53. Frederick Lloyd to Arthur Ashe, May 22, 1992, Ashe papers, box 2, folder: correspondence L; Steve Milano to Arthur Ashe, September 2, 1992, Ashe papers, box 2, folder: correspondence M.

54. Richard Keen to Arthur Ashe, April 8, 1992, Ashe papers, box 2, folder: correspondence K; Stanley Mandel to Arthur Ashe, June 8, 1992, Ashe papers, box 2, folder: correspondence M; M.C. to Arthur Ashe, April 12, 1992, Ashe papers, box 2, folder: correspondence C.

55. Eileen Leonard to Arthur Ashe, April 14, 1992, Ashe papers, box 2, folder: correspondence L; Vicky Marty to Arthur Ashe, May 27, 1992, Ashe papers, box 2, folder: correspondence M; George W. Haywood to Arthur Ashe, April 23, 1992, Ashe papers, box 2, folder: correspondence H.

56. Jean Paul to Arthur and Jeanne Ashe, April 10, 1992, Ashe papers, box 2, folder: correspondence P; Reva Quitt to Arthur Ashe, April 18, 1992, Ashe papers, box 2, folder: correspondence Q; Alix Ehlers to Arthur Ashe, April 19, 1992, Ashe papers, box 2, folder: correspondence E.

57. Melissa Mercer to Arthur Ashe, May 1, 1992, and Pat McCord to Arthur Ashe, April 15, 1992, Ashe papers, box 2, folder: correspondence M; Chauntey Thompson

to Arthur Ashe, n.d., and Jean Smallwood to Arthur Ashe, n.d., Ashe papers, box 2, folder: correspondence, schoolchildren.

58. Stephen B. Thomas and Sandra C. Quinn, "The Tuskegee Syphilis Study, 1932–1972: Implications for HIV Education and AIDS Risk Education Programs in the Black Community," *American Journal of Public Health* 81 (1991): 1498–1505.

59. Ashe discussed Kemron in *Days of Grace*, pp. 144–51. See also Ashe's speech to Neighbor Care Pharmacies, Baltimore, October 1, 1992, Ashe papers, box 2, folder: speaking engagements, 9–12/92.

60. Ashe and Rampersad, *Days of Grace*, p. 151.

61. Ibid., p. 139; Kenny Moore, "The Eternal Example."

62. Ashe and Rampersad, *Days of Grace*, pp. 284, 303.

63. Speech to Community Health Centers, Atlanta, September 20, 1992, Ashe papers, box 2, folder: speaking engagements, 9–12/92; speech to Harvard Medical School commencement, June 4, 1992, Ashe papers, box 2, folder: speaking engagements, 1–8/92; Ashe and Rampersad, *Days of Grace*, p. 301.

64. Speech at Niagara Community College, October 13, 1992, Ashe papers, box 2, folder: speaking engagements, 9–12/92; Gemma Mazeak to Arthur Ashe, April 8, 1992, Ashe papers, box 2, folder: correspondence M; Ashe and Rampersad, *Days of Grace*, pp. 321, 326.

65. "Man of Grace and Glory," *People*, February 22, 1993, pp. 66–72; Dick Schaap, *ABC World News Tonight*, February 7, 1993.

66. Lewis, *NBC Nightly News*, December 3, 1994.

67. Susie Zeegen, interview by the author, February 9, 2004; Chau Lam, "Classmates, Admirers Remember AIDS Fighter," *Newsday (Long Island)*, February 6, 1995, p. A21.

Chapter 12. The Last Angry Man and Woman

1. Russell Miller, "Lorenzo's Oil," *Sunday Times Magazine* (London), January 28, 1990, pp. 26–32.

2. Lena Berman and Hugo W. Moser, "Incidence of X-linked Adrenoleukodystrophy and the Relative Frequency of Its Phenotypes," *American Journal of Medical Genetics* 76 (1998): 415–19.

3. Michael Ryan, "Trying to Will a Miracle," *People*, September 22, 1991, pp. 88–93; David Kronke, "Medical Detectives: Parents' Search for Son's Cure Detailed in 'Lorenzo's Oil,'" *Los Angeles Daily News*, January 2, 1993, courtesy of Paula Brazeal; Miller, "Lorenzo's Oil," p. 29.

4. Miller, "Lorenzo's Oil," p. 28; Odone quoted in Jerry Adler with Mary Hager, "They Won't Let Their Son Die," *Newsweek*, November 16, 1987, pp. 98–100.

5. Miller, "Lorenzo's Oil," p. 29. Hugo Moser has never seen this medical journal article.

6. Miller, "Lorenzo's Oil," p. 30; Ryan, "Trying to Will," p. 92.

7. Miller, "Lorenzo's Oil," p. 30.

8. Adler, "They Won't Let Their Son Die," p. 99.

9. Hugo Moser, M.D., interview by the author, November 19, 2002.

10. Lucy Atkins, "Lorenzo's Trial," *Guardian* (London), October 15, 2002, p. 10; Odone quoted in Miller, "Lorenzo's Oil," p. 32.

11. Miller, "Lorenzo's Oil," p. 32; William Lowther, "After Fifteen Years and 2,000 Nurses, Lorenzo's Oil Boy Is Still Not Cured," *Mail* (London), August 22, 1999, courtesy of Hugo Moser.

12. Augusto and Michaela Odone, "The Interplay of Monounsaturated and Saturated Fatty Acids: Therapeutic Applications in ALD," unpublished manuscript, April 30, 1985, and "Update of Our Efforts to Normalize Lorenzo's VLCFA," unpublished manuscript, June 1987, both courtesy of Augusto Odone.

13. Carollyn James, "Fighting Diseases No One Knows," *Insight*, December 2, 1985, pp. 62, 63.

14. Augusto Odone, interview by the author, December 18, 2002; Gina Kolata, "Lorenzo's Oil: A Movie Outruns Science," *New York Times*, pp. B5, B8; Paula Brazeal, interview by the author, July 8, 2003.

15. Augusto and Michaela Odone to ALD Family, January 18, 1985, courtesy of Hugo Moser, M.D.

16. Hugo W. Moser to Augusto and Michaela Odone, January 29, 1985, courtesy of Augusto Odone.

17. Odone interview, December 18, 2002.

18. Hugo W. Moser, "Status Report on a New Nutritional Approach to Adrenoleukodystrophy," unpublished manuscript, May 31, 1985, courtesy of Augusto Odone.

19. W. B. Rizzo et al., "Dietary Erucic Acid Therapy for X-Linked Adrenoleukodystrophy," *Neurology* 39 (1989): 1415–22.

20. Hugo W. Moser, "Suspended Judgment: Reactions to the Motion Picture 'Lorenzo's Oil,'" *Controlled Clinical Trials* 15 (1994): 161–64; Ron Brazeal to editors, *Chicago Tribune*, February 11, 1993, courtesy of Paula Brazeal.

21. Adler, "They Won't Let Their Son Die"; Amy Berger, "They Had to Find the Cure Themselves," *Woman's World*, July 24, 1990, p. 30; Miller, "Lorenzo's Oil," p. 28; J. R. Sargent at degree conferment ceremony, University of Stirling, March 2, 1991, courtesy of Augusto Odone.

22. Geraldine O'Brien, "The Doctor and 'Lorenzo's Oil,'" *New York Times*, January 24, 1993, Arts and Leisure sect., pp. 13, 17.

23. Terrence Rafferty, "Force of Nature," *New Yorker*, January 11, 1993, pp. 101–3.

24. O'Brien, "The Doctor," p. 13.

25. Alex McGregor, "Miller's Tale," *Time Out* (London), February 17–24, 1993, p. 16; O'Brien, "The Doctor," p. 17.

26. O'Brien, "The Doctor," p. 17; Mal Vincent, "Sarandon Stars as Fiercely Devoted Mom," *Virginia-Pilot/Ledger Star*, January 24, 1993, pp. G1, G5.

27. Paul Willistein, "Fate Led Susan Sarandon to Role in 'Lorenzo's Oil,'" *Allentown (Pennsylvania) Morning Call*, January 10, 1993, p. F1.

28. Rafferty, "Force of Nature," p. 101; Janet Maslin, "Parents Fight Ignorance to Keep Their Child Alive," *New York Times*, December 30, 1992, pp. B1, B2; Susan Wloszczyna, "Courageous 'Lorenzo's Oil' Strikes It Rich," *USA Today*, December 30, 1992, p. 1D; Jeffrey Westhoff, "'Lorenzo's Oil' Highly Inspiring," *Northwest Herald (Illinois)*, January 29, 1993, p. 5.

29. Maslin, "Parents Fight Ignorance," p. B1; Joanna Connors, "Film Does Justice to Parents' Passion, Pain," *Cleveland Plain Dealer*, January 22, 1993, courtesy of Paula Brazeal.

30. Lowther, "After Fifteen Years"; Moser, "Suspended Judgment," pp. 162, 163.

31. Reuben Matalon to Ron Brazeal, January 27, 1993, courtesy of Paula Brazeal; Barranger quoted in Christopher Snowbeck, "The Legacy of Lorenzo's Oil," *Pittsburgh Post-Gazette*, May 8, 2001, pp. G1, G2.

32. Brazeal interview; Mary Ann Wilson, "Lorenzo's Oil: ALD Featured in Family Saga," *Mid-Atlantic Regional Genetics Information Newsletter*, summer 1993, p. 13; "Real-Life Family Helped Ill Son Beat the Odds," *Virginia-Pilot/Ledger Star*, January 24, 1993, pp. G1, G5.

33. Cheryl K. Danner, "'Lorenzo's Oil' Portrays Parent Group Inaccurately," *Elgin (Illinois) Courier-News*, March 2, 1993, p. A6; Susan O'Donnell O'Toole to editor, *Chicago Tribune*, January 18, 1993; David Edwin to Ron, Paula, and ULF Friends, January 28, 1993, courtesy of Paula Brazeal.

34. Fred S. Rosen, "Pernicious Treatment," *Nature* 361 (1993): 695.

35. Ella Taylor, "Absolution on the Rocks," *L.A. Weekly*, January 1–7, 1993, p. 27.

36. "Lorenzo's Oil and Ethics," www.macalester.edu/~psych/whathap/diaries/diariesf96/kristi/diary2.htm (accessed November 30, 2004).

37. Rosen, "Pernicious Treatment," p. 695.

38. Snowbeck, "Legacy," p. G2; Odone quoted in Kolata, "Lorenzo's Oil," p. B8.

39. Adler, "They Won't Let Their Son Die," p. 98.

40. Susan Sarandon, interview by the author, February 13, 2004; Sidney Zion, interview by the author, June 18, 2003.

41. Lisa Priest, "Lorenzo's Curing Oil 'Misleading' Critics Say," *Toronto Star*, February 21, 1993, courtesy of Paula Brazeal.

42. Kolata, "Lorenzo's Oil," p. B8.

43. Augusto Odone, interview by the author, February 25, 2005.

44. Hugo W. Moser, "Status Report about Adrenoleukodystrophy and Its Therapy," unpublished manuscript, December 1992, courtesy of Augusto Odone.

45. Both quoted in Lisa J. Atkins, "Searching for a Miracle," *Asbury Park (New Jersey) Press*, February 2, 1993, pp. B1, B2.

46. Moser, "Status Report about Adrenoleukodystrophy."

47. Moser interview; Moser, "Status Report about Adrenoleukodystrophy."

48. David Concar, "Lorenzo's Oil Finally Proven to Work," *New Scientist*, September 26, 2002, www.myelin.org/newssci092602.htm (accessed January 4, 2005).

49. Moser, e-mails to the author, January 14, 2004, and October 26, 2005; Hugo W.

Moser et al., "Follow-up of 89 Asymptomatic Patients with Adrenoleukodystrophy Treated with Lorenzo's Oil," *Archives of Neurology* 62 (2005):1073–80.

50. Concar, "Lorenzo's Oil"; "Lorenzo's Oil Vindicated," press release by the Myelin Project, September 26, 2002, www.myelin.org/lopr092602.htm (accessed December 16, 2002); Moser interview.

51. Atkins, "Lorenzo's Trial," p. 10; Elizabeth Cohen reporting on *Connie Chung Tonight*, CNN, December 2, 2002; *The Montel Williams Show*, Paramount Domestic Television, December 10, 2002; Benton quoted in John McKenzie, "Homegrown Medicine Worked," *ABC News.com*, September 27, 2002, http://printerfriendly.abcn .etchFromGLUE=true&GLUEService=ABCNewsCom (accessed October 3, 2002).

52. David Concar, "Lessons from Lorenzo," *New Scientist*, January 26, 2002, www .myelin.org/newsci.htm (accessed January 4, 2005); Moser, "Suspended Judgment," p. 161.

53. William A. Silverman to Hugo W. Moser, April 15, 1993, courtesy of Hugo Moser; Kolata, "Lorenzo's Oil," p. B8.

54. Augusto and Michaela Odone, "Addendum," unpublished manuscript, June 10, 1985, courtesy of Augusto Odone.

Conclusion

1. Lance Armstrong with Sally Jenkins, *It's Not About the Bike: My Journey Back to Life* (New York: Berkley, 2001), p. 69; Lance Armstrong with Sally Jenkins, *Every Second Counts* (New York: Broadway Books, 2003), p. 3.

2. Armstrong, *It's Not About the Bike*, p. 268; Armstrong, *Every Second Counts*, p. 194; quotation from www.lancearmstrongfanclub.com/lancequotes.html (accessed December 7, 2004).

3. Quotations from www.allreaders.com/Topics/Info_1040.asp (accessed December 7, 2004); www.personal.psu.edu/users/k/a/ka1306/assign3.htm (accessed March 1, 2005); and www.sirwes.net/blogs/sirwes/archives/2003_07.html (accessed November 12, 2003).

4. David Shaw, "Medical Miracles or Misguided Media?" *Los Angeles Times*, February 13, 2000, www.aegis.com/news/lt/2000/LT000206.html (accessed December 31, 2004); Dorothy Nelkin, *Selling Science: How the Press Covers Science and Technology*, rev. ed. (New York: W. H. Freeman, 1995).

5. Neal Gabler, *Life: The Movie. How Entertainment Conquered Reality* (New York: Vintage Books, 1998); Daniel J. Boorstin, *The Image: A Guide to Pseudo-Events in America*, 25th anniv. ed. (New York: Vintage Books, 1987). See also David Greenberg, *Nixon's Shadow: The History of an Image* (New York: W. W. Norton, 2003), p. 291.

6. On the search for truth in history, see Richard J. Evans, *In Defense of History* (New York: W. W. Norton, 2000), pp. 65–87.

7. David M. Lubin, *Shooting Kennedy: JFK and the Culture of Images* (Berkeley: University of California Press, 2003), p. 153; Mark Ebner and Lisa Derrick, "Star Sick-

ness," *Salon*, November 29, 1999, www.salon.com/health/feature/1999/11/29/celeb_ disease (accessed December 30, 2004).

8. Armstrong, *It's Not About the Bike*, p. 267.

9. Ebner and Derrick, "Star Sickness."

10. Armstrong, *Every Second Counts*, p. 12; *The Oprah Winfrey Show*, ABC Television, April 4, 2002 (I thank Sara Siris for this reference); "Michael J. Fox: Miracle Cure! His New Treatments Banish Parkinson's Symptoms," *Star*, March 29, 2004.

11. Boorstin, *The Image*, p. ix; Richard Schickel, *Intimate Strangers: The Culture of Celebrity in America* (Chicago, Ivan R. Dee, 2000), p. xi.

12. "'Magic' Johnson Touts HIV Drug," *Atlanta Journal-Constitution*, January 21, 2003, p. 2D.

13. Lawrence Goodman, "Well, If Kathleen Turner Says It Works," *Guardian* (London), July 23, 2002, sect. G2, p. 8; Alex Kuczynski, "Treating Disease with a Famous Face," *New York Times*, December 15, 2002, sect. 9, pp. 1, 15.

14. Steven Epstein, *Impure Science: AIDS, Activism, and the Politics of Knowledge* (Berkeley: University of California Press, 1996).

15. Armstrong, *It's Not About the Bike*, p. 90.

16. Greenberg, *Nixon's Shadow*, pp. xxiv, xxv, xxxii.

17. Ron Rosenbaum, *Explaining Hitler: The Search for the Origins of His Evil* (New York: Random House, 1998), p. xlvi; Joseph Campbell, *The Hero with a Thousand Faces* (Princeton, NJ: Princeton University Press, 1968), p. 11; Gabler, *Life: The Movie*, pp. 239–41. Jim Cullen has argued that persistent myths express what Abraham Lincoln termed "the better angels of our nature." See Cullen, *The Civil War in Popular Culture: A Reusable Past* (Washington, DC: Smithsonian Institution, 1995), p. 7. For an excellent discussion of the different myths that pervade medical storytelling, see Anne Hunsaker, *Reconstructing Illness: Studies in Pathography* (West Lafayette, IN: Purdue University Press, 1999).

18. Eva Hoffman, *After Such Knowledge: Memory, History, and the Legacy of the Holocaust* (New York: Public Affairs, 2004), p. 173; Gina Kornspan Levin, "Heroics among the 'Ordinary,'" *Philadelphia Inquirer*, September 3, 1982, Morris Abram papers, Robert W. Woodruff Library, Emory University, Atlanta, box 7, loose letter; Paula Brazeal, interview by the author, July 8, 2003.

19. Harry M. Marks, *The Progress of Experiment: Science and Therapeutic Reform in the United States, 1900–1990* (Cambridge: Cambridge University Press, 1997); Evidence-Based Medicine Working Group, "Evidence-Based Medicine: A New Approach to Teaching the Practice of Medicine," *Journal of the American Medical Association* 268 (1992): 2420–25.

20. Barron H. Lerner, *The Breast Cancer Wars: Hope, Fear and the Pursuit of a Cure in Twentieth-Century America* (New York: Oxford University Press, 2003), pp. 175–81.

21. Ibid., pp. 297–301 (postscript to paperback edition).

22. "Some of the Many Views of Mammography," *New York Times*, February 5, 2002, p. F3. See also Sheryl Gay Stolberg, "Senators Hear from Experts, Then Support Mammography," *New York Times*, March 1, 2002, p. A20.

23. There is a growing literature in narrative medicine, which seeks to make sense out of patients' stories. For a comprehensive review of the field, see Rita Charon, *Narrative Medicine: Honoring the Stories of Illness* (New York: Oxford University Press, 2006). See also Arthur W. Frank, *The Wounded Storyteller: Body, Illness, and Ethics* (Chicago: University of Chicago Press, 1995).

24. Stephen Jay Gould, "The Median Isn't the Message," *Discover*, June 1985, www .phoenix5.org/articles/GouldMessage.html (accessed November 7, 2002).

25. Jonathan Sadowsky has provocatively argued that historians need to examine the actual efficacy of past medical interventions in order to understand the history of how they were debated, used, and evaluated. While such an argument is beyond the scope of this book, it would be worth considering the history of something like Lorenzo's Oil, which turned out to "work," within this context. See Sadowsky, "Electroconvulsive Therapy and the Question of Progress in Medical History," work in progress. For a historical example of patients promoting "therapeutic activism," see Colin Talley, "The Treatment of Multiple Sclerosis in Los Angeles and the United States, 1947–1960," *Bulletin of the History of Medicine* 77 (2003): 874–99. For a modern example, see Denise Grady, "The Paths They Took: Five Gambles, Five Altered Lives," *New York Times*, December 28, 2004, pp. F1, F6.

26. Peter Cram et al., "The Impact of a Celebrity Promotional Campaign on the Use of Colon Cancer Screening," *Archives of Internal Medicine* 163 (2003): 1601–5; Jerome Groopman, "The Reeve Effect," *New Yorker*, November 10, 2003, pp. 80–93.

27. Jack D. Pressman, *Last Resort: Psychosurgery and the Limits of Medicine* (Cambridge: Cambridge University Press, 1998), p. 433.

28. Lisa M. Schwartz and Steven Woloshin, "The Media Matter: A Call for Straightforward Medical Reporting," *Annals of Internal Medicine* 140 (2004): 226–27; Vivienne Parry, "Health: A Matter of Life and Death," *Guardian* (London), July 6, 2004, features sect., p. 10; Rebecca Dresser, *When Science Offers Salvation: Patient Advocacy and Research Ethics* (New York: Oxford University Press, 2001), pp. 159–65.

29. Felicia Ackerman, "A Dying Patient's Decision," *New York Times*, October 15, 2002, p. F3; Chuck Klosterman, "Culture Got You Down?" *Esquire*, January 2005, pp. 38–41.

30. Charlie Tolchin, *Blow the House Down: The Story of My Double Lung Transplant* (New York: Writers Club Press, 2000); Jane E. Brody, "A Conversation with Charlie Tolchin: Beating the Odds, with New Lungs and a Zeal for Life," *New York Times*, January 14, 2003, p. F5.

31. Brody, "Conversation with Charlie Tolchin," p. F5. Tolchin died of cystic fibrosis on August 7, 2003, almost seven months after Brody's story.

Arnold, Dan, 114, 116
asbestos, 142–43
Ashe, Arthur, 14, 113, 222–45, 271; activism of, 222, 236, 241–42; and blood transfusions, 222–23; and going public, 225, 237–38, 240, 244; as HIV positive, 16–17, 222, 226; letters to, 239–41; outing of, 236, 238, 239; and race, 222, 224–25, 240–41
Ashe, Camera, 226–27, 236
Ashman, Hyman, 121, 132
Astaire, Adele, 166
Astaire, Fred, 160
attitudes: fear, 49–50, 52, 53; fighting, 75–76, 114, 116, 124, 157, 270–71; hope, 31–33, 35, 69, 76, 79–80, 94–95, 135, 219, 235, 274; and mental illness, 50, 52, 53; optimism, 86–89, 114–15, 122, 132; and survival, 131–32, 135; will to live, 131–32, 133–34, 135, 269
autonomy, 8, 15–16, 128, 180–81, 199, 279
Axelrod, David, 209
AZT (azidothymidine), 227–32, 236

Bacall, Lauren, 165
Bak, Richard, 40
Balde, Myrna, 203, 204
Bankhead, Tallulah, 35
Banks, Ernie, 109
Barnum, P. T., 8
Barranger, John A., 259
Barrow, Edward G., 25, 26–27, 35
Barton, Ernesta, 93, 99
Baruch, Bernard, 6
Beattie, Edward J. (Ted), 108, 111, 113–15, 125
Belafonte, Harry, 226
Bell, Bertrand M., 209, 218
Bensel, Francis P., 213
Benton, Michael, 266
Berenson, Claudia K., 193–95
Bernays, Edward, 8, 235
Bernstein, Barton J., 192
Bias, Len, 212
bioethicists, 180–81, 186, 191–92, 280
bipolar illness. See manic-depression
Blinn, William, 102, 105
Block, Terence, 181, 187
blood transfusions, 113–14, 122, 222–25
Bollettieri, Nick, 226
Boorstin, Daniel, 7, 9, 270, 272
Boston Globe, 45, 135

Boudreau, Lou, 44, 45
Bourke-White, Margaret, 14, 61, 62–80; as activist, 62, 65, 79–80; and brain surgery, 15, 66–71; and going public, 70–73, 75–77, 79; letters to, 70–75; and physical therapy, 64–65, 75, 78
Bowen, Catherine Drinker, 93
Bradlee, Benjamin, 88
Braudy, Leo, 8, 24
Brazeal, Ron and Paula, 252, 259–60, 263–64, 275
Brenna, Tony, 144
Brian Piccolo: A Short Season (Morris), 100, 106, 114, 116
Brian's Song (film), 13, 15, 100, 102–6, 112, 114, 116–18
Broad, William J., 184
Brody, Jane E., 281
Brown, Guillermo, 46, 48–49, 51–52, 56
Bull, Ronnie, 102
Burnett, Carol, 165, 171
Butkus, Dick, 111
Butler, Robert, 174

Caan, James, 103, 105, 116–17
Campbell, Joseph, 257, 274
cancer, 9, 122; alternative treatments for, 91–94, 139–58; breast, 118, 134, 178, 276–77; colon, 15, 70–71, 80–99; embryonal cell carcinoma, 107, 113–14, 118; individualized treatment for, 146–47; and Mexican clinics, 146, 148, 156; pancreatic, 158; public knowledge of, 84–85, 89–90; testicular, 1, 118, 268–69
Cansino, Richard, 176
Caplan, Arthur I., 192
Capote, Truman, 168
Carlson, Stanley W., 21
Carter, Jimmy, 136
Carter, Lynda, 273
Cedars-Sinai Medical Center, 142, 144, 149, 223–24
celebrities, 76–77; bonding with, 7, 8, 77, 272; ulterior motives of, 272–73
Centers for Disease Control (CDC), 223
Chambers, Robert, 213
Charen, Mona, 238
chemotherapy, 94–95, 108, 111, 124, 158; aggressive, 122, 126; cytosine arabinoside (Ara-C), 126; daunorubicin, 126; and infection, 125–26; 7 + 3, 126, 134

Cher, 229, 233
Churchill, Winston, 98, 99, 150
Church of Latter-Day Saints (LDS). *See* Mormonism
civil rights, 121, 205, 225
Clark, Barney, 14, 16, 18, 137, 179, 180–200; complications for, 181, 183–84, 187, 190, 196; death of, 182, 185, 186, 188, 192, 195; and informed consent, 180–82, 185, 187–88; media coverage of, 182, 184, 193–94; and Mormon influence, 190–91; and quality of life, 191–97; suicidal ideation of, 185–86, 193–94; surgeries for, 182, 184, 196
Clark, Gary, 181
Clark, Stephen, 181, 196
Clark, Una Loy Mason, 181, 184, 188, 190, 191, 196, 198
clinical trials, 17, 30, 155, 266–67, 275–76
CML. *See under* leukemia
cocaine, 201, 202, 211–12
Colleta, Morey, 106
communism, cancer of, 81, 97
confidentiality, 3, 9–10
Connors, Joanna, 258
consumerism: in medicine, 148, 209, 227; and sick role, 64, 68, 261
Cooley, Denton A., 183, 184
Cooper, Gary, 34, 38
Cooper, Irving S., 66–79
Corum, Bill, 33
Corzatt, Dick, 107
Couric, Katie, 278
Crawford, "Wahoo" Sam, 25
Crowther, Bosley, 39
Crystal, Billy, 234
Cuomo, Mario M., 209
cures, 6, 56, 92, 99
Cushing, Harvey, 5
Cuttner, Janet, 127, 130
cystic fibrosis, 280–81
cytosine arabinoside (Ara-C), 126

Dahlgren, Babe, 25
Daley, Arthur, 45
Danner, Cheryl K., 260
daunorubicin, 126
The Day Is Short (Abram), 123, 125, 128, 130–31, 137
Days of Grace (Ashe), 225, 236
Dean, James, 141
death and dying, 3, 15, 31, 149; of Clark, 182,

185, 186, 188, 192, 195; of McQueen, 153, 155; media coverage of, 35, 97–98
deception, 32–33, 83
decision-making, 3, 17, 100, 180; basis for, 18, 70, 277–79; for patients, 116, 188. *See also* informed consent
Deford, Frank, 237
DeLaurentis, Susan, 232, 233
dementia, 163. *See also* Alzheimer's disease
dementia praecox (schizophrenia), 161
Demerol, 203, 206, 210–12, 215, 218
Dempsey, Jack, 7
denial, 26, 33, 45, 170–71, 173
depression, 193; medications for, 202, 206, 210, 212, 215, 218. *See also* manic-depression
DeVries, William C., 180–82, 184–93, 196, 199
diabetes, 4, 27
diagnoses, 16; concealment of, 64, 83, 171; of Hayworth, 159, 161, 170; of Zion, 203, 214–15
Dickey, Bill, 27, 33, 35
didanosine (ddI), 236
Dimaggio, Joe, 23
Dinkins, David, 237
diseases: and activism, 16–18, 40, 77, 80, 177, 234, 244, 277; fighting, 75–76, 114, 116, 124, 157, 270–71; labeling of, 6, 163; randomness of, 30, 201, 214
Doctor X, 207
Domagk, Gerhard, 4
Douglas, R. Gordon, Jr., 210, 212
Dresser, Rebecca, 280
Drinker, Cecil, 93
Drinker, Philip, 93
drug interactions, 206, 208, 215, 218
Dryden, John, 225
Dukakis, Olympia, 273
Duke, Shearlean, 173
Dulles, Allen, 92–94, 99
Dulles, Avery, 98
Dulles, Clover, 96
Dulles, Eleanor Lansing, 97
Dulles, Janet, 82, 95
Dulles, John, 98
Dulles, John Foster, 14, 15, 80, 81–99, 239; letters to, 81, 89–93, 95; openness from, 83–84, 88; prognosis for, 86–87, 91; strength of, 89, 95–96; and unorthodox treatments, 94–95
DuPont, Ethel, 2